Modern Trends in Vascular Surgery

Carotid Artery Disease

Mark K. Eskandari, M.D.
Associate Professor of Surgery, Radiology, and Cardiology
Division of Vascular Surgery
Department of Surgery
Northwestern University
Feinberg School of Medicine
Chicago, IL

William H. Pearce, M.D.
Violet R. and Charles A. Baldwin
Professor of Vascular Surgery
Chief, Division of Vascular Surgery
Department of Surgery
Northwestern University
Feinberg School of Medicine
Chicago, IL

James S. T. Yao, M.D., Ph.D.
Professor Emeritus
Division of Vascular Surgery
Department of Surgery
Northwestern University
Feinberg School of Medicine
Chicago, IL

2010
PEOPLE'S MEDICAL PUBLISHING HOUSE—USA
SHELTON, CONNECTICUT

People's Medical Publishing House–USA
2 Enterprise Drive, Suite 509
Shelton, CT 06484
Tel: 203-402-0646
Fax: 203-402-0854
E-mail: info@pmph-usa.com

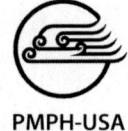

PMPH-USA

09 10 11 12 13/PMPH/9 8 7 6 5 4 3 2 1

13-digit ISBN: 978-1-60795-052-3
10-digit ISBN: 1-60795-052-9

Printed in China by People's Medical Publishing House of China
Copyeditor/Typesetter: Spearhead Global, Inc.; Cover Designer: Mary McKeon

LOC to come

Notice: The authors and publisher have made every effort to ensure that the patient care recommended herein, including choice of drugs and drug dosages, is in accord with the accepted standard and practice at the time of publication. However, since research and regulation constantly change clinical standards, the reader is urged to check the product information sheet included in the package of each drug, which includes recommended doses, warnings, and contraindications. This is particularly important with new or infrequently used drugs. Any treatment regimen, particularly one involving medication, involves inherent risks that must be weighed on a case-by-case basis against the benefits anticipated. The reader is cautioned that the purpose of this book is to inform and enlighten; the information contained herein is not intended as, and should not be employed as, a substitute for individual diagnosis and treatment.

Sales and Distribution

Canada
McGraw-Hill Ryerson Education
Customer Care
300 Water Street
Whitby, Ontario L1N 9B6
Canada
Tel: 1-800-565-5758
Fax: 1-800-463-5885
www.mcgrawhill.ca

Foreign Rights
John Scott & Company
International Publisher's Agency
P.O. Box 878
Kimberton, PA 19442
USA
Tel: 610-827-1640
Fax: 610-827-1671

Japan
United Publishers Services Limited
1-32-5 Higashi-Shinagawa
Shinagawa-ku, Tokyo 140-0002
Japan
Tel: 03-5479-7251
Fax: 03-5479-7307
Email: kakimoto@ups.co.jp

United Kingdom, Europe, Middle East, Africa
McGraw Hill Education
Shoppenhangers Road
Maidenhead
Berkshire, SL6 2QL
England
Tel: 44-0-1628-502500
Fax: 44-0-1628-635895
www.mcgraw-hill.co.uk

Singapore, Thailand, Philippines, Indonesia,
Vietnam, Pacific Rim, Korea
McGraw-Hill Education
60 Tuas Basin Link
Singapore 638775
Tel: 65-6863-1580
Fax: 65-6862-3354
www.mcgraw-hill.com.sg

Australia, New Zealand
Elsevier Australia
Locked Bag 7500
Chatswood DC NSW 2067
Australia
Tel: +61 (2) 9422-8500
Fax: +61 (2) 9422-8562
www.elsevier.com.au

Brazil
Tecmedd Importadora e Distribuidora
de Livros Ltda.
Avenida Maurilio Biagi 2850
City Ribeirao, Rebeirao, Preto SP
Brazil
CEP: 14021-000
Tel: 0800-992236
Fax: 16-3993-9000
Email: tecmedd@tecmedd.com.br

India, Bangladesh, Pakistan, Sri Lanka, Malaysia
CBS Publishers
4819/X1 Prahlad Street 24
Ansari Road, Darya Ganj, New Delhi-110002
India
Tel: 91-11-23266861/67
Fax: 91-11-23266818
Email:cbspubs@vsnl.com

People's Republic of China
PMPH
Bldg 3, 3rd District
Fangqunyuan, Fangzhuang
Beijing 100078
P.R. China
Tel: 8610-67653342
Fax: 8610-67691034
www.pmph.com

Contents

Preface

Carotid Artery Disease is a compilation of presentations on topics relating to carotid artery disease from the last five symposia sponsored by the Division of Vascular Surgery, Feinberg School of Medicine, Northwestern University, Chicago, Illinois, USA. The Vascular Symposium is a continuing education event that has been held in December each year since December 2, 1976. Each year, approximately 40 leading vascular surgeons from the US and overseas serve as faculty to address topics of their special interest. A compendium book is published as a permanent record of their contributions. Unlike previous years, the last five symposium books were published by a private publisher. They were distributed only to participants of the symposia and are not commercially available. We soon recognized that the lack of worldwide circulation of the books has done an injustice to the faculty members and to the medical community because these chapters represent a real contribution to the medical literature. When we were approached by People's Medical Publishing House-USA to republish some of the chapters, we seized the opportunity to formulate a book of chapters on carotid artery that were published in the last five symposium books and *Carotid Artery Disease* was born. The book highlights the advances of diagnosis and management of carotid artery disease in recent years.

 Carotid Artery Disease begins with several chapters on critical issues related to diagnosis and management of carotid artery disease. In recent years, one of the major changes in vascular surgery is the advent of catheter-based endovascular technology. Stent technology has changed the landscape of treatment of carotid stenosis. Angioplasty with stent placement is now a viable alternate treatment to open surgery. Several leading experts in carotid stenting were invited to address the symposia on issues related to this new technology. These include acquisition of the technology for vascular surgeons, selection of candidates for stent, the techniques—especially cerebral protection, and, finally, the results of current clinical trials of stent versus open surgery. New technology brings new problems and we devoted a section to perioperative care of patients who have undergone stent placement including surveillance of the result of the stent placement using duplex scan.

 While stent technology provides a new approach, open carotid revascularization procedures remain an important part of the treatment armamentarium. Carotid endarterectomy, even re-do operation, is an effective and durable procedure. The performance of carotid endarterectomy must be measured and the result can be enhanced by statin therapy. For carotid arteries with kinks and coils, stent placement would be a difficult and risky undertaking so open surgical technique is needed. Other surgical problems that need attention include revascularization of the vertebral and subclavian arteries. For supra-aortic trunk lesions, a hybrid procedure offers a new combined endovascular and open technique. Other carotid pathology of interest includes carotid dissection and carotid body tumor; both conditions present a surgical challenge to vascular surgeons.

The book ends with a special section on the debate of carotid stent versus carotid endarterectomy by two leading experts. We hope the debate highlights the pros and cons of both techniques and provides helpful advice for surgeons who must determine which technique is best-suited for their patients. Most importantly, the surgeons who treat carotid disease must be equipped to offer either stent or open surgery for their patients. Treatment of vascular disease is changing and surgeons must make changes accordingly.

Contributors

Thomas A. Abbruzzese, M.D.
Critical Surgery Care
Vascular Surgeon
General & Vascular Specialists
Boynton Beach, Florida

Saad Ali, M.D.
Resident
Department of Radiology
University of Iowa Hospitals and Clinic
Iowa City, Iowa

Gary M. Ansel, M.D.
Assistant Clinical Professor of Medicine
Medical University of Toledo
Director, Center for Critical Limb Care
Riverside Methodist Hospital
Columbus, Ohio

Paul A. Armstrong, D.O., F.A.C.S.
Division of Vascular and Endovascular
    Surgery
Universtiy of South Florida College of
    Medicine
Chief, Vascular Surgery
James A. Haley Veterans Hospitals
Tampa, Florida

Dennis F. Bandyk, MD.,F.A.C.S.
Professor of Surgery
Chief, Division of Vascular & Endovascular
    Surgery
Universtiy of South Florida College of
    Medicine
Tampa, Florida

Michel A. Bartoli, M.D.
Faculté de Médecine de Marseille
Université de la Méditerranée
Assistance Publique Hôpitaux de Marseille –
Hôpital de la Timone,
Service de Chirurgie Vasculaire
Marseille, France

Ramon Berguer, M.D., Ph.D.
Frankel Professor of Surgery,
Divisions of Vascular and Cardiac Surgery
University of Michigan Health System
Ann Arbor, Michigan

Giorgio M. Biasi, M.D.
Professor of Vascular Surgery
Chief of the Vascular Surgery Unit
University of Milano Bicocca
San Gerardo University Hospital
Milano, Italy

Benjamin S. Brooke, M.D.
Resident
Johns Hopkins University College of
    Medicine
Johns Hopkins Hospital
Baltimore, Maryland

Katherine E. Brown, D.O.
Associate professor in Surgery
University of California at San Diego
San Diego, California

Richard P. Cambria, M.D.
Professor of Surgery
Harvard Medical School
Chief, Division of Vascular and
    Endovascular Surgery,
Massachusetts General Hospital
Boston, Massachusetts

Valter Camesasca, M.D.
Vascular Surgeon, Vascular Surgery Unit
University of Milano Bicocca
San Gerardo University hospital
Milano, Italy

James C. Carr, M.D.
Co-Director of Cardiac MRI
Program Director of Cardiovascular Imaging
Department of Radiology
Northwestern University's Feinberg School
    of Medicine
Northwestern Memorial Hospital
Chicago, Illinois

Timothy J. Carroll, Ph.D.
Associate Professor
Biomedical engineering; Radiology
Northwestern University's Feinberg School
    of Medicine
Northwestern Memorial Hospital
Chicago, Illinois

Seemant Chaturvedi, M.D.
Professor of Neurology
Director, Comprehensive Stroke Program
Wayne State University and Detroit
    Medical Center
Detroit, Michigan

Jae-Sung Cho, M.D.
Division of Vascular Surgery
University of Pittsburgh Physicians
UPMC Shadyside
Pittsburgh, Pennsylvania

Jayer Chung, M.D.
Vascular Fellow,
Division of Vascular and Endovascular
    Surgery
Emory University School of Medicine
Emory University Hospital
Atlanta, Georgia

Alberto Cremonesi, M.D.
Chief, Interventional Cardiology
Villa Maria Cecilia Hospital
Cotignola, Italy

Gaetano Deleo, M.D.
Vascular Surgeon, Vascular Surgery Unit
University of Milano Bicocca
San Gerardo University Hospital
Milano, Italy

Mark K. Eskandari, M.D.
Assoicate Professor in Surgery-Vascular
Northwestern University's Feinberg School
    of Medicine
Northwestern Memorial Hospital
Chicago, Illinois

Cindy Felty, C-ANP
Assistant Professor
Mayo Medical School
Mayo Clinic
Rochester, Minnesota

Alberto Froio, M.D.
Assistant Professor, Vascular Surgery Unit
University of Milano Bicocca
San Gerardo University Hospital
Milano, Italy

Mark W. Fugate, M.D.
Assistant Professor, Department of Surgery
University of Tennessee Chattanooga
Chattanooga, Tennessee

William A. Gray, M.D.
Associate Professor of Clinical Medicine,
Director of Endovascular Services
Columbia University Medical Center
New York, New York

Robert W. Hobson, II, M.D.
(Former) Professor
Department of Surgery, Division of
  Vascular Surgery
UMDNJ-NJMS, the University
  Hospital
Newark, New Jersey
(Former) Director of the Vascular
  Institute
Gagnon Heart Hospital
Morristown Memorial Hospital
Morristown, New Jersey

Luigi Inglese, M.D.
Professor of Interventional Radiology
Chief Dept. of Haemodynamics
San Donato University Hospital
Milano, Italy

Glenn R. Jacobowitz, M.D.
Associate Professor
New York University Langone Medical
  Center
NYU Vascular Surgery Associates
New York, New York

William D. Jordan, Jr., M.D.
Professor of Surgery
University of Alabama
Birmingham, School of Medicine
Chief, Section of Vascular Surgery,
University of Alabama, Birmingham,
  Hospital
Birmingham, Alabama

Vikram R. Kalakuntla, M.D.
Vascular Surgeon
Northeast Ohio Vascular Associates
Willouby, Ohio

K. Craig Kent, M.D.
A.R. Curreri Professor of Surgery,
Chairman, Department of Surgery,Section
  of Vascular Surgery
University of Wisconsin School of Medicine
  and Public Health
University of Wisconsin Hospital
Madison, Wisconsin

Ioannis Koktzoglou, Ph.D.
Center for Advanced Imaging
Evanston Hospital
Evanston, Illinois

Timothy F. Kresowik, M.D., F.A.C.S.
Professor Department of Surgery
Division of Vascular Surgery
University of Iowa Health Care
Iowa City, Iowa

Russell C. Lam, M.D.
Allopathic & Osteopathic Physicians
  Surgery
Vascular Surgery
Dallas, TX

Debiaco Li, Ph.D.
Professor, Biomedical Engineering
Northwestern University
Evanston, Illinois

Angela Liloia, M.D.
Vascular Surgeon, Vascular Surgery Unit
University of Milano Bicocca
San Gerardo University Hospital
Milano, Italy

G. Matthew Longo, M.D.
Assistant Professor, Department of Surgery
Section of General Surgery - Vascular
  Surgery
University of Nebraska, College of
  Medicine
University of Nebraska Medical Center
Omaha, Nebraska

Douglas W. Massop, M.D.
Heart & Vascular Clinic, Iowa Clinic
Des Moines, Iowa

Jon S. Matsumura, M.D.
Professor of Surgery, Chief, Vascular
  Surgery
University of Wisconsin School of Medicine
  and Public Health
University of Wisconsin Hospital
Madison, Wisconsin

Michael Monge, M.D.
Resident, General Surgery
Northwestern University's Feinberg School
  of Medicine
Chief, Division of Vascular Surgery
 Northwestern Memorial Hospital
Chicago, Illinois

Wesley S. Moore, M.D.
Professor Emritus
UCLA David Geffen School of Medicine at
  UCLA
Los Angeles, California

Mark D. Morasch, M.D.
Associate Professor in Surgery-Vascular
Northwestern University's Feinberg School
  of Medicine
Practice Director
Northwestern Memorial Hospital
Chicago, Illinois

Xian Mang Pan, M.D.
Vascular Surgery Service
San Francisco VA Medical Center
San Francisco, California

Juan C. Parodi, M.D.
Professor of Surgery
University of Buenos Aires
Clinical Vascular Surgery
FLENI Institute
Buenos Aires, Argentina

Federico E. Parodi, M.D.
Vascular Surgery Resident
University of South Florida,
Tampa, Florida

Mark A. Patterson, M.D.
Assistant Professor
University of Alabama, Birmingham School
  of Medicine
University of Alabama, Birmingham Hospital
Birmingham, Alabama

William H. Pearce, M.D.
Violet R. and Charles A. Baldwin Professor
  in Vascular Surgery
Northwestern University's Feinberg School
  of Medicine
Chief, Division of Vascular Surgery
Northwestern Memorial Hospital
Chicago, Illinois

Bruce A. Perler, M.D.
Julius H. Jacobson II, Professor of Surgery
Johns Hopkins University College of
  Medicine
Chief, Division of Vascular Surgery
Johns Hopkins Hospital
Baltimore, Maryland

Claudia Piazzoni, M.D.
Vascular Surgeon, Vascular Surgery Unit
University of Milano Bicocca
San Gerardo University Hospital
Milano, Italy

Richard J. Powell, M.D.
Professor of Surger - Vascular Surgery
Dartmouth Medical School
Section Chief, Vascular Surgery
Dartmouth-Hitchcock Medical Center
Lebanon, New Hampshire

Amritha Ragunathan, M.D.
ER Resident
Stanford University Medical School
Stanford University Hospital
Stanford, California

Joseph H. Rapp, M.D.
Professor of Surgery
University of California at San Francisco
School of Medicine
Chief of Vascular Surgery Service
San Francisco VA Medical Center
San Francisco, California

Daniel J. Reddy, M.D.
Henry Ford Hospital
Detroit, Michigan

Robert S. Rhodes, M.D.
Associate Executive Director for Vascular
    Surgery
American Board of Surgery
Philadelphia, Pennsyvania

John J. Ricotta, M.D.
Chair, Department of Surgery
Washington Hospital Center
Washington, DC

Thomas S. Riles, M.D.
Frank C. Spencer Professor of Cardiac
    Surgery
Associate Deanfor Medical Education &
    Technology
New York University Medical Center
NYU Vascular Surgery Associates
New York, New York

Sean P. Roddy, M.D.
Professor of Surgery
Albany Medical College, Albany Medical
    Center
The Institute for Bascualr Disease
Albany, New York

Thom W. Rooke, M.D.
John and Posy Krehbiel Professor of
    Vascular Medicine
Mayo Medical School
Mayo Clinic, Gonda Vascular Center
Rochester, Minnesota

Kenneth Rosenfield, M.D.
Director, Cardiac and Vascular Invasive
    Service
Massachusetts General Hospital
Boston, Massachusetts

Dhiraj M. Shah, M.D.
Professor
Albany Medical College
Albany Medical Center
Albany, New York

Ali Shaibani, M.D.
Associate Professor of Radiology and
    Neurosurgery
northwestern University's Feinberg School
    of Medicine
Northwestern Memorial Hospital
Chicago, Illinois

Anton N. Sidawy, M.D., M.P.H.
Professor
Georgetown and George Washington
    Universities
Chief, Surgical Services, VA Medical Center
Washington, DC

Daniel Surdell, M.D.
Assistant Professor
Department of Surgery - Neurosurgery
University of Nebraska, College of
    Medicine
University of Nebraska Medical Center
Omaha, Nebraska

Lawrence R. Wechsler, M.D.
Director, UPMC Stroke Institute,
Vice-Chair Clinical Affairs, Department of
    Neurology
University of Pittsburgh Medical School
Pittsburgh, Pennsyvania

Thomas A. Whitehill, M.D.
Associate Professor of Sugery
Division of Vascular Surgery
University of Colorado Health Sciences
    Center
Denver, Colorado

James S. T. Yao, M.D., Ph.D.
Professor Emeritus
Northwestern University's Feinberg School
    of Medicine
Northwestern Memorial Hospital
Chicago, Illinois

SECTION **I**

Issues in Carotid Artery Disease

Screening Program for Stroke Prevention

Thomas S. Riles, M.D.
and Glenn R. Jacobowitz, M.D.

Stroke is the third leading cause of death in the United States, following heart disease and cancer. Although more than 150,000 die each year from stroke, an estimated 750,000 people suffer a new or recurrent stroke annually leaving an estimated four million stroke survivors in the U.S. Given the fact that 15–30% of stroke survivors are permanently disabled, the estimated costs for acute and long-term care are near $50 billion a year.[1] Clearly stroke is a devastating illness both to patients, their families, and to the health care system.

For decades, the focus has been on understanding the causes of stroke and treating stroke victims. Specialized hospital units and nursing homes have been created to provide for the acute and chronic care. Therapies to reverse the neurological injury of stroke have been disappointing. For acute presentations of stroke, medical regimens have been developed to minimize infarction of brain tissues or to minimize zones of cerebral ischemia. Catheter directed thrombolysis has proven to be effective in improving the outcome for individuals suffering from thrombotic strokes.[2] Unfortunately, this is helpful only for a select population able to reach a skilled facility within the first few hours of symptoms. Although these therapies have improved the outcome and survival for stroke victims, they have had negligible effect on the prevalence of stroke.

Inasmuch as the interval between being entirely asymptomatic to having irreversible brain injury from a stroke is a matter of hours, the likelihood of developing a program that will be effective in diagnosing and treating individuals before permanent injury is sustained is most unlikely. Clearly, prevention of stroke is a better strategy. To date, stroke prevention has been limited to one of two main areas. At one end of the spectrum are those individuals fortunate enough to have been diagnosed as having a condition that could cause a stroke, and have been given appropriate therapy by their physician. An example would be the individual with palpitations who is found to have atrial fibrillation and placed on Warfarin, or the hypertensive patient who is under careful blood pressure control with medication. Unfortunately, diagnosis of the underlying conditions has been opportunistic and often dependent on the

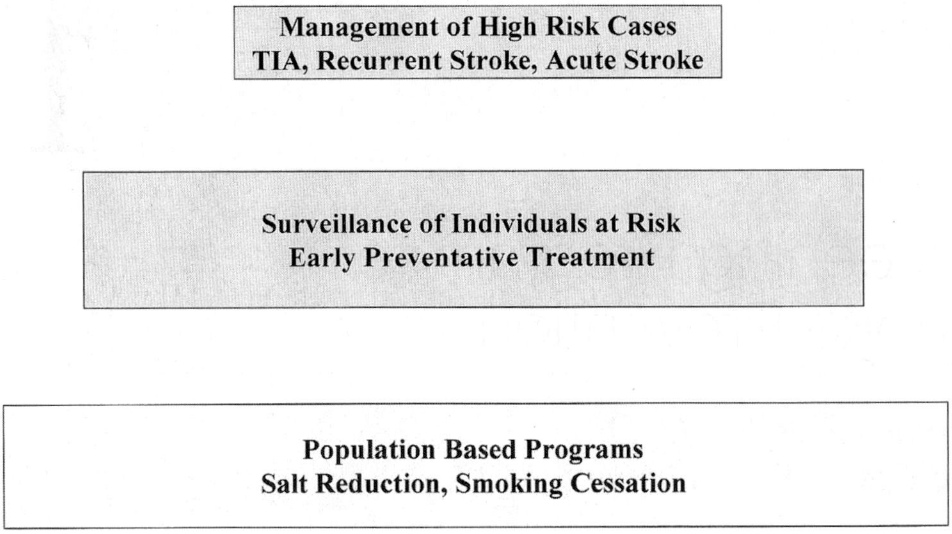

Management of High Risk Cases
TIA, Recurrent Stroke, Acute Stroke

Surveillance of Individuals at Risk
Early Preventative Treatment

Population Based Programs
Salt Reduction, Smoking Cessation

Figure 1-1. Stroke Prevention Methods

quality of medical care an individual can afford. The second preventive strategy has been broad public awareness efforts such as programs to reduce smoking, salt intake, or cholesterol in our diets. Although helpful, the ineffectiveness of these efforts to date is evident from the fact that stroke remains at epidemic proportions in the U.S. and other developed countries.

Lacking is a screening program to identify individuals at risk of stroke due to some underlying condition. Since most individuals do not know they are at risk until they become victims, a program to identify those with conditions that could lead to stroke and to provide preventative treatment seems sensible (Figure 1–1). In a health conscious country such as ours that embraces preventative programs for cancers of the breast, prostate, and colon, and prevention of osteoporosis and a host of other conditions, it is curious that we do not have a focused stroke prevention program, particularly since the mortality, morbidity, and cost of stroke exceeds all of the other mentioned illnesses. In this chapter, we will explore some of the historical problems to stroke prevention, and some views on the development of an effective and cost-saving program to reduce the risk of stroke for our society.

CAUSES OF STROKE

To plan a program for the prevention of stroke, it is necessary to understand the causes of stroke and the effectiveness of specific management programs for each. Strokes are generally divided into two main categories: ischemic and hemorrhagic. Hemorrhagic strokes include intracerebral bleeding as well as subarachnoid hemorrhage. The cause of these strokes is predominately hypertension, although bleeding from cerebral artery aneurysms and arteriovenous malformations, trauma, and bleeding from coagulation disorders or anticoagulant therapy must be included among the differential. Ischemic strokes are generally due to emboli from the carotid arteries, arch vessels, or the heart, or due to occlusive diseases of the intracranial vasculature. The latter is often related to diabetes or chronic hypertension.

In the United States, 84% of strokes are ischemic, and of those, the major causes are atheroemboli from the carotid arteries and cardioemboli.[3] The underlying conditions in these cases are atherosclerotic disease at the carotid bifurcation, and atrial fibrillation or recent myocardial infarction. The distribution of causes of stroke in the U.S. is shown in Figure 1–2. It should be noted that in other societies, although the prevalence of stroke may be similar, the causes of stroke may be different. In Korea, for example, half of the strokes are hemorrhagic as compared to only 16% in the U.S. (Figure 1–3).[4]

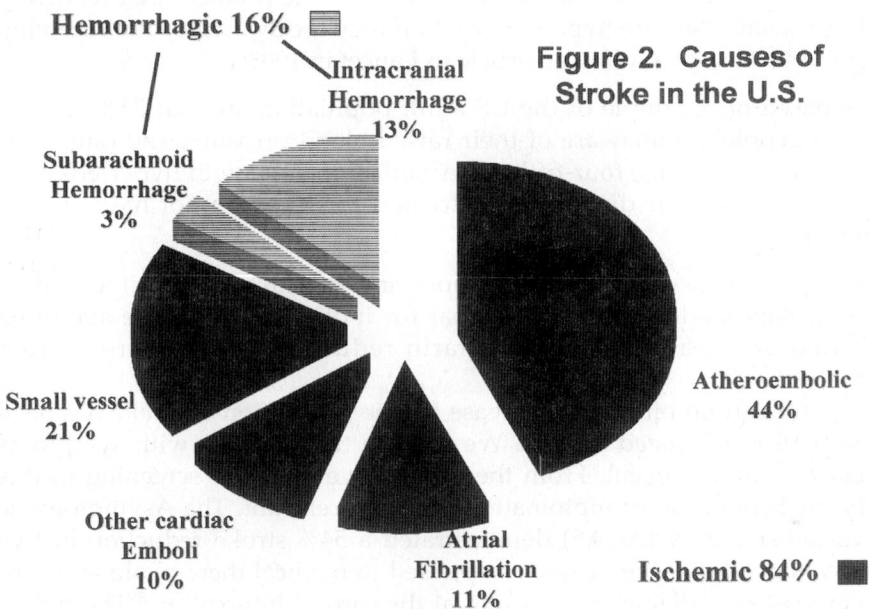

Figure 2. Causes of Stroke in the U.S.

Figure 1-2. Causes of Stroke in the United States

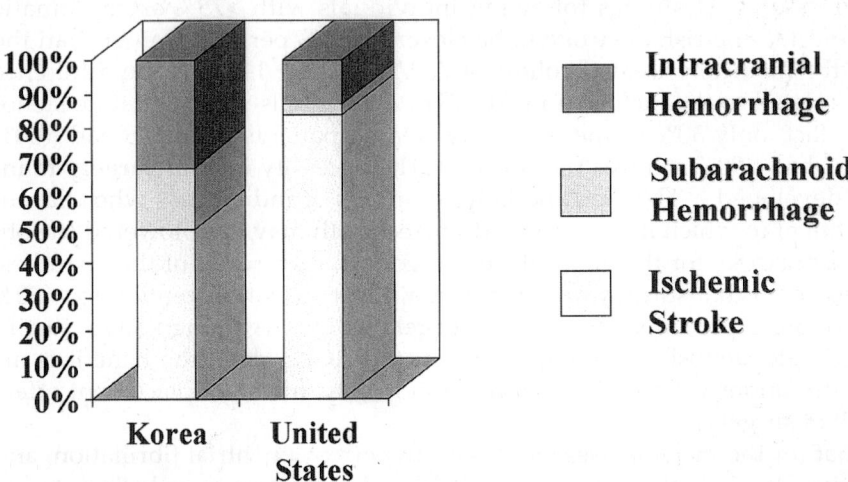

Figure 1-3. Comparison of Causes of Stroke: Korea and U.S

TREATMENTS FOR THE PREVENTION OF STROKE

It is important to recognize that hypertension, atrial fibrillation, and carotid bifurcation are the underlying causes of 75% of strokes in the United States. For each, there is strong evidence that if the medical condition is effectively treated, the risk of stroke is significantly reduced. For hypertension, numerous studies have shown a direct correlation between the level of the diastolic and systolic blood pressure and the risk of stroke. MacMahon and associated, reporting on collected studies, showed the risk of stroke increases five-fold if the diastolic blood pressure is above 100 mm.Hg, and is 13 times greater if the diastolic pressure is above 110 mm.Hg.[5] Clearly, if hypertension is controlled, the risk of stroke can be dramatically reduced. The problem that relatively few individuals are aware they are hypertensive, or if they are aware, are not receiving proper treatment. As stated by Wolf in an article in Lancet in 1998:

> "Estimates based on a sample of the US adult population are that 35% of hypertensive people are unaware of their raised blood pressure, and only half are on treatment. Thus, four-fifths of American people with hypertension are unaware of their disorder, not treated for it, or do not have it under control."[6]

Likewise, the risk of stroke for atrial fibrillation can be greatly reduced if identified and treated. Controlled studies have shown that for individuals over the age of 65 with atrial fibrillation, treatment with Warfarin reduce the risk of stroke from 4.3–1.1%, a 74% decrease.[7]

The treatment for carotid bifurcation disease for the prevention of stroke has been the subject of several randomized studies. We assume that patients with symptoms would seek treatment in any event. From the perspective of stroke screening in this discussion, only the benefit for asymptomatic patients is relevant. The Asymptomatic Carotid Atherosclerosis Study (ACAS) demonstrated a 54% stroke reduction in five years with surgical removal of the plaque as apposed to medical therapy alone for individuals with at least 60% diameter reduction at the carotid bifurcation.[8] The reduction, from 11–5.1%, or approximately 1% per year, was disappointing to some who expected an even larger benefit from surgical therapy.

Earlier nonrandomized studies following individuals with >75% asymptomatic stenosis had indicated the risk of stroke to be closer to 5.4% per year, rather than the 2.2% shown in the medically treated cohort of ACAS (Figure 1–4).[9-15] The difference may have been related to the inclusion in ACAS of individuals with moderate stenosis (60–80%). In fact, only 30% of the medically treated patients in ACAS had >80% stenosis; only 5% had >90% stenosis (Figure 1–5). The necessity to offer surgery to individuals who developed a TIA, and the large numbers of individuals who did not receive the treatment to which they were randomized, both may have lowered the observed incidence of stroke for the medical treated cohort. As a result of these studies, it is generally accepted that surgery does offer significant stroke prevention for >80% asymptomatic stenosis provided the risk of surgery is low. Although some justify surgery for moderate stenosis (60–80%) based on the ACAS data, the benefit is arguable. Studies are underway to see if carotid angioplasty and stent placement offers the same benefit of surgery.

It is clear that for the major causes of stroke—hypertension, atrial fibrillation, and carotid bifurcation disease—therapies are available and effective in reducing stroke.

Study		Patients (#)	Follow-up (mos.)	Strokes (%)
Roederer	1984	25	36	16.0
Bogousslavsky	1986	38	37	13.2
Hertzer	1986	195	35	9.2
Moneta	1987	73	24	19.0
Hennerici	1987	36	29	8.3
Caracci	1989	62	21	17.7
Hobson	1993	107	48	9.3

Average rate of stroke = 5.4% per year

Figure 1-4. Pre-ACAS Studies of Natural History of >75% Asymptomatic Carotid Stenosis

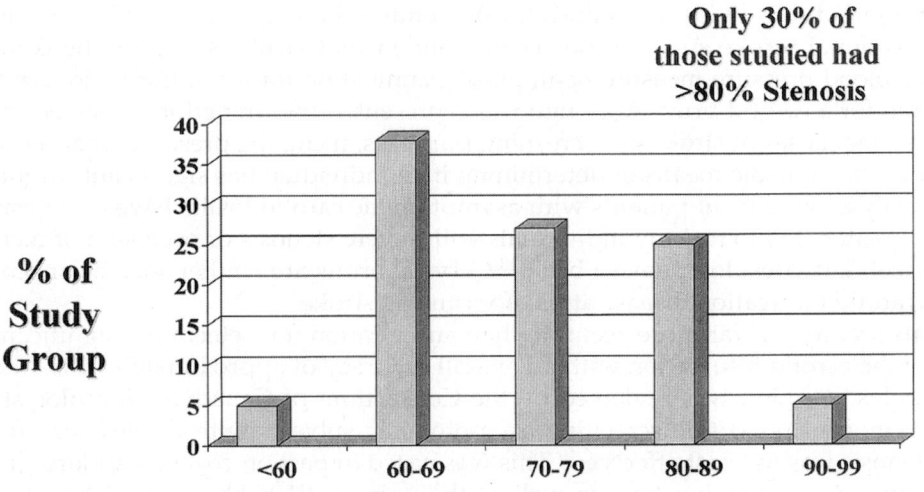

Only 30% of those studied had >80% Stenosis

% of Study Group

Carotid Stenosis by Prerandomized Angiogram

Figure 1-5. ACAS - Percent Carotid Stenosis

Why is it, then, that stroke continues to be a major affliction of our society? As Vladimir Hachinski, M.D. stated in his presidential address to the Stroke Council of the American Heart Association:

> "The hope is that up to 75% of cardiac and cerebrovascular disease can be prevented by the successful management of the known risk factors. The disappointment is that only about 25% of those with known risk factors have them controlled."[16]

SCREENING FOR STROKE

The basic tenets for any screening test are that the test must have a high degree of specificity and sensitivity, the risk to individuals being tested must be minimal, and the costs must be reasonable. Ultimately, it must be proven to be effective in reducing the mortality and/or morbidity of the disease to which it is targeted. For stroke, there is the additional problem of multiple causes. Testing, therefore, might need to include a battery of tests, or else be limited to focusing on one type of stroke. As in all types of screening, it is important to identify a population at risk to increase the likelihood that testing will yield an acceptable percentage of positive results, making the effort worthwhile.

Although efforts have been made to provide screening for diseases related to stroke such as hypertension, vascular disease, and heart disease, to date few attempts have been made to provide screening specifically focused at prevention of stroke. Stroke prevention initiatives by the American Stroke Association have been largely confined to risk factor modification and identification and control of hypertension. Hart et al found that current stroke prevention guidelines do not provide adequate methodologic information to permit assessment of their quality and clinical applicability.[17]

In an attempt to provide guidelines for preventing the major causes of stroke, in 1994 the National Stroke Association recommended that stroke screening be comprised of a blood pressure measurement, pulse examination for atrial fibrillation, and auscultation for a carotid bruit. Although this represented the first effort to screen for the three major causes of stroke, for screening purposes, using the presence or absence of a bruit is not a reliable means of determining if an individual has significant carotid stenosis. Only about 25% of patients with asymptomatic carotid bruits have a stenosis of 75% or greater, and that many individuals with severe stenosis or occlusion of their internal carotid arteries don't have a bruit.[18] Cervical bruits are neither specific or sensitive for carotid bifurcation disease at risk for causing stroke.

Duplex scanning is far more accurate than auscultation for detecting a significant stenosis at the carotid bifurcation with an overall accuracy of approximately 97%. The use of Duplex scanning was reviewed by the Consortium of Canadian Neurologists in 1997. They concluded that screening asymptomatic subjects with duplex scan for carotid stenosis was not cost effectve.[19] This was based in part on cost of standard duplex scanning as a screening test, as well as the opinion that there would be additional costs for conventional angiography to confirm the Duplex findings before recommending surgical therapy for asymptomatic high-grade carotid stenosis. Given the cost of Duplex scans, more than $400 each in many areas, the assumption was correct. If one adds the cost of a consultation with a physician to have an ECG and blood pressure evaluation *before* the referral for the Duplex scan, the total cost could easily exceed $650 a person. If all 35 million persons over age 65 in the U.S. were screened, this would be a cost of $22.7 billion in the first year. Even if 50% of strokes were prevented by screening, this would not be cost-effective (Figure 1–6). Magnetic resonance angiography, CT angiography, and conventional angiography are even more expensive and not appropriate for screening. The latter, conventional angiography also carries some significant risk, limiting its use for all forms of assessment of individuals suspected of being at risk for stroke.

The concept of developing an abbreviated Duplex scan for screening purposes was first suggested by Lavenson.[20] In this study, the carotid bulb was examined by

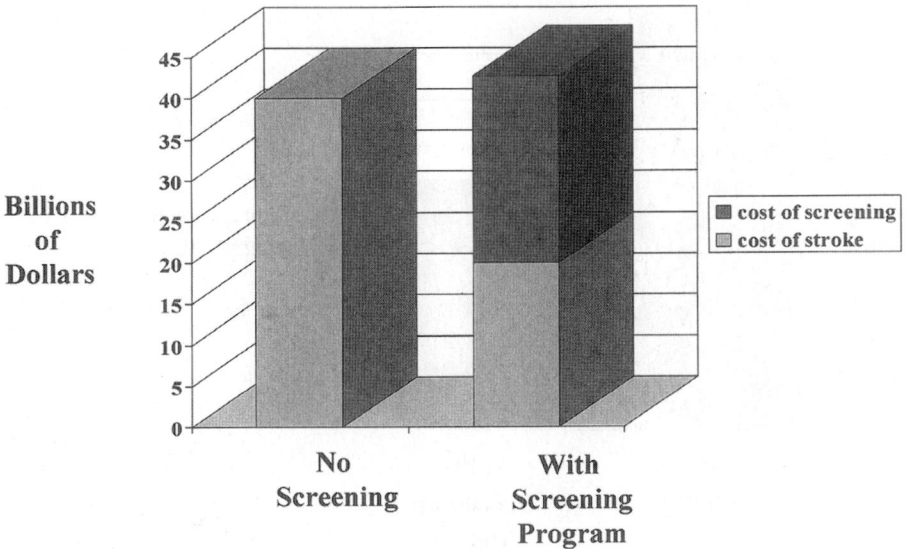

Figure 1-6. Cost of Stroke with Screening at $650 per subject >65 years of age

B-mode ultrasound. A color shift identified defined areas of stenosis. Further evaluation would be performed if the test were positive. A negative finding excluded the carotid bifurcation as being a potential source for stroke. The important factor was that the test could be performed within minutes, reducing costs without compromising on accuracy. Carsten et al., using color-flow duplex imaging and an immediate Doppler-derived velocity of the segment of the internal carotid artery with the most turbulent flow, could screen individuals in an average of 3.2 minutes. Their positive and negative predictive values were greater than 89% when the abbreviated scans were compared to standard complete duplex scans in the same patients.[21]

A similar test was developed at New York University in which ultrasound imaging of the distal common carotid artery, bulb, and proximal internal and external carotid arteries was performed, evaluating the Doppler signal for three to five beats in each location. Positive predictive value was 100% and negative predictive value was 97% when compared to standard duplex examinations. The average scan time for this test was about 1.5 minutes.[22] The initial direct cost of this test plus a blood pressure evaluation and two lead ECG was less than $75 per patients.[23] With increased efficiency and experience, this cost has dropped to less than $40 per person.

Clearly, cost reduction is important to making screening available to our populace. If all individuals over the age of 65 could be screened for $40 per person per year, the cost would be only $2.65 billion a year. Assuming that screening would lead to effective treatment for individuals unaware they had hypertension, atrial fibrillation, and/or asymptomatic carotid stenosis, it is possible that the incidence of stroke could be reduced by at least 50%.[4, 7, 8, 24] If applied on a large scale, the cost savings to our society from the prevention of stroke could be enormous (Figure 1–7). It is likely that experience would lead to more precise selection criteria for individuals to be screened. Also, most individuals would not require annual screening. Factoring these two into the equation, the cost of mass screening would be even less.

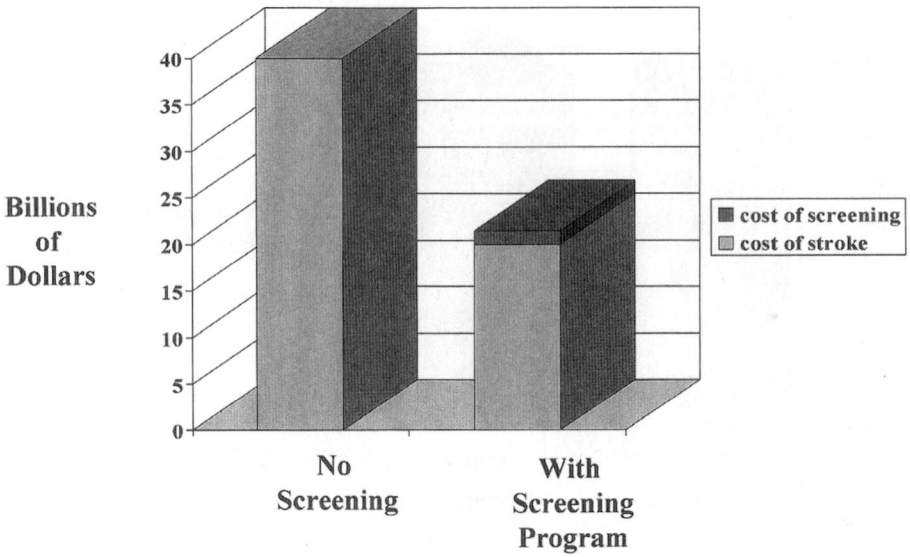

Figure 1-7. Cost of Stroke with Screening at $40 per subject >65 years of age

SELECTION OF INDIVIDUALS FOR SCREENING

Holloway et al reviewed multiple studies on the cost-effectiveness of stroke evaluation and concluded that the cost-effectiveness improved when subjects with a higher prevalence of the underlying disease were tested.[25] Others have commented that screening would be most cost-effective if applied to a population known to be at high risk.[26-27] Therefore, the goal of a stroke screening program should be to use effective, low-cost tests in a group of subjects with a high prevalence of disease.

Although strokes can occur at any age, the vast majority occur among the elderly.[28] Age, therefore, is an important first criterion in the selection of individuals for screening. Many authors have identified populations with an increased prevalence of carotid artery stenosis among those with other known vascular disease such as peripheral artery disease, aortic aneurysms, and coronary artery disease.[29-34] Also, associated medical conditions such as elevated serum cholesterol, diabetes, hypertension, and smoking have been shown to carry a higher risk of carotid bifurcation disease. In a subset of the Framingham Study involving 1,116 patients ages 66 to 93, multivariate analysis revealed that age, cigarette smoking, systolic blood pressure, and cholesterol were independently related to the presence of significant carotid atherosclerosis.

The overall prevalence of significant carotid atherosclerosis in the general population was about 8%.[35]

In the Tromso Study from Norway, 6,727 persons aged 25 to 84 years were screened for extracranial carotid stenosis with Duplex ultrasound of the right carotid artery. The overall prevalence of carotid stenosis was 3.3%, but gradually increased by age in both men and women. Cholesterol, systolic blood pressure, and current smoking were independently associated with carotid artery stenosis in both women and men.[36] Qureshi et al. evaluated 1,331 unselected volunteers without previous stroke, transient ischemic attack, or carotid artery surgery by personal interview and Duplex ultrasound. The main outcome measure was carotid artery stenosis >60% by duplex ultrasound.[37] Age >65 years, current smoking, coronary artery disease, and hypercholesterolemia were significantly associated with asymptomatic carotid artery stenosis. Posttest probability for asymptomatic carotid artery stenosis ranged from 7% in a low-risk group to 35% in a high-risk group. The authors concluded that duplex ultrasound screening in the subgroup of high-risk patients might prove cost effective and have an effect on stroke-free survival.[37]

In all of these studies on unselected populations, increased age, cigarette smoking, and hypercholesterolemia were risk factors for carotid stenosis. Systolic blood pressure was a risk factor in the two studies in which it was measured and coronary artery disease was also identified.[35-37] Much work is yet to be done to determine how to use these data to determine who would most benefit from a stroke screening program.

RESULTS OF STROKE SCREENING PROGRAMS

To date, there have been several model programs for stroke screening that have provided sufficient data to determine their effectiveness in discovering previously undiagnosed hypertension, atrial fibrillation, and carotid bifurcation disease; all conditions, if properly monitored and treated, could significantly reduce the risk of stroke.

Lavenson established the Central California Screening program in 1997. This program was open to all participants, but included mostly elderly individuals. In the past eight years, he has screened 2,559 individuals. Remarkably, of the individuals screened, 29.3% had a blood pressure >140/90 mm.Hg., 5.1% had atrial fibrillation, and 7.5% had >50% stenosis of at least one carotid artery. His cost for screening is $15 per person.[38]

New York University has run a stroke screening program limited to individuals over the age of 65 and with at least one risk factor; i.e., smoking, hypertension, coronary artery disease, diabetes, or a family history of stroke. Of the 610 individuals screened, 10.8% had previously undiagnosed carotid stenosis (>50%), 2.6% were hypertensive, and 0.5% had atrial fibrillation.[23]

Recently, the American Vascular Association, a foundation of the Society for Vascular Surgery, has sponsored a vascular screening day at a number of institutions across the country. Stroke screening has been a part of the program. In the first two years of the program, 2,446 individuals were screened. Previously undiagnosed carotid disease was found in 7.6%, atrial fibrillation in 2.9%, and hypertension >140/90 in 22.8% (Table 1–1).[39]

In summary, the time is right to develop a comprehensive stroke screening program in this country. Ample data is available to demonstrate the following:

1. Stroke is one of the major causes of morbidity and mortality in the U.S.
2. The cost of stroke in the U.S. is staggering, upward of $50 billion a year.
3. The major causes of stroke are clearly defined.
4. Evidence-based treatments of the major causes of stroke—hypertension, atrial fibrillation, and carotid bifurcation disease—show that if treated, the risk of stroke can be reduced by more than half for each.
5. The vast majority of individuals with one of the above conditions are unaware or untreated.

TABLE 1-1. RESULTS OF STROKE SCREENING PROGRAMS

Study	# Screened	HBP	AF	CAS > 50%
Lavenson (38)	2557	29.3%	5.1%	7.5%
NYU (23)	610	2.6	0.5	10.8
AVA 2002 (39)	859	22.6	3.4	7.8
AVA 2003 (39)	1587	22.9	2.7	7.4

6. Pilot stroke screening programs have demonstrated effective, accurate assessment at low cost, and a remarkably high yield of positive results among participants.

As yet, the pilot programs have been too small and too early to demonstrate an impact on the incidence of stroke. This would take a much larger study with a control group and long-term follow-up. Nonetheless, it would seem logical to launch a mass screening program even while a randomized study is being organized. It addition to the obvious benefit for stroke prevention, the conditions that lead to stroke are also closely related to heart disease, the number one cause of death in our country. The benefits of diagnosing and treating underlying conditions early could have multiple benefits.

Although at some point the Medicare system will need to provide funding for stroke screening, it would seem appropriate for the medical profession to take the lead in establishing programs for this purpose. Programs could be run through philanthropy, as a public service effort by hospitals or medical organizations, or even for profit. It is important, however, that we make stroke screening available for our minority populations and for the underprivileged as the prevalence of stroke among these groups is exceptionally high. Clearly, the time is ripe for a major initiative to reduce the ravages of stroke in this country. The need is great. The solutions are available. With good leadership and resolve, we can make a significant change in the health of our society by coupling effective treatments to those at risk through a stroke prevention program.

REFERENCES

1. American Heart Association. *2002 Heart and Stroke Statistical Update*. Dallas: The American Heart Association; 2001.
2. Clark WM, Wissman S, Albers GW, et al. Recombinant tissue-type plasminogen activator (Alteplase) for ischemic stroke 3 to 5 hours after symptom onset. The ATLANTIS Study; a randomized controlled trial. *JAMA*. 1999;282:2019–2026.
3. Taylor TN, Davis, PH, Torner JC, et al. Lifetime cost of stroke in the United States. *Stroke*. 1996;27:1459–1466.
4. Korean Neurological Association. Epidemiology of cerebrovascular disease in Korea: a collaborative study, 1989-1990. *J Korean Med Sci*. 1993;8:281–289.
5. McMahon S, Peto R, Cutler J et al. Blood pressure, stroke, and coronary heart disease: Part 1, prolonged differences in blood pressure: prospective observational studies corrected for the regression dilution bias. *Lancet*. 1990;35: 765–774.
6. Wolf, PA. Prevention of stroke. *Lancet*. 1998;352 (supplII):15–18, 28.

7. Atrial Fibrillation Investigators. Risk factors for stroke and efficacy of antithrombotic therapy in atrial fibrillation: analylsis of pooled data from five randomized controlled trials. *Arch Intern Med*. 1994;154:1449–1457.

8. Executive Committee for the Asymptomatic Carotid Atherosclerosis Study. Endarterectomy for asymptomatic carotid artery stenosis. *JAMA*. 1995;273:1421–1428.

9. Bofousslavsky J, Displand PA, Regli F. Asymptomatic tight stenosis of internal carotid artery: Long-term progress. *Neurology*. 1986;36:861–863.

10. Hennerici M, Hulsbomer MB, Hefter H, et al. Noninvasive assessment of stroke risk in asymptomatic and nonhemispheric patients with suspected carotid disease. *Ann Surg*. 1985;202:491–504.

11. Roederer GO, Langlois YE, Jager KA, et al. The natural history of carotid arterial disease in asymptomatic patients with cervical bruits. *Stroke*. 1984;15:605–613.

12. Moneta GL, Taylor DC, Nicholls SC et al. Operative vs. nonoperative management of asymptomatic high-grade internal carotid artery stenosis: Improved results with endarterectomy. *Stroke*. 1987;18:1005–1010.

13. Caracci BF, Zukowski AJ, Hurley JJ et al. Asymptomatic severe carotid stenosis. *J Vasc Surg*. 1989;9:361–366.

14. Hertzer NR, Flanagan RA, Beven EG, et al. Surgical versus nonoperative treatment of asymptomatic carotid stenosis. 290 patients documented by intravenous angiography. *Ann Surg*. 1986;204:221–227.

15. Hobson RW, Weiss DG, Fields WS, et al. Efficacy of carotid endarterectomy for asymptomatic carotid stenosis. *N Engl J Med*. 1993;328:221–227.

16. Hachinski V. Stroke: the next 30 years. *Stroke*. 2002;33:1–4.

17. Hart RG, Bailey RD. An assessment of guidelines for prevention of ischemic stroke. *Neurology* 2002; 59:977–982.

18. Chambers RB, Norris JW. Outcome in patients with asymptomatic neck bruits. *N Eng J Med*. 1986;315:860–865.

19. Perry JR, Szalai JP, Norris JW for the Canadian Stroke Consortium. Consensus against both endarterectomy and routine screening for asymptomatic carotid artery stenosis. *Arch Neurol*. 1997;54:25–28.

20. Lavenson GS Jr. A new accurate, rapid and cost-effective protocol for stroke-prevention screening. *Cardiovasc Surg*. 1998; 6:590–593.

21. Carsten CG III, Elmore JR, Franklin DP, et al. Use of limited color-flow dulex for a carotid-screening project. *Am J Surg*. 1999;178:174–177.

22. Jacobowitz GR, Rockman CB, Gagne PJ, et al. A model for predicting occult carotid artery disease: screening is justified in a selected population. *J Vasc Surg*. 2003;38:705–709.

23. Rockman CB, Jacobowitz GR, Gagne PJ, et al. Focused screening for occult carotid artery disease: patients with known heart disease are at high risk. *J Vasc Surg*. 2004;39:44–51.

24. Weinberger J. Prevention of ischemic stroke. *Curr Cardiol Rep*. 2002;4:164–171.

25. Holloway RG, Benesch CT, Rahilly CR, Courtright CE. A systematic review of cost-effectiveness research of stroke evaluation and treatment. *Stroke*. 1999;30:1340–1349.

26. Lee TT, Solomon NA, Heidenrich PA, et al. Cost-effectiveness of screening for carotid stenosis in asymptomatic patients. *Circulation*. 1996;94:194–198.

27. Yin D, Carpenter JP. Cost-effectiveness of screening for asymptomatic carotid stenosis. *J Vasc Surg*. 1998;27:245–255.

28. Sacco RL, Benjamin EJ, Broderick JP, et al. Risk Factors Panel - American Heart Association Prevention Conference IV. *Stroke*.1997;28:1507–1517.

29. Marek J, Mills JL, Harvich J, et al. Utility of routine carotid duplex screening in patients who have claudication. *J Vasc Surg*.1996;24:572–577.

30. Axelrod DA, Diwan A, Stanley JC, et al. Cost of routine screening for carotid and lower extremity occlusive disease in patients with abdomoinal aortic aneurysms. *J Vasc Surg*. 2002;35:754–758.

31. de Virgiliio C, Toosie K, Arnell T, et al. Asymptomatic carotid artery stenosis screening in patients with lower extremity atherosclerosis: a prospective study. *Ann Vasc Surg*. 1997;11:374–377.

32. Ascher E, Hingorani A, Yorkovich W, et al. Routine preoperative carotid duplex scanning in patients undergoing open-heart surgery: is it worthwhile?" *Ann Vasc Surg*. 2001;15:669–678.

33. Berens ES, Kouchoukos NT, Murphy SF, Wareing TH. Preoperative carotid artery screening in elderly patients undergoing cardiac surgery.*J Vasc Surg*.1992;15:313–23.

34. Simons PCG, Algra A, Eikelboom BC, et al for the SMART study group. Carotid artery stenosis in patients with peripheral arterial disease: The SMART study. *J Vasc Surg*. 1999;30:519–525.

35. Fine-Edelstein JS, Wolf PA, O'Leary DH, et al. Precursors of extracranial carotid atherosclerosis in the Framingham Study. *Neurology*. 1994; 44:1046–1050.

36. Mathieson EBl, Joakimsen O, Bonaa KH. Prevalence of and risk factors associated with carotid artery stenosis: the Tromso Study. *Cerebrovasc Dis*. 2001;12:44–51.

37. Qureshi AI, Janardhan V, Bennett SE, et al. Who should be screened for asymptomatic carotid artery stenosis? Experience from the Western New York Stroke Screening Program. *J Neuroimaing*. 2001;11:105–111.

38. Lavenson GS Jr, Pantera RL. Stroke prevention screening development and implementation [abstract]. Presented at the 26th World Congress of the International Cardiovascular Society. Maui, Hawaii, March 22, 2004.

39. Flinn WR. National screening program for abdominal aortic aneurysm. In: Pearce WH, Matsumura JS, Yao JST. *Trends in Vascular Surgery 2003*. Precept Press: Chicago, IL; 2004:153–161.

2

Controversies in Vascular Screening

Thom W. Rooke, M.D. and
Cindy Felty, R.N., M.S.N., C.N.P.

Screening programs for various medical conditions share certain characteristics. The participants typically have no signs, symptoms, objective evidence, or personal history of the disease in question. The diseases sought by screening usually pose a significant risk to health. Effective treatments for screenable diseases must be available, and when used in those with early disease, these treatments should improve outcome. Screening is ideally part of a cost-effective approach to disease management. Finally, individuals must be willing to pay extra for screening because these tests are generally *not* covered by Medicare or other forms of health insurance.

Issues relating to the appropriateness, risk-benefit balance, accuracy, cost, and quality of screening mix nicely to form a toxic cocktail of controversy that is now rising to the lips of the vascular community. Vascular screening has already become a "big business" that will unquestionably grow in the future, and as it grows, so will the controversies surrounding it.

It is beyond the scope of this presentation to address all of the controversies associated with vacular screening, so discussion will be limited to four specific areas:

1. Should we screen?
2. What to screen for, and how?
3. Who to screen?
4. Standards for screening

SHOULD WE SCREEN?

The rationale for disease screening seems intuitive. "Why not identify and treat disease early, before it has a chance to produce significant harm? Why wait until it is *too late*?" The logic to this approach is all but irrefutable, and in other disciplines, this type of thinking has led to widely accepted screening programs for diseases like breast cancer, colon cancer, prostate cancer, and many others. While the justification for screening may appear to be a "no-brainer," the reality is that screening requires at least three elements to be effective: 1) it must be possible to detect occult disease "early;" 2) effective therapy (for occult disease) must be available; and 3) early treatment of the occult disease must lead to better outcomes. When applied to vascular screening, are these three criteria met?

Can Occult Disease be Detected "Early"?

There is ample evidence to suggest that simple noninvasive imaging and/or functional tests can detect occult vascular disease before it becomes clinically apparent. The 2004 American Vascular Association (AVA) National Screening Program, an initiative involving 132 centers in 40 states and more than 8,000 Americans 55 and older, demonstrated that *ultrasound imaging* and *ankle-brachial index measurement* can detect occult abdominal aortic aneurysms, carotid artery disease, peripheral arterial disease, and hypertension.[1] Specific findings included the following.

Abdominal Aortic Aneurysm (AAA).   Aneurysms were identified in 2.5% of the screened population. Although the majority was small (3 to 5 cm), 16% were 5 cm or more in diameter.

Carotid Artery Disease.   7.6% of those screened had an internal carotid artery stenosis of 50% or more.

Peripheral Arterial Disease (PAD).   10.5% of those screened had an ankle-brachial index of less than 0.85, consistent with hemodynamically significant PAD.

Hypertension.   Brachial artery pressure was measured as part of the ankle-brachial index, and it was incidentally noted that 22% of those screened had systolic blood pressures over 160 mmHg, consistent with systemic hypertension.

According to the AVA Web site, the national screening program demonstrates ". . . that there is a significant amount of undiagnosed noncardiac vascular disease in a broad segment of the population. . . ." This disease can be detected using standard, widely available, simple technologies. The possibility that more sophisticated approaches such as assessment of arterial intimal thickening, brachial reactivity, and others can lead to even earlier detection of occult disease will be addressed later, but in general, there does not appear to be any controversy regarding the ability of routine vascular screening tests to detect silent disease "early."

Is Effective Therapy Available?

Most health care practitioners believe that the progression and severity of atherosclerosis can be reduced with simple lifestyle modifications. Smoking cessation, management of risk factors (hypercholesterolemia, diabetes, obesity, etc.), exercise or increased physical activity, diet modification, and many others can statistically reduce the burden of vascular disease in the population. But, as some argue, shouldn't these measures be implemented for everyone, not just those with evidence of early atherosclerosis? Aggressive medical regimens involving statins, platelet inhibitors, antihypertensives, hypoglycemic agents, and others offer even more opportunity to influence the natural history of arterial disease. But when should they be initiated? When does the predicted effectiveness of these agents justify their potential risk and cost? If we assume that aggressive risk-factor management and/or certain medical therapies are appropriate for patients with occult disease, the results of the 2004 AVA screening program suggest that many patients with occult disease are not properly managing their risk factors. Thirty percent of those with unsuspected abdominal aortic aneurysms were hypertensive at the time of their evaluation, and of these, a third were not taking antihypertensive medications. Half of the patients with undiagnosed carotid disease or peripheral arterial disease were not taking antiplatelet or lipid-lowering agents. To the extent that antihypertensives, lipid-lowering agents, and antiplatelet drugs are generally considered "effective," there are "effective" therapies that could be given to many of those with occult vascular disease.

It should be noted that there are still controversies regarding the absolute effectiveness of "standard" medical treatments for vascular disease, although this topic remains taboo in polite medical circles and is rarely discussed. While it is generally accepted that lifestyle modifications or aggressive medical regimens offer a *statistical* benefit for populations with vascular disease, it is difficult to know whether (or how much) a particular *patient* will benefit from a specific *therapy*. For example, certain cancers (breast, colon, prostate, etc.) may be surgically removed and thus completely "cured" when detected and treated early, but once it has become established, vascular disease (like PAD or carotid disease) is never "cured" by risk factor modification or medical therapy. Worse, it tends to progress despite aggressive therapy. How do we know that therapeutic efforts to alter the natural history of atherosclerosis or aneurysm are effective in a particular patient when progression occurs despite treatment?

The "effectiveness" issue is equally perplexing when advanced occult vascular disease is discovered for which an interventional therapy is indicated.[2] Therapies such as carotid artery stenting and endovascular repair of AAAs are themselves controversial, and become even more so when administered in the setting of asymptomatic, previously unsuspected vascular disease.

For these reasons, the effectiveness of therapy for occult vascular disease remains surprisingly controversial.

Does Early Treatment Lead to Better Outcomes?

Even for relatively well-accepted approaches to disease screening (like mammography for breast cancer, or rectal examinations/PSA for prostate cancer), there is some uncertainty about the influence of early detection on improvement and outcome. According to the National Cancer Institute, screening mammography (in woman age 40 to 70) will decrease breast cancer mortality, but the absolute benefit is only on the order of 1% overall.[3] The situation is less rosy for rectal examination/prostate specific antigen in men; the American Cancer Society acknowledges that "these tests *may* eventually prove to have a clinically important benefit on life expectancy."[4] The cost-effectiveness of tests such as PSA screening remains uncertain. If the relationship between screening and outcome seems vague for a disease in which the role of screening is apparently well established, it should come as no surprise that the effect of screening on outcomes remains controversial for vascular disorders. Specific vascular screening problems need to be assessed individually, but the dilemma can be illustrated by contrasting the situations for abdominal aortic aneurysm versus PAD.

With regard to AAA screening, all major national vascular societies and selected industry groups (at least those with a financial interest in aneurysm detection and repair) contend that screening is valuable and could save more than 15,000 American lives every year. These groups have joined together to form the National Aneurysm Alliance (NAA) which has been a major force advocating for aneurysm screening.[5] A separate group, the U.S. Preventive Services Task Force, has independently concluded that ultrasound screening for abdominal aneurysms in elderly male smokers could reduce aneurysm-related mortality by 43% (in men age 65 to 75) and have deemed it to be a cost-effective endeavor.[6] This determination, along with lobbying efforts by the NAA and others, led Congress to pass the SAAVE bill, a controversial act that covers the cost of one-time AAA screening in selected high-risk populations.

Contrast this with the case for peripheral arterial disease screening. The U.S. Preventive Services Task Force also addressed this situation and concluded that routine screening of asymptomatic persons is *not* recommended (although this is only a "D" recommendation).[7] While recognizing that the early detection of PAD offers some potential benefit, the task force noted that risk reduction measures such as increased physical activity, smoking cessation, and the like, should already be offered to all patients, not necessarily just to those with early evidence of PAD. Using this logic, it was argued that early detection of PAD will have little effect on the eventual outcome from the disease.

WHAT TO SCREEN FOR, AND HOW?

There is general agreement that certain vascular conditions can be detected simply, safely, and at relatively low cost using everyday technology. Abdominal aortic aneurysms and carotid disease can be screened for using duplex ultrasonography, and peripheral arterial disease is easily identified with a noninvasive ankle-brachial index. There is little controversy regarding these assessments.

Perhaps not surprisingly, a plethora of new technologies purported to improve the detection of occult vascular disease are appearing and metastasizing. There are too many of these tests to cover each in detail, but the controversy can be appreciated by considering three relatively well-known members of this club. *Intimal thickness*, as measured using high-resolution ultrasound equipment (particularly in the carotid artery) has been correlated with increased risks of stroke and myocardial infarction.[8] *Brachial artery reactivity*, a technique using real-time ultrasound analysis of nitric oxide-mediated flow-induced vasodilation to assess intimal health, may offer an even earlier way to detect incipient vascular disease.[9] *Rapid CT scanning* to look for calcification in the coronary arteries (or perhaps other vessels?) is now a widely used screening technique for identifying patients at increased risk of coronary atherosclerotic disease. Perhaps genetic techniques will someday allow us to examine the DNA of individuals (at birth? or even before birth?) and identify those at risk for the development of vascular disease? With regard to techniques that are currently available (intimal thickness, brachial reactivity, CT calcification, etc.), it remains controversial as to whether these methods provide meaningful information above and beyond that which can already be obtained using conventional ultrasound imaging or pressure (index) measurement techniques.

Vascular medicine now teeters on the precipice of another potential "what to screen for" controversy of biblical proportions. In January of 2006, the results of a pilot screening program sponsored by the American Venous Forum were announced at the

Venous Forum's national meeting in Miami.[10] This study, which involved 154 patients, utilized a limited duplex evaluation to screen for venous obstruction and incompetence. The information was coupled with a questionnaire to determine an individual's risk for venous thromboembolic disease during "high-risk" situations. The screening study revealed one occult popliteal DVT and a venous incompetence rate of approximately 30%. The conclusion of the presentation was that ". . . the risk and incidence of venous disease in a target group . . . is surprisingly high. . . ." While these findings are promising, there remains considerable controversy as to the value of venous screening as it relates to whether "silent" venous disease can be detected "early," whether effective therapy is available, and whether early treatment will lead to better outcomes. Although it seems intuitive that these criteria will be met, we do not have the proof at this time. Other issues related to the cost effectiveness of venous screening, the true danger of occult disease, and so on remain unknown.

WHO TO SCREEN?

Conventional wisdom suggests that there are certain populations for which screening is appropriate. In general, we try to identify subgroups of patients for screening that are likely to be at high risk for the disease, or are likely to benefit from early treatment. For example, it does not make sense to screen third graders for occult vascular disease using the controversial methods of ultrasound and pressure measurement (although some might argue that intimal thickness, brachial reactivity, and other methods could conceivably identify children at risk for vascular disease). Conversely, it is of questionable value to screen very high-risk populations in whom the potential to meaningfully alter the course of the disease with treatment may be limited (do we really want to screen elderly patients in nursing homes for vascular disease?).

At present, most patients presenting for screening are self-selected; screening programs are offered in church basements, shopping mall parking lots, or other locations, and patients who are interested in identifying their own personal risk for vascular disease can attend the screening. It is in this group of patients that one of the biggest controversies in vascular screening resides. Specifically, what is the appropriate role of screening in the "affluent worried-well"? These are patients who have a low pretest risk of vascular disease, ample disposable income, and a significant fear of occult vascular disease. A typical example might be a 35-year-old woman with no cardiovascular risk factors who presents for vascular screening. Given her extremely low risk of abdominal aortic aneurysm, significant carotid disease, or PAD, is it even ethical to take her money in exchange for vascular screening? At one end of the spectrum are those who feel that it is morally irresponsible to screen in a situation like this. The argument is often accompanied by unfounded claims that private testing agencies, industry sources, or others hype the risk of vascular disease and create an environment in which the general population is scared not to be screened. At the other end of the spectrum are those capitalism purists who believe that we live in a free country and that people should be allowed to spend their money any way they want. We let folks buy booze, cigarettes, and music by Ashley Simpson—why not let them waste their money on unnecessary vascular screening? Sure, it is unnecessary, but those other things are also unnecessary, and we don't stop people from spending their money on them. If screening helps somebody sleep better at night, why not do it? Naturally, screening of extremely low-risk individuals will occasionally turn up an unsuspected, sometimes significant finding, which only serves to bolster the argument for "screening anyone who wants it. This aspect of screening may be the most controversial—and ultimately most difficult—of all issues to resolve.

STANDARDS FOR SCREENING

Should there be standards for vascular screening? Should the ability to perform screening examinations be limited only to those who can demonstrate proficiency with vascular screening studies in other settings, or does the "free enterprise" aspect of screening (i.e., it is not affecting private insurers or Medicare) justify a "wide open" marketplace? Should all physicians be allowed to operate screening programs? Should nonphysicians be allowed to screen for disease? And if screening standards are to be developed, who should be responsible for this activity?

These questions may ultimately prove less controversial than others. The Intersocietal Commission for the Accreditation of Vascular Laboratories (ICAVL) has already established a screening credential for existing, accredited vascular laboratories. These standards address issues such as the type of equipment that must be used for screening exams, training and credentialing of physicians and technologists, numbers of exams to be performed, and so on. A similar screening credential is being developed for free-standing entities through an ICAVL-affiliated organization called the Accreditation of Vascular Screening Services (AVSS).[11] It seems obvious that credentialing and standards are important for maintaining the integrity and legitimacy of the screening process in this country, but as with everything else related to screening, it is likely that controversy will develop as these programs proliferate.

CONCLUSIONS

Vascular screening has arrived and is here to stay. How widespread it ultimately becomes will largely depend on the resolution of the controversies noted above. Will screening be limited to those situations where silent disease can be detected early, effective therapy is available, and early treatment leads to better outcomes? Will it prove to be cost-effective? Standard technologies such as duplex ultrasound and ankle-brachial index measurements are at the forefront of screening operations now, but what role will assessment of intimal thickness, brachial reactivity, vessel calcification, and other tests play? Will venous screening prove to be a valuable endeavor? Are there other types of vascular disease for which screening will emerge? Can we identify populations that will optimally benefit from screening? How do we handle the "worried well" who demand screening but have a very low risk of the disease? Finally, will we be able to establish and enforce meaningful standards for screening operations?

So many questions, so few answers.

REFERENCES

1. American Vascular Association Screening Program. Retrieved from http://www.vascularweb.org/_CONTRIBUTION_PAGES/AVA_Screening/AVA_Screening_Report_2004.html

2. Bettmen MA, Dake MD, Hopkins LN, et al. Atherosclerotic Vascular Disease Conference: Revascularization. *Circulation*. 2004;109:2643–2650.
3. Pisano E, Gatsonis C, Hendrick E, et al. Diagnostic Performance of Digital versus Film Mammography for Breast Cancer Screening – The Results of the American College of Radiology Imaging Network (ACRIN) Digital Mammographic Imaging Screening Trial (DMIST). NEJM, published online September 16, 2005 and in print on October 27, 2005. Retrieved from www.cancer.gov/newscenter/pressreleases/DMISTrelease
4. Coley CM, Barry JM, Mulley AG, was developed for the Health and Public Policy Committee by the Clinical Efficacy Assessment Subcommittee. Clinical Guideline: Part III: Screening for Prostate Cancer. Annals of Internal Medicine. March 1997; 126(6):480–484. Retrieved May 2, 2006, from www.annals.org/cgi/content/full
5. Retrieved from www.vascularweb.org
6. Fleming C, Whitlock EP, Beil TL, Lederle FA. Screening for Abdominal Aortic Aneurysm: A Best-Evidence Systematic Review. *Ann Internal Medicine* 2005; 142:203–11. Retrieved May 4, 2006, from www.ahcpr.gov/clinic/uspstf05/aaascr/aaarev.htm
7. U.S. Preventive Services Task Force Report on Screening for Peripheral Arterial Disease. Release date: August 2005. Retrieved May 1, 2006, from http://www.ahrq.gov/clinic/uspstf05/pad/padup.htm
8. Allison MA, Tiefenbrun J, Langer RD, Wright CM. Atherosclerotic calcification and intimal medial thickness of the carotid arteries. *Inter J Cardio*. 2005;103:98–104.
9. Moens AL, Goovaerts I, Claeys MJ, Vrints CJ. Flow-Mediated Vasodilation. A Diagnostic Instrument or an Experimental Tool? *Am Coll Chest Physicians*. 2005;127:2254–2263.
10. McLafferty RB, Lohr JM, Padberg FT, et al. Results of a Pilot Screening program for Venous Disease by the American Venous Forum. Abstract presented at 18th Annual American Venous Forum Meeting. February 23, 2006. Intercontinental Hotel – Miami, Florida.
11. Retrieved May 6, 2006, from http://www.icavl.org/icavl/news/vascularnews.htm

3

The Leapfrog Recommendations in Vascular Surgery

William H. Pearce, M.D.

The Leapfrog group was established in November of 2002 to improve the quality of health care delivery. The goal of the Leapfrog group was to improve hospital care by "rewarding hospitals that implemented significant improvements in quality and safety." The group chose the name to reflect the underlying philosophy that leaps could be made in the improvement of the delivery of the health care of employees and retirees through this mechanism. The Leapfrog group gained national attention by acquiring the support of many Fortune 500 companies with the intent of reducing health care costs by improving quality. Similarly, the purchasers of health care and other consumer groups could use the data from the Leapfrog group as benchmarks to compare hospitals and physicians. Currently, the Leapfrog group publishes the results of their surveys and studies at www.leapfroggroup.org. This site, like other consumer sites, attempts to compare the quality of hospitals and physicians. The basis of quality in the Leapfrog survey reflects the impact of both hospital volume and processes that have been associated with good outcomes.

The quality of health care is difficult to define, particularly in surgical procedures. The standard surgical outcome measure is 30-day mortality. But other outcome measures of a procedure may be better reflected by in-hospital mortality, length of stay, one-year survival, and quality of life metrics such as the SF-36. In addition, it is important to remember that not all procedures carry the same risk, nor are the patients necessarily similar. To determine a difference in the outcome of a patient undergoing a hernia repair may be very difficult because the incidence of a complication is very low and late outcome (recurrence) may be difficult to detect. However, in patients with ruptured abdominal aortic aneurysms (rAAA), there is a high in-hospital mortality rate, and the differences in outcome may be easily detected based simply on mortality statistics. This chapter will briefly review the data behind the Leapfrog group's recommendations for carotid endarterectomy (CEA) and abdominal aortic aneurysm (AAA) repair. In addition, the chapter will discuss the contradictory positions of volume-related based outcome measures and propose additional measures of outcomes.

VOLUME-BASED OUTCOMES

More than 20 years ago, Luft and colleagues reported that surgical operations should be regionalized since surgical volume determines outcome.[1] In this landmark paper in the *New England Journal of Medicine* in 1979, Luft documented the inverse relationship between volume and mortality. High-volume surgeons were found to have lower mortalities than low-volume surgeons. The authors suggested that this difference in outcome was based either on a "selective referral pattern" or that "practice makes perfect." A selective referral pattern developed when referring physicians recognized excellent outcomes and preferentially referred patients to surgeons with good outcomes. In the other view (practice makes perfect), high-volume surgeons learn techniques to improve care. Unfortunately, both points of view excluded the possibility that other factors outside of the surgeon may be important such as patient selection and hospital resources. In the era of managed care, these concepts became important since physician referral was no longer dictated by the patient or physician desires, but based on administrative decisions by the insurer. Thus, patients would be referred to centers based on expenses rather than excellence or higher volume centers.

Numerous studies have been published by vascular surgeons and others assessing outcomes of CEA, AAA repair, and repair of ruptured AAAs.[2-10] These studies share similar methodology. Large Medicare or hospital discharge databases are studied using univariable and multivariable analysis. Risk adjustment is variable and verification of data nonexistent. In addition, the studies are unable to accurately distinguish between indications for the procedure. For example, the results of CEA are highly dependent on the indication. The periprocedural complication rate is significantly different for asymptomatic patients (<2%) versus symptomatic patients (5.6%).[11] In this example, case mix is the major determinant of outcome.

Outcome studies demonstrate that surgical outcomes are better with increased surgeon or hospital volume. The effect is greatest with rAAA and least with CEA. To systematically test the methodologic rigors of these studies, Halm and colleagues reviewed more than 272 studies to examine the relationship between outcome and physician or hospital volume.[12] The authors concluded that "high volume was associated with better outcomes across a wide range of procedures and conditions, but the magnitude of the association varied greatly." The investigators found that the greatest differences existed in patients undergoing high-risk procedures including those for rAAA, pancreatectomy, and esophogectomies. There was an increased association with CEA, although the association was small. Twenty-one studies examined the relationship between physician and hospital volume, and 12 of these found a significant independent effect for both, four found a significant independent effect for hospital volume, and four a significant independent effect for physician volume. Surgeon volume appeared to be more important in determining outcome than hospital volume in cases of coronary artery bypass grafting (CABG), CEA, and surgery for rAAA and colorectal cancer. However, hospital volume effect is important for repair of nonruptured AAA.

In our own studies of California and Florida databases, we found that surgeon volume and certification were significantly related to better patient outcome in patients undergoing CEA and AAA.[13,14] However, hospital volume played an important role, particularly in high-risk and resource-intensive procedures such as AAA and rAAA. In a detailed study by Ebaugh of 16,000 admissions in Northern Illinois for lower extremity bypasses, he found that the mortality and outcomes of lower extremity procedures were superior at high capability hospitals (i.e., hospitals with cardiac cath labs, noninvasive vascular laboratories, intensive care units, and vascular fellowship training programs).[15] This study was one of the first to look beyond surgeon or hospital volume to hospital structure.

While volume is associated with better outcomes, the threshold for minimum volume is difficult to determine for vascular surgery. In a study of surgical case volume and certification, the minimal annual volume for AAA and CEA was 15 and 25, respectively.[14] However, some low-volume surgeons had excellent results while some high-volume surgeons had poor results. Halm concluded from his review of the literature that the definition of high- and low-volume procedures and surgeons varied dramatically. By overemphasizing volume at the expense of quality, unintended consequences may arise. If volume becomes the sole determinant of quality, surgeons may respond by increasing the volume of a procedure by liberalizing indication. Finally, what is the important impact of high-volume versus low-volume in a low-risk procedure such as a carotid endarterectomy? Is a relative difference of <1% in mortality and stroke important clinically?

PROCESS AND OUTCOMES

An alternative to using mortality and morbidity as a measure of quality of care, there has been a recent trend to focus on identifiable processes associated with high quality care. The strategy is to identify a process that is associated with good outcomes and then generalize the process to all hospitals. Protocols for the management of certain patients would be developed and compliance measured. This process is the current basis of the pay for performance G codes that are being promoted by Centers for Medicare and Medicaid (CMS). While processes such as prophylactic antibiotics and perioperative beta blockers are easy to measure, the true quality of care is more difficult to measure because of the enormous number of other variables that impact patient outcome. The fact that a surgeon uses beta blockers does not guarantee that the surgeon is competent, nor does it guarantee a good outcome. Process alone will not improve quality without a feedback system to alter physician performance. This process was employed by the Northern New England Cardiovascular Study Group (NNECOSG),[16] National Surgical Quality Improvement Project,[17] and CMS 10-State Peer Review Organization (PRO).[18] Northwestern Memorial Hospital was a participant in the CMS PRO CEA review program. Previously, identified measures of CEA quality (1995) antiplatelet use, carotid patching, and intraoperative heparin were collected and reported semiannually and compared with peers for two years. The follow-up article by Kresowik reported significant increases in carotid patching and other processes, but the overall improvement in the stroke death rate was only 0.6%.[19] However, the overall stroke rate in asymptomatic patients was 3.8%, which is unacceptable. To reduce this rate to Asymptomatic Carotid Artery Stenosis (ACAS) levels (1.7%), it would be expensive and time-consuming to identify outlier surgeons. Of the 10 states, Georgia had an overall stroke rate of 4.2% and was 1.4% in asymptomatic patients (consistent with ACAS). Georgia has an ongoing quality improvement program and its success should be studied.

The Multistate Quality Program provided many insights on how a governmental review process may work. There was clearly an improvement in process (i.e., the surgeons were complying) but the net benefit was small, with Georgia being the exception. Quality improvement programs (like Georgia and the NNECDSG) were successful because of smaller scale and direct physician feedback. In addition, it is likely that the observed changes in process in the multistate program will disappear as the program is no longer functioning (Hawthorne effect). Without the specter of outside monitoring, outcomes may decline.

In summary, physicians will respond by complying with processes, but the result may not necessarily lead to better outcomes. Continued monitoring of outcomes appears to be a better approach, but costly. An alternative is to publish surgical outcomes as was done in New York (surgeon-specific) or on Healthgrades.com (hospital-specific). Unfortunately, if the published results are not accurately risk-adjusted, surgeons caring for the sickest patients will be penalized. A sophisticated and monitored system such as the Society for Thoracic Surgery (STS) database is needed in vascular surgery. Recently, direct patient marketing of outcomes has been used by hospitals and health care systems. These un-audited results are either mailed directly to patients or physicians, usually comparing outstanding single-center results with national statistics in an effort to attract patients.

THE LEAPFROG RECOMMENDATIONS

The Leapfrog group selected two vascular procedures (CEA and AAA). The Leapfrog group utilized ZYNX Research group, which recruited expert panels consisting of members of the Society for Vascular Surgery to recommend processes thought to be important as quality indicators for both operations. The ZYNX group then reviewed the relevant literature and provided a draft of proposed recommendations on which the expert panel could comment. At the conclusion, the following recommendations were made for CEA and AAA repairs. For the most part, randomized clinical trials played the greatest role followed by prospective quality improvement programs such as the multistate CEA program. For all patients undergoing carotid endarterectomies, the patients should:

- receive aspirin or antiplatelet agent for within 48 hours prior to CEA.
- receive aspirin or another antiplatelet agent if aspirin allergic on hospital discharge.
- receive carotid patch angioplasty.
- receive heparin during carotid clamping.

For unknown reasons, the Leapfrog group does not report CEA compliance on its Web site. For AAA repair, the only recommendations were the use of perioperative beta blockers. The number of patients receiving beta blockers both before and after repair is documented and compared to the total number of patients undergoing AAA repair. In addition, based on their analysis of volume studies, the Leapfrog group categorized hospitals into those performing fewer than 17, 17–49, and 50 or greater. In order to achieve the highest Leapfrog rating, the hospital had to have taken part in the Leapfrog survey, had a greater than 80% adherence to the process (use of perioperative beta blockers), and monitor and perform more than 50 procedures.

COMMENTS

Since the Leapfrog group bases its quality measures on volume and compliance with a recommended process, moderate volume centers may be impacted, even though they have excellent outcomes and even if they have 100% compliance with process. These hospitals and surgeons may feel pressure to increase volume. Likewise, high-volume hospitals with 100% compliance may have a low-volume surgeon with poor outcomes, and yet the hospital will receive the highest rating. The Leapfrog group has missed its goal. The Leapfrog group and others concerned with quality care should recommend internal data registries and ongoing quality monitoring of indications, case mix, severity indexing, and outcomes. The Leapfrog group or other health organizations would count this feature as a plus. These databases then could be randomly reviewed for accuracy. Such a program is not so far-fetched. CMS has mandated such registries as a condition to be approved for reimbursement for carotid artery stenting (www.cms. hhs.gov/coverage/carotid_stent_facilities.asp). All hospitals must ensure periodic review and CMS access to the carotid artery stenting registry.

Other strategies to improve surgical outcomes have been proposed to improve quality. One strategy employed by the State of New York was to publish surgeon-specific outcomes of patients undergoing CABGs. The publication of surgeon-specific results may lead to changes in practice that may be harmful to the patient (i.e., avoiding difficult cases). Other public data (including www.healthgrades.com) contains risk-adjusted data for a variety of surgical procedures including lower extremity bypass procedures, aortic aneurysm repair, and CEAs. Currently, these databases are only hospital-specific and are not surgeon-specific. The reported results are based on Medicare discharge data and are risk-adjusted based on coded complications. Unfortunately, these databases are not validated for accuracy.

The multistate improvement program and NNECOSG provided baseline data that assess procedures associated with good outcomes. Physician results are monitored and feedback given. Unfortunately, these programs are costly and difficult to sustain. However, it is unclear whether the adoption of a process leads to better outcomes or was simply the result of the surgeons knowing that their results were to be scrutinized by peers.

As fewer open procedures are being performed, new quality measures will be needed. Indications may change (liberalized). Mortality will decrease but long-term outcomes may be difficult to monitor. Vascular surgeons and endovascular surgeons must establish internal registries that are audited. The Society for Vascular Surgery has registries for both AAA and CEA/carotid artery stenting, but they are rarely used. Vascular surgeons must participate in these programs or an outside organization will impose a program as the Leafrog group has done and miss the mark.

REFERENCES

1. Luft HS, Bunker JP, Enthoven AC. Should operations be regionalized? The empirical relation between surgical volume and mortality. *N Eng J Med*. 1979;301:1364–1369.
2. Perler BA, Dardik A, Burleyson GP, et al. Influence of age and hospital volume on the results of carotid endarterectomy: a statewide analysis of 9918 cases. *J Vasc Surg*. 1998; 27:25–31.

3. Wennberg DE, Lucas FL, Birkmeyer JD, et al. Variation in carotid endarterectomy mortality in the Medicare population: trial hospitals, volume, and patient characteristics. *JAMA*. 1998;279:1278–1281.

4. Katz DJ, Stanley JC, Zelenock GB. Operative mortality rates for intact and ruptured abdominal aortic aneurysms in Michigan: an eleven-year statewide experience. *J Vasc Surg*. 1994;19:804–815.

5. Hannan EL, Kilburn H Jr, O'Donnell JF, et al. A longitudinal analysis of the relationship between in-hospital mortality in New York State and the volume of abdominal aortic aneurysm surgeries performed. *Health Serv Res*. 1992;27:517–542.

6. Wen SW, Simunovic M, Williams JI, Johnston KW, Naylor CD. Hospital volume, calendar age, and short term outcomes in patients undergoing repair of abdominal aortic aneurysms: the Ontario experience, 1988–92. *J Epidemiol Community Health*. 1996;50:207–213.

7. Kazmers A, Jacobs L, Perkins A, et al. Abdominal aortic aneurysm repair in Veterans Affairs medical centers. *J Vasc Surg*. 1996;23:191–200.

8. Dardik A, Burleyson GP, Bowman H, et al. Surgical repair of ruptured abdominal aortic aneurysms in the state of Maryland: factors influencing outcome among 527 recent cases. *J Vasc Surg*. 1998;28:413–420.

9. Hannen EL, Popp AJ, Tramner B, et al. Relationship between provider volume and mortality for carotid endarterectomies in New York state. *Stroke*. 1998;29:2292–2297.

10. Cebul RD, Snow RJ, Pine R, et al. Indications, outcomes and provider volumes for carotid endarterectomy. *JAMA*. 1998;279:1282–1287.

11. Hertzer NR. Presidential address: Outcome assessment in vascular surgery - Results mean everything. *J Vasc Surg*. 1995;21:6–15.

12. Halm EA, Lee C, Chassin MR. Is volume related to outcome in Health Care? A systematic review and methodologic critique of the literature. *Ann Intern Med*. 2002;137:511–520.

13. Manheim LM, Sohn MW, Feinglass J, et al. Hospital vascular surgery volume and procedure mortality rates in California, 1982–1994. *J Vasc Surg*. 1998;27:25–31.

14. Pearce WH, Parker MA, Feinglass J, et al. The importance of surgeon volume and training in outcomes for vascular surgical procedures. *J Vasc Surg*. 1999;29:768–778.

15. Ebaugh JL, Feinglass J, Pearce WH. The effect of hospital vascular operation capability on outcomes of lower extremity arterial bypass graft procedures. *Surgery*. 2001;130:561–567.

16. O'Connor GT, Plume SK, Olmstead EM. A regional intervention to improve the hospital mortality associated with coronary artery bypass graft surgery. The Northern New England Cardiovascular Disease Study Group. *JAMA*. 1996;275:841–846.

17. Khuri SF, Daley J, Henderson WG. The comparative assessment and improvement of quality of surgical care in the Department of Veteran Affairs. *Arch Surg*. 2002;137:20–27.

18. Kresowik TF, Bratzler DW, Karp HR, et al. Multistate utilization, processes, and outcomes of carotid endarterectomy. *J Vasc Surg*. 2001;33:227–235.

19. Kresowik TF, Bratzler DW, Kresowik RA, et al. Multistate improvement in process and outcomes of carotid endarterectomy. *J Vasc Surg*. 2004;39:372–380.

4

The Significance of Silent Infarctions of the Brain

Joseph H. Rapp, M.D., Amritha Ragunathan, B.A., and Xian Mang Pan, M.D.

Neuroanatomists have long described areas of infarction in elderly patients' brains without antecedent history of stroke. With the advent of widely disseminated access to brain imaging, both by CT and MRI, a great deal of epidemiologic evidence has been gained regarding these so called "silent infarcts." As with clinically apparent stroke, these lesions are undoubtedly manifestations of a variety of pathologic entities. For this reason, there are a variety of findings regarding etiology, undoubtedly reflecting a variety of populations studied. It is our belief that micro atheroemboli are an important etiologic factor. In the course of this review, we will summarize current literature on the size, location and frequency of silent infarctions; their associated demographics, and the evidence primarily in animal studies that implicates micro atheroemboli in the pathologic process leading to silent infarction in the brain.

The location of silent infarctions is primarily subcortical. The Cardiovascular Health Study examined 3647 elderly subjects.[1] On MRI scan, they found that for patients with single silent infarcts, 8% were in the cortex, 72% were subcortical, and 7% were found in the posterior fossa. This report also noted that silent infarctions are far more common among patients with a separate lesion that corresponded to a clinically evident stroke. These silent infarctions were overwhelmingly lacunar type infarctions. That is not surprising, given the high prevalence of subcortical lesions among silent infarcts.

Among patients with a previous history of stroke, up to 68% of MRI scans will show at least one silent infarction. When elderly patients without an antecedent history of stroke were scanned, approximately 30% were shown to have at least one lesion of 3 mm or greater. While lacunar strokes may be the most common type in the Cardiovascular Health Study, these lesions were not necessarily small. The diameter of the largest silent infarct was over 15 mm in 19%, 3 to15 mm in 66%, and less than 3 mm in 15% of patients presenting with no antecedent history of neurologic event.

In addition to being far more prevalent among patients with an antecedent history of stroke, silent infarcts are far more common as patients age. They are also found more commonly among patients with impaired cognitive function, as discussed below, and with minor neurologic abnormalities. Patients who have silent infarctions on MRI are also likely to have visual field defects and weakness with walking. It seems clear that the term silent infarction is not descriptively accurate. It may be more appropriate to describe patients suffering these lesions as having had strokes creating a low level of symptomatology.

Increased age, hypertension, smoking, diabetes, and carotid artery stenosis have been associated with silent infarctions that were not preceded by clinically evident stroke. These are also associated conditions in those silent infarcts noted in patients with stroke. In addition, male gender is associated with a higher incidence among those with prior stroke. Of the multiple factors associated with silent infarctions, increased age appears to be the most dominant factor for silent infarction. The incidence of these lesions in patients with no prior stroke increases steadily from age 60 until age 85, 40% of patients have evidence of an infarction. In those patients who have had a clinically evidenced stroke, there is no such progression, causing these authors to consider that this represents a different disease process.

Given the location of the majority of silent infarctions, it is not surprising that there is a strong association of high blood pressure with these lesions. A high rate of silent infarction has been shown in the Rotterdam Scan Study to be associated with diastolic and systolic blood pressure.[2] Patients with elevated diastolic blood pressure were three times more likely to have unrecognized cerebral infarctions. A higher risk is also independently associated with systolic blood pressure. Not surprisingly, pulse pressure also was significantly associated with silent infarctions. Whether this is a primary factor or simply a result of the influence of systolic hypertension is speculative. Interestingly, in this population-based study, hypertension was not a risk factor for silent infarctions in patients with symptomatic strokes.

In population-base studies such as the Rotterdam Scan Study, smoking is not significantly associated with the incidence of silent infarction.[2] However, among patients who have had a clinically evidenced stroke, smoking is related to silent lesions,[3] once again suggesting different etiologic factors among these patients as noted in the Cardiovascular Health Study publication[1]. Similar segregation in risk exists for carotid artery stenosis and diabetes.

The relationship of silent infarcts to carotid atherosclerosis is quite strong in patients who have had a symptomatic stroke. In patients with TIAs, the frequency of clinically silent infarcts found on scans was 47%. The frequency was 30% in patients with asymptomatic carotid stenosis, and 19% in patients with transient ischemic attack but without carotid stenosis.[4] This clear association does not hold up in other studies, however. In some cases, while the incidences in silent infarcts was associated with carotid stenosis, more than half of the lesions were on the side of the more severe of the carotid lesions.[5] The variable results may reflect variations in severity of atherosclerotic carotid plaque examined in the study populations.

Atrial fibrillation also is a potent risk factor for silent infarcts as well as for stroke. The incidence of silent infarcts in patients with atrial fibrillation is as high as 48%[6]. The data is particularly impressive when MRI scanning is used among patients who have already suffered a clinical stroke. In one study, a full 85% of these individuals have had evidence of silent, or at least previously unrecognized, infarcts in the brain.[7] The silent lesions were more typically cortical when associated with atrial fibrillation,[8] but certainly not exclusively. Once again, demonstrating that while microemboli may preferentially affect the cortex, they are also likely to travel down the smaller vessels such as the lenticular striate arteries that feed the subcortical areas.

SILENT BRAIN INFARCTIONS FROM MICROATHEROEMBOLI AS A CAUSE OF VASCULAR DEMENTIA

Work in our laboratory has focused on the ability of microatheroemboli to cause lacunar type strokes by damage to the small artery wall and not by necessarily occluding the artery primarily. These lesions would eventually lead to lacunar type infarctions but also set up a local inflammatory reaction that results in a microdisruption of the blood brain-barrier. Thus, emboli would set in motion the very disease process thought to be responsible for "hypertensive strokes." As noted previously, this type of lesion may not be completely asymptomatic. Rather, it may cause a subtle disruption in intellectual functioning: a vascular dementia.

Vascular dementia (VaD) can occur in the setting of multiple strokes[9] but it may be much more common than generally recognized to occur in the setting of few other neurologic signs (i.e., as a result of multiple small, "silent" infarctions in either the cortical or subcortical areas).[10-11] In the former setting, atheroemboli are recognized as a frequent cause while in the latter setting atheroemboli are thought to be less common than hypertension as the etiologic agent.

Along with lacunar infarcts, small areas of deterioration within the white matter, or leukoaraiosis, are recognized as important causes of cognitive decline.[12-14] Diffusion-weighted imaging by MRI has shown local disruptions of the BBB in the areas of leukoaraiosis.[15] These lesions also are thought to be due to focal ischemia resulting from microvascular disease with hypertension regarded as the etiologic agent. The pathophysiology of this process is thought to include a degeneration of the small cerebral artery wall termed lipohyalinosis and characterized by intrusion of a thickened vessel wall on the vessel lumen resulting in near or complete occlusion.[16]

There is strong epidemiologic evidence that there are other etiologies of lacunar lesions and leukoaraiosis besides hypertension. First, these lesions frequently occur in patients without hypertension or diabetes.[17] Second, the incidence of hypertension is no higher in patients with lacunar infarcts and leukooaraiosis than those with presumed atheroembolic strokes.[18] Finally, the blood pressure elevations required to create these lesions in experimental animals are uncommon in clinical practice.[19]

Recently, Wardlaw and colleagues have suggested that a primary deterioration of small penetrating vessels with disruption of the BBB and perivascular leakage of blood products may initiate the arterial wall thickening characteristic of lipohyalinosis.[20] Experimentally localized edema of the vessel wall with perivascular leakage of plasma into the brain initiates fibinoid necrosis, the acute phase of lypohyaninosis.[21] Indeed, simply injecting plasma proteases into the brain can initiate arterial wall damage and disrupt the BBB.[22] But is this primary event initiating CNS artery wall damage always hypertension? We suggest that in many cases it is microatheroemboli, creating focal areas of inflammation and disrupting the BBB.

FREQUENCY OF MICROEMBOLI IN PATIENTS WITH CEREBROVASCULAR ATHEROSCLEROSIS

Random transcranial doppler (TCD) studies in patients with cerebrovascular atherosclerosis have shown that microembolic signals are frequently observed within intracranial arteries. The incidence of spontaneous microemboli detected during a 30-60 minute monitoring session ranges from 21% to 60%.[23-27] Monitoring for four hours can nearly double the number of patients with detectable emboli,[28] suggesting that the true incidence of spontaneous microemboli in a population with cerebrovascular atherosclerosis is quite high. The frequency of emboli detected can reach impressive levels. Droste reported over 100 embolic signals per hour in several patients who recently had experienced a TIA-like event.[23]

Further evidence of the brain's ability to tolerate emboli without tissue infarction comes from TCD monitoring in patients undergoing carotid angioplasty. Several hundred emboli have been documented during this procedure,[29-31] yet the incidence of stroke is low.[32] The lower size threshold for TCD detection of microemboli is in the range of 70μm,[33] indicating that there is great potential for these fragments to lodge in the small penetrating arteries (50-200μm) of the brain.

Inflammatory Response to Atheroemboli in the Artery Wall

When atheroemboli lodge in the arterial tree, they initiate a localized inflammatory response that damages the local artery wall. This includes a cellular infiltrate, a chronic inflammatory response, and eventual scarring. This process has been studied extensively in the kidney[34-36] but there is evidence that a similar process occurs in the human brain.[37] The reaction begins within 24 hours of embolization with a panarteritis characterized by hyperplasia and an accumulation of monocytes that engulf cholesterol crystals. By three days, the reaction is characterized by an accumulation of eosinophils, and by seven days, a fibrotic response is initiated with cellular proliferation and extracellular matrix formation. At this later stage, cholesterol crystals are seen within giant cells. Several investigators have described that progressive arteriolar sclerosis caused by atheroemboli can result in end-organ ischemia.[38-40]

In areas with extensive collaterals such as the cerebral cortex, these changes may not create end-organ ischemia.[41] This extensive collateral network may be an important factor in the brain's ability to tolerate large numbers of microemboli. However, in the lenticulostriate arteries or in other areas that are less well collateralized, such changes would lead to localized ischemia.

Evidence that Microatheroemboli Can Cause Subcortical and White Matter Infarction

Although microatheroemboli are not considered to be a common cause of brain small artery disease,[20,42] they do lodge in the small penetrating arteries of the brain and cause distal ischemia.[43] Atheroemboli have been found occluding the leptomeningeal and small penetrating arteries proximal to lacunar infarctions.[44-45] In 16 autopsy cases, Soloway and Arenson found all but one supratentorial infarction to be correlated with occluded terminal branches, and that 52 of the 71 occluded arteries were between 50 and 200μm.[45] Masuda et al. examined 15 cases and found atheroemboli were occluding vessels 50μm–3 mm in size, including perforating and leptomeningeal arteries that ranged from 50–300μm in diameter.[37]

There also is an association between cerebrovascular atherosclerosis and lacunar infarcts, further suggesting that the involvement of microatheroemboli in subcortical and white matter infarction may be common. For example, among the 23%–50% of patients with lacunar infarcts who have neither hypertension nor diabetes, there is a high prevalence of cerebrovascular and/or cardiac atherosclerosis,[43,46-47] and in patients with severe carotid atherosclerosis, the risk of lacunar infarction is increased 10-fold.[48]

Evidence Linking Microemboli to Dementia in Humans

Evidence linking dementia and microemboli comes from three clinical scenarios where large numbers of cerebral emboli have been noted on TCD, coronary artery bypass (CABG), prosthetic valve placement, and atrial fibrillation, Manipulation of the aortic arch during CABG can dislodge atherosclerotic debris, resulting in hundreds of embolic signals.[49-50] The risk of embolization is greater if the aorta is calcified[51]. Embolic fragments 20–300μm in diameter are commonly found lodged in the small penetrating arteries of the brain and retina post CABG,[52-53] often occluding vessels in the 100–200 micron range.[53] As is common with microemboli, the incidence of acute neurologic deficits is low, 6% after routine CABG54 increasing to 15.8% when valve repair is added to the procedure.[51] However, there can be subtle deficits. When greater than 1,000 emboli were noted on TCD, Pugsley found the incidence of neuropsychiatric deterioration post-CABG to be over 40%.[49] Other authors also have reported a correlation between higher rates of emboli and decline in intellectual function.[50] Unlike the expected clinical improvement after cardiopulmonary bypass, cognitive deficits associated with high rates of CNS emboli were not transient and became more pronounced when the patients were tested again eight weeks after surgery.[49] Furthermore, patients who showed neurocognitive deterioration early post-CABG had greater cognitive decline five years after the procedure.[55]

Cumulative effects of chronic microembolization to the brain have been reported with prosthetic cardiac valves and atrial fibrillation. Deklunder et al. compared the results of TCD and neuropsychiatric testing two years postoperatively in patients with prosthetic valves, compared to patients with biologic valves and patients post-CABG with no valve repair, and found decreased working memory in the prosthetic valve patients.[56] Microembolic signals were found in every patient with a prosthetic cardiac valve at a rate of 12–60/hr. No signals were detected in the other groups. Prosthetic valves create N_2 bubbles as flow through the valve can create cavitation. These can be eliminated by breathing 100% oxygen. Performing TCD in prosthetic valve patients, Nadeareishvili et al. found that the lower performance on neuropsychiatric testing correlated with emboli on TCD after inhaling O_2 (i.e., microthrombotic emboli).[57] In patients with atrial fibrillation, embolus detection has been shown to correlate with a reduction in cognitive function independent of stroke, hypertension, or diabetes.[58]

Statins, Hypercholesterolemia, and Neuronal Injury

Statin therapy has been shown to reduce the risk of stroke both clinically and experimentally.[59] The effects of statins are multiple. They can reduce the inflammatory response by a measurable reduction in several inflammatory cytokines[60], reduce lymphocyte binding and adhesion[61], and decrease platelet activation.[62] Furthermore, a statin has been shown to reduces neurologic deficit and induce angiogenesis, neurogenesis, and synaptogenesis in the rat after brain ischemic injury[63] and brain trauma.[64]

Statins also cause vasodilation secondary to an increase in the expression of eNOS.[65] This may be influential in modifying injury from emboli to the microcirculation. This vasodilation effect is independent of cholesterol level although hypercholesterolemic subjects have impaired vasodilation, increasing their risk of vasospasm.[66] It is not clear whether the statin effect removes or counteracts the hypercholesterolemic effect. Vasospasm in the area of an embolus could be a critical feature determining the extent of injury. The relative contributions of hypercholesterolemia and atherosclerotic lesions to disruption of the BBB with a given embolic challenge and the effect of statin treatment in these settings have not been examined.

RESEARCH EVIDENCE THAT MICROATHEROEMBOLI CAN CAUSE LACUNAR TYPE INFARCTIONS

To date, we have shown that microemboli can create focal CNS injury without infarction. This causes perivascular disruption of the BBB with subsequent activation of microglia and astrocytes. Since the microcirculation of the rat is quite similar to that of humans,[67] these findings have implications for the clinical setting.

In our initial experiments examining the relationship between atheroemboli and cerebral injury, we made no attempt to differentiate the risk posed by emboli of varying composition. Stimulated by a case of extensive neurological injury following the angioplasty of a heavily calcified carotid plaque, we asked if the composition as well as size of atheroemboli could determine the extent of neurological injury.

Carotid plaques that were either heavily calcified or plaques that were primarily fibrous (containing little calcium and minimal or no necrotic core) were identified by high resolution MRI. These plaques were wrapped in PTFE and subjected to ex vivo angioplasty. The resulting fragments of calcified or fibrous atheroma were sized at 100–200μm and 60–100μm, respectively. Rats were injected with 100 fragments, imaged with a 7T SMIS System (T2 weighted SE sequences, 12 slices/mm), and immunohistochemistry was performed on brain sections to identify brain ischemia by the presence of heat shock protein (HSP) and neuronal cell death by loss of NeuN staining.

Calcified atheroembolic fragments caused infarction more frequently and with significantly larger areas of infarction by MRI than did fibrous atheroembolic fragments $(p = 0.04)$. However, the fibrous fragments caused injury without infarction in nine out of the 11 animals injected (Table 4-1). These areas of injury were generally small, presumably localized to the area where the embolus lodged in the vascular bed.

TABLE 4-1. BRAIN INJURY ASSESSED BY MRI, HSP70 AND NEUN IMMUNOSTAINING AFTER INJECTING 60–100 MICRON FRAGMENTS FROM CALCIFIED OR FIBROTIC CAROTID PLAQUES

	Sham	Ca2$^+$	Fibrous
Total No. of rats	5	12	11
MRI Total no. rats with positive T2 lesion	N/A	7	1
Total infarct volume (mm^3)**	N/A	766.6	137.7
Hsp70 Total no. rats with positive staining	0	9	9
Total score*	0	48	26
Average score**	0	4.0 ± .26	2.35 ± 1.69
NeuN Total no. rats with loss of staining	0	5	4
Total score*	0	225	10
Average score**	0	2.27 ± 3.38	0.91 ± 1.51

*Scoring criteria: 0: no positive staining; 1: the diameter of positive staining area less than 0.5 mm and no necrotic tissue. 2: the diameter of positive staining area more than 0.5 mm or the diameter of necrotic tissue less than 0.5mm; 3: the diameter of necrotic tissue area more than 0.5 mm. The score was determined in striatum, cortex, septum, hippocampus, thalamus, and corpus callosum separately. Total scores include all of the above six areas; the maximal total scores in one animal was 18.

**p = 0.04 for MRI. Average score of hsp70 and NeuN staining was obtained and expressed as mean ± sem. The average score for HSP and NeuN indicated a more severe injury caused by calcified emboli than fibrotic emboli; however, Mann-Whitney nonparatric test did not find significant difference between the groups (p = 0.24 and p = 0.29, respectively).

Conclusions: a. Embolus composition as well as size is a factor in determining the risk of brain injury for any given embolic shower. b. Fibrous atheroemboli 60–100 ?m commonly caused focal areas of injury without causing acute neuronal cell death.

TABLE 4-2. ACTIVATION OF MICROGLIA AND ALBUMIN LEAKAGE AFTER CHOLESTEROL CRYSTAL INJECTION IN ANIMALS WITHOUT INFARCTION

Group	Rats	CD11b		ED-1		Albumin Staining
		Positive	Total scores*	Positive		Total scores*
4d	4	4	18	4	18	3
1 week	4	3	10	2	7	2
2 weeks	4	3	8	3	4	1
4 week	6	4	8	4	5	Not done
2 months	3	0	Not done	0	Not done	Not done
4 months	3	1	Not done	1	Not done	Not done
Control	5	0	Not done	0	Not done	Not done

**Scoring criteria are the same as Table 4-1

Conclusions: a. After the embolizations of cholesterol crystals alone, there are focal breaks in the BBB and activation of inflammatory cells (microglia) in animals without cerebral infarction. b. The microglia remain activated for at least four weeks after the injury from cholesterol crystal injection

Free cholesterol crystals, called cholesterol clefts, were seen in the necrotic core of carotid plaques. These slender crystals are 60–140μm in length and 10–20μm in width. USP crystalline cholesterol (Sigma Pharmaceutical) was suspended in saline sized with 60 and 100μm filters, and 300 crystals (60–100μm) were injected into the internal carotid artery of SD rats. All animals underwent T_2-weighted MRI studies. Animals were sacrificed at four days, one week, two weeks, four weeks, two months, and four months. A control group was sacrificed at the one-week time point. Immunohistochemical stains were performed to identify both the presence (CD11b) and activation (ED-1) of microglia, and for the presence of albumin.

Six of the 30 animals injected had infarcts seen on MRI and were eliminated from the study. Table 4-2 summarizes the findings in animals that had *no infarct* seen on

MRI. Albumin staining was focal showing small disruptions in the BBB around two cross-sectioned vessels. The vessels affected had a range of diameters from 25–60μm and a mean diameter of 42μm.

CONCLUSION

There is much work to be done to clarify both the incidence and importance of silent brain infarctions. In the setting of carotid stenosis, there is growing evidence that these lesions, whether in the cortex or subcortical areas, are related to microatheroembli. Furthermore, their presence not only suggests that the atherosclerotic lesions are shedding particulates, but also suggests that the individual is at increased risk for dementia. Additional clinical research will need to be done to determine whether therapies directed at stabilization of the plaques or removal of the atherosclerotic burden at the carotid bifurcation will impact this process and prevent dementia as removal of the carotid atheroma will prevent clinically apparent stroke.

REFERENCES

1. Price TR, Manolio TA, Kronmal RA, et al. Silent brain infarction on magnetic resonance imaging and neurological abnormaolties in community-dwelling older adults: The cardiovascualr health study (chs) collaborative research group. *Stroke.* 1997;28:1158–1164
2. Vermeer SE, den Heijer T, Koudstaal PJ, et al. Incidence and risk factors of silent brain infarcts in the population-based rotterdam scan study. *Stroke.* 2003;34:392–396
3. Corea F, Tambasco N, Luccioli RC, et al. Brain ct scan in acute styroke patients: Silent infarcts and relatio to outcome. *Clin Exper Hypertension.* 2000;8:669–676
4. Norris JW, Zhu CA. Silent stroke and carotid stenosis. *Stroke.* 1992;23:483–485
5. Tanaka H, Sueyoshi D, Nishino M, et al. Silent brain infarction and coronary artery disease in japanese patients. *Arch Neurol.* 1993;50:706–709
6. Petersen P, Madsen EB, Brun B, et al. Silent cerebral infarction in chronic atrial fibrillation. *Stroke.* 1987;18:1098–1100
7. Okada Y, Fujishima M. Silent stroke. *Adv Neuro Imag.* 1989;34:641–646
8. Boone A, Lodder J, Heuts-van Raak L, Kessels F. Silent brain infarcts in 755 consecutive patients with a first-ever supratentiorial ischemic stroke. Relation ship with index-stroke subtype, vascular risk factors and mortality. *Stroke.* 1994;25:2384–2390
9. Hachinski VC, Lassen NA, Marshall J. Multi-infarct dementia. A cause of mental deterioration in the elderly. *Lancet.* 1974;2:207–210
10. Tomlinson BE, Blessed G, Roth M. Observations on the brains of demented old people. *J Neurol Sci.* 1970;11:205–242
11. Gorelick PB, Mangone CA. Vascular dementias in the elderly. *Clin Geriatr Med.* 1991;7: 59–615
12. Jellinger KA. The pathology of ischemic-vascular dementia: An update. *J Neurol Sci.* 2002; 203-204:153–157
13. van Gijn J. White matters: Small vessels and slow thinking in old age. *Lancet.* 2000;356: 612–613
14. Garde E, Martensen L, Krabbe K, et al. Relation between age-related decline in intelligence and cetebral white-matter hperintensities in healthy octogenarians: A longitudinal study. *Lancet.* 2000;356:628–634
15. Starr JM, Wardlaw JM, Ferguson K, et al. Increased blood-brain barrier permeability in type ii diabetes demonstrated by gadolinium magnetic resonance imaging. *J Neurol Neurosurg Psychiatry.* 2003;74:70–76
16. Fisher CM. Lacunar strokes and infarcts: A review. *Neurology.* 1982;32:871–876
17. Baumgartner RW, Sidler C, Mosso M, Georgiadis D. Ischemic lacunar stroke in patients with and without potential mechanism other than small-artery disease. *Stroke.* 2004;34: 653–659
18. Schulz UGR, Rothwell PM. Differences in vascular risk factors between etiological subtypes of ischemic stroke. Importance of population-based studies. *Stroke.* 2003;34:2050–2059
19. Gustafsson F. Hypertensive arteriolar necrosis revisited. *Blood Pressure.* 1997;6:71–77
20. Wardlaw JM, Sandercock PAG, Dennis MS, Starr J. Is breakdown of the blood-brain varrier responsible for lacunar stroke, leukoaraiosis, and dementia? *Stroke.* 2003;34:806–812
21. Johansson BB. Who satellite symposium: Hypertension mechanisms causing stroke. *Clin Exp Pharmacol Physiol.* 1999;26:563–565
22. Armao D, Kornfeld M, Strada EY, et al. Neutral proteases and disruption of the blood-brain barrier in the rat. *Brain Res.* 1997;767:259–264
23. Droste DW, et al. Oxygeninhalation can differentiate gaseous from nongaseous imicroemboli detected by transcranial doppler ultrasound. *Stroke.* 1997;28:2453–2456
24. Babikian VL, et al. Cerebral microembolism and early recurrent cerebral or retinal ischemic events. *Stroke.* 1997;28:1314–1318
25. Grosset DG, et al. Doppler emboli signals vary according to stroke subtype. *Stroke.* 1994;25:382–384

26. Wijman CAC, Babikian VL, Matjucha ICA, et al. Cerebral microembolism in patients with retenal ischemia. *Stroke.* 1998;29:1139–1143
27. Del Sette M, et al. Microembolic signals with serial dtranscranial doppler monitoring in acute focal ischemic deficit - a local phenomenon? *Stroke.* 1997;28:1311–1313
28. Mackinnon AD, Aaslid R, Markus HS. Long-term ambulatory monitoring for cerebral emboli using transcranial doppler ultrasound. *Stroke.* 2004;35:73–78
29. Markus HS, et al. Carotid angioplasty. Detection of emboli signals during and after the procedure. *Stroke.* 1994;25:2403–2406
30. Crawley F, et al. Comparison of hemodynamic cerebral ischemia and microembolic signals detected during carotid endarterectomy and carotid angioplasty. *Stroke.* 1997;28:2460–2464
31. Jordan WD, Jr., et al. Microemboli detected by transcranial doppler monitoring in patients during carotid angioplasty versus carotid endarterectomy. *Cardiovasc Surg.* 1999;7:33–38
32. Lovblad KO, et al. Diffusionweighted mri for monitoring meurovascular interventions. *Neuroradiology.* 2000;42:134–138
33. Moerhing MA, Spencer MP. Power M-mode doppler for observing cerevbral blood flow and tracking emboli. *Ultrasound Med Biol.* 2002;28:49–57.
34. Snyder HE. A correlative study of atheromatous embolism in human beings and experimental animals. *Surgery.* 1961;49:195–203
35. Gore I, McCombs HL, Lindquist RL. Observations on the fate of cholesterol emboli. *J Atheroscler Res.* 1964;4:527–535
36. Otken LB. Experimental production of atheromatous embolization. *Arch Path.* 1959;68:105–109
37. Masuda J, Yutani E, Ogata J, et al. Atheromatous emboli to the brain: A clinicopathologic analysis of 15 autopsy cases. *Neurology.* 1994;44:1231–1237
38. Dahlberg PJ, Frecentesese DF, Cogbill TH. Cholesterol embolization: Experience with 22 histologically proven cases. *Surgery.* 1989;105:737–746
39. Thurlbeck WM, Castleman B. Atheromatous emboli to the kedneys after aortic surgery. *NEJM.* 1957;257:242–247
40. Kassirer J. Atheroembolic renal disease. *NEJM.* 1969;280:812–818
41. Reina-de la Torre F, Rodrequez-Baeza A, Sahuquillo-Barris J. Morphological characteristics and distribution pattern of the arterial vessels in human cerebral cortex: A scanning electron microscope study. *Anat Rec.* 1998;251:87–96
42. Mead GM, Lewis SC, Wardlaw JM, et al. Severe ipsilateral crotid stenosis and middle cerebral artery disease in lacunar ischaemic stroke: Innocent bystanders? *J Neurol.* 2002;249:266–271
43. Milikan C, Futrell N. The fallacy of the lacune hypothesis. *Stroke.*1990;21:1251–1257
44. Laloux P, Brucher J-M. Lacunar infarctions due to cholesterol emboli. *Stroke.* 1991;22:1440–1444
45. Soloway HB, Aronson SM. Atheromatous emboli to central nervous system: Report of 16 cases. *Arch Neurol.* 1964;11:657–667
46. Bogousslavsky J, Van Melle G, Regli F. The lausanne stroke registry: Analysis of 1,000 consequetive pateints with first stroke. *Stroke.* 1988;19:1083–1092
47. Horowitz DR, Tuhrim S, Weinberger JM, Rudolph SH. Mechanisms of lacunar infarction. *Stroke.*1992;23:325–327
48. Hollander M, Bots ML, Del Sol AI, et al. Carotid plaques increase the risk of stroke and subtypes of cerebral infarction in asymptomatic elderly: The rotterdam study. *Circulation.* 2002;105:2872–2877
49. Pugsley W, Klinger L, Paschalis C, et al. The impact of microemboli during cardiopulmonary bypass on neuropsychological functioning. *Stroke.* 1994;25:1393–1399
50. Padayachee TS, et al. The detection of microemboli in the middle cerebral artery during cardiopulmonary bypass: A transcranial doppler untrasound investigation using membrane and buble oxygenators. *Ann Thor Surg.* 1987;44:298–302

51. Wolman RL, et al. Cerebral injuy after cardiac surbgery: Identification of a group at extraordinary risk. Multicenter study of perioperative ischemia research group and the ischemia research foundation investigators. *Stroke.* 1999;30:514–522

52. Blauth CI, Arnold JV, Schulenberg WE, et al. Cerebral microembolism during coardiopulmonary bypass. *J Thorac Cardiovasc Surg.* 1988;95:668–676

53. Price DL, Harris J. Cholesterol emboli in cerebral arteries as a complication of retrograde aortic perfusion during cadiac surgery. *Neurology.* 1970;20:1209–1214

54. Roach GW, et al. Adverse cerebral outcomes ftar coronary bypass surbery. Multicenter strudy of perioperative ischemia research group and the ischemia research and education foundation investigators. *NEJM.* 1996;335:1857–1863

55. Newman MF, Krchner JL, Phillips-Bute B, et al. Longitudinal assessment of neurocognitive function after coronary artery bypass surgery. *NEJM.* 2001;344:395–402

56. Deklunder G, Roussel M, Lecroart J-L, et al. Microemboli in cerebral circulation and alteration of cognitive abilities in patiens with mechanical prosthetic heart valves. *Stroke.* 1998;29:1821–1826

57. Nadareishmili ZG, Beletsky M, Black SE, et al. Is cerebral microembolism in mechanical prosthetic heart valves clinically relevant? *J Neuroimaging.* 2002;12:310–315

58. Kilander L, Andren B, Nyman H,et al. Atrial fibrillation is an independent determinant of low cognitive function: A cross-sectional study in elderly men. *Stroke.* 1998;29:1816–1820

59. Vaughan CJ. Prevention of stroke and dementia with statins. *Amer J Cardiol.* 2003;91(4), Suppl1:23–29.

60. Pahan K, Sheikh FG, Namboodiri AM, Singh I. Lovastatin and phenylacetate inhibit the induction of nitric oxide synthase and cytokines in rat primary astrocytes, microglia, and macrophages. *J Clin Invest.* 1997;100:2671–2679.

61. Weitz-Schmidt G, Welzenbach K, Brinkmann V, Kamata T, Kallen J, Bruns C, Cottens S, Takada Y, Hommel U. Statins selectively inhibit leukocyte function antigen-1 by binding to a novel regulatory integrin site. *Nat Med.* 2001;7:687–692.

62. Laufs U, Gertz K, Huang P, Nickenig G, Bohm M, Dirnagl U, Endres M. Atorvastatin upregulates type III nitric oxide synthase in thrombocytes, decreases platelet activation, and protects from cerebral ischemia in normocholesterolemic mice. *Stroke.* 2000;31:2442–2449.

63. Chen J, Zhang ZG, Li Y, Wang Y, Wang L, Jiang H, Zhang C, Lu M, Katakowski M, Feldkamp CS, Chopp M. Statins Induce Angiogenesis, Neurogenesis and Synaptogenesis after Stroke. *Ann Neurol.* 2003;53:743–751.

64. Lu D, Goussev A, Chen J, Pannu P, Li Y, Mahmood A, Chopp M. Atorvastatin Reduces Neurological Deficit and Increases Synaptogenesis, Angiogenesis, and Neuronal Survival in Rats Subjected to Traumatic Brain Injury. *J. Neurotrauma* 2004;21(1):21–32.

65. Endres M, Laufs U, Huang Z, Nakamura T, Huang P, Moskowitz MA, Liao JK. Stroke protection by 3-hydroxy-3-methylglutaryl (HMG)-CoA reductase inhibitors medicated by endothelial nitric oxide synthase. *Proc Natl Acad Sci USA.* 1998;95:8880–8885.

66. Chowienczyk PJ, Watts GF, Cockcroft JR, Ritter JM. Impaired endothelium-dependent vasodilation of forearm resistance vessels in hypercholesterolaemia. *Lancet.* 1992; 340(8833):1430–2.

67. Lange W, Halata Z. Comparative studies on the pre-and postterminal blood vessels in the cerebellar cortex of the rhesus monkey, cat and rat. Anat Embryol. 1979;158:51–62.

5

Magnetic Resonance Imaging of Atherosclerotic Plaque

Ioannis Koktzoglou, M.S.,
James C. Carr, M.D.,
Timothy J. Carroll, Ph.D.,
and Mark D. Morasch, M.D.

Atherosclerosis, a systemic disease associated with lipid infiltration and fibrous proliferation in the intimal layer of medium and large sized arteries, accounts for nearly three fourths of cardiovascular disease related deaths in the United States.[1] In the early stages of atherosclerotic disease, enlargement of the affected artery may compensate for atherosclerotic thickening, thereby avoiding luminal stenosis despite the presence of disease.[2-3] This compensatory arterial process, also referred to as positive or outward arterial remodeling, may make detection of atherosclerotic plaques difficult with conventional X-ray angiography and other luminographic techniques.[4] Early stage plaques, however, may still be clinically important since acute atherothrombotic complications including stroke and myocardial infarction can result.[5-6]

Clearly, direct imaging of plaque is desired to properly assess the extent and severity of atherosclerotic disease. Direct imaging of atherosclerotic plaques can be performed with computed tomography (CT), intravascular ultrasound, and echocardiography. However, these imaging modalities suffer from limitations including ionizing radiation, invasiveness, and poor soft tissue contrast. In the past decade, magnetic resonance imaging (MRI) has emerged as the most promising noninvasive imaging modalities for atherosclerotic plaque detection and characterization.[7] MRI does not use ionizing radiation, and thus may be used to serially monitor the progression and regression of atherosclerotic, and its response to lipid lowering therapy.[8-9] Furthermore, due to its excellent soft tissue contrast, MRI has demonstrated the ability to characterize plaque composition.[10-11] Through further research, MRI may ultimately be capable of determining unstable plaques predisposed to rupture and thrombosis.

In this chapter, we will introduce current MRI methods that allow direct imaging of atherosclerotic plaque, describe how MRI can be used to characterize plaque composition, and comment on possible future directions of the field.

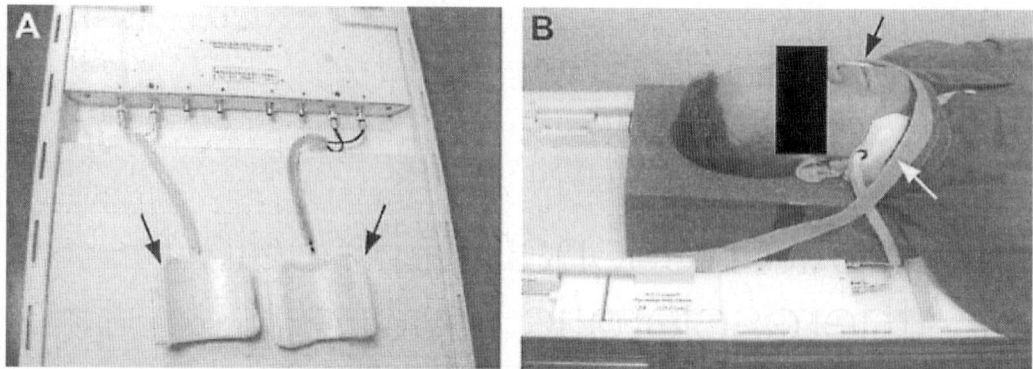

Figure 5-1. A. Phased array surface reception coils (arrows) used for carotid artery wall imaging. **B.** Coils are placed on both sides of the neck (arrows) to facilitate imaging of both the left and right carotid arteries.

MR PLAQUE IMAGING METHODS

To image the thin arterial wall, submillimeter spatial resolution is required. In MRI images, the signal-to-noise ratio (SNR) is reduced in proportion to the increase of spatial resolution. To compensate for the low SNR associated with high spatial resolution, dedicated surface reception coils placed near the arteries of interest are used (Figure 5-1).[12-13] Suppression of arterial blood signal (i.e., black-blood imaging) is also desired during MR imaging to clearly delineate the arterial wall from the arterial lumen.[14-15]

The standard MRI plaque imaging sequence is black-blood prepared multiecho spin-echo pulse sequence referred to as "Turbo Spin-Echo" (TSE) or "Fast Spin-Echo" (FSE) (Figure 5-2). In general, blood flowing into an image will appear bright. To achieve high contrast between the blood flowing in a vessel and the arterial wall, the signal from blood must be eliminated with a technique called "black-blood" imaging. Black-blood MR imaging is achieved by application of a double inversion-recovery (DIR) radiofrequency (RF) preparation, followed by a delay time (TI) before data acquisition.[14] The TI, which provides the optimal suppression of the signal from flowing blood, is given by the relation:

$$TI = T_1 \ln \left(\frac{2}{1 + e^{-TR/T_1}} \right)$$

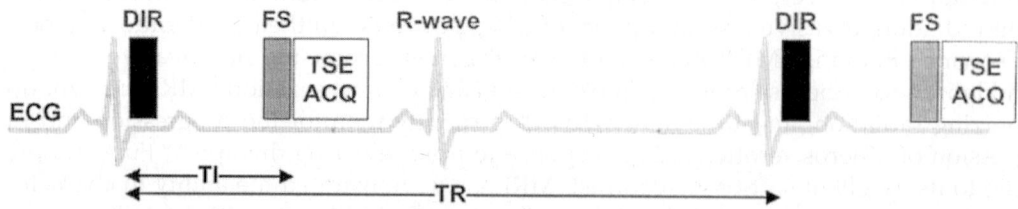

Figure 5-2. Typical timing diagram for a black-blood turbo spin-echo (TSE) vessel wall imaging sequence. A double inversion-recovery (DIR) preparation is followed by and inversion delay time (TI) to render blood black. TSE acquisition is preceded by a fat saturation (FS) pulse to remove subcutaneous fat signal. The repetition time (TR) of the sequence is the time between acquisition periods. Electrocardiographic (ECG) gating may be used to remove cardiac motion and/or arterial wall pulsatility. In this example the TR used is equal to 2 R-R periods.

where TR is the repetition time of the TSE sequence and T_1 is the longitudinal relaxation time of blood. For a typical TR of 2000 ms and given the T_1 of blood is 1250 ms at 1.5 T, the TI used to suppress blood is roughly 635 ms. A fat suppression RF prepulse is also generally applied before data acquisition to suppress subcutaneous fat signal, thereby improving arterial plaque conspicuity.[13,16]

In arteries that experience significant cardiac motion and/or pulsatility such as the coronary arteries, electrocardiographic (ECG) gating is used during MR imaging to limit data acquisition to the quiescent period within the cardiac cycle, generally diastole. When ECG gating is used, the DIR preparation is typically applied in systole soon after detection of the ECG R-wave (Figure 5-2).[17] A coronary artery wall image acquired using an ECG-gated, DIR-prepared, TSE imaging sequence is shown in (Figure 5-3).

Another approach to black-blood imaging is to saturate (i.e., eliminate) the signal from blood as is flows into the image. Spatial presaturation applies spatially selective RF pulses to eliminate the signal from blood upstream from the imaging slice.[18] Plaque imaging with spatial presaturation is more time efficient than with the DIR method since several imaging slices may be acquired within the repetition time (TR), while DIR is inherently a single slice technique.[19] The timing diagram of a 12-slice spatially presaturated TSE carotid artery wall imaging sequence is shown in (Figure 5-4). While the spatial presaturation approach is less effective than the DIR method for suppressing luminal blood signal,[20] it generally performs well and remains a valuable option when fast, multislice assessment of arterial wall is desired.

Under conditions of slow or turbulent blood flow, black-blood imaging with both DIR and spatial presaturation methods may be difficult to achieve since both rely on inflow of tagged blood into the imaging slice to render blood black. This is especially true in the carotid bifurcation, where blood can reside in flow vortices within the carotid bulb for several cardiac cycles.[15,21] To identify lumen boundaries in presence of slow and/or recirculating blood flow, bright-blood imaging (i.e., 3-D time-of-flight [TOF] angiography) may be performed in conjunction with black-blood imaging.[22-23]

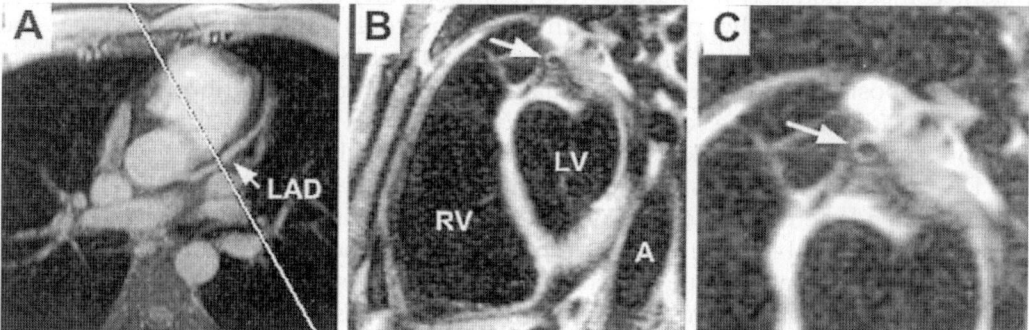

Figure 5-3. A. Coronary magnetic resonance angiogram depicting the left anterior descending coronary artery (LAD). B Cross sectional image through the LAD acquired using an ECG-gated, DIR-prepared, TSE imaging sequence. The slice position is shown in **A.** (solid line). The coronary vessel wall is well depicted (arrow), and excellent suppression of blood signal is realized in the right ventricle (RV), left ventricle (RV), and in the descending thoracic aorta **A, C,** Close up of **B,** depicting the LAD coronary artery wall.

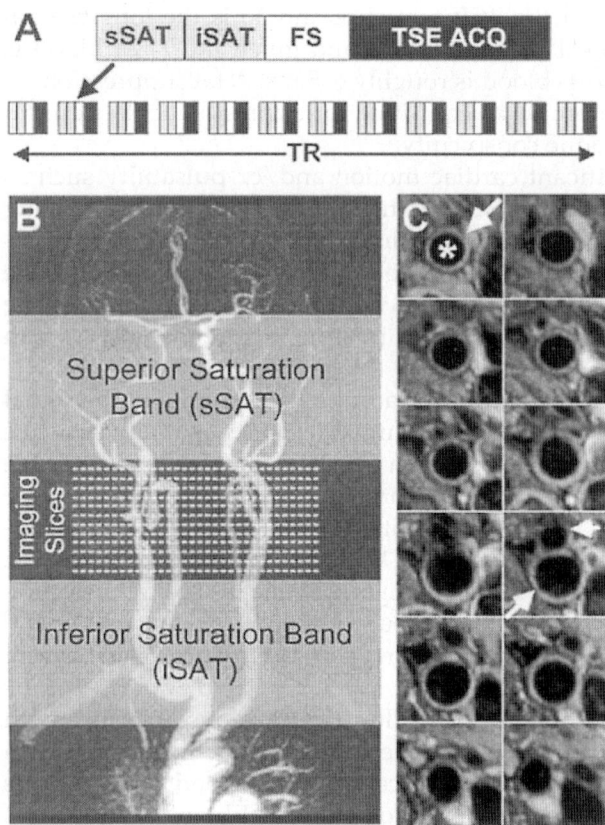

Figure 5-4. A. Timing diagram of a twelve-slice spatial presaturation TSE imaging sequence. Superior and inferior spatial presaturation bands (sSAT and iSAT, respectively) are applied continuously throughout the sequence to suppress blood. **B.** Example placement of imaging slices and saturation bands relative to a contrast enhanced magnetic resonance angiogram. **C.** Acquired MR images depicting the common (thick solid arrow), internal (thin solid arrow), and external (thin dashed arrow) carotid artery walls. The asterisk indicates the arterial lumen.

CHARACTERIZATION OF PLAQUE COMPOSITON WITH MRI

Atherosclerotic plaques consist of several tissues including collagen, lipid, calcium, intraplaque hemorrhage, and thrombus. Varying proportions of these constituents are found in plaques, thus giving rise to a wide range of lesion types.[6] Research has shown that plaque composition may be indicative of plaque stability and risk of atherothrombotic complications. Specifically, plaques with large lipid cores (relative to plaque area) and thin fibrous caps are generally accepted to be less stable (i.e., more prone to rupture and thrombosis) than plaques with small lipid cores and thick fibrous caps.[5,7,24-27] Characterization of plaque composition with in vivo MRI may, therefore, allow identification of unstable, high-risk lesions before they lead to clinical events.

Due to their large size, superficial location, lack of physiologic motion, and accessibility via endarterectomy, the carotid arteries have provided the most profound insights into how MRI may be used to assess atherosclerotic plaque composition.[12-13] To accurately differentiate plaque constituents, it has become apparent that acquisition of several MR imaging sequences, each of which elicit a distinct image appearance and soft tissue contrast, is necessary.[7,28-31] This type of imaging, referred to as "multisequence MRI" or "multispectral MRI," has been reported to characterize plaque components with high sensitivity and specificity.[28,32]

Three imaging sequences are typically acquired during multisequence MRI to characterize plaque composition: (1) Proton density-weighted (PDW) TSE, (2) T_2-

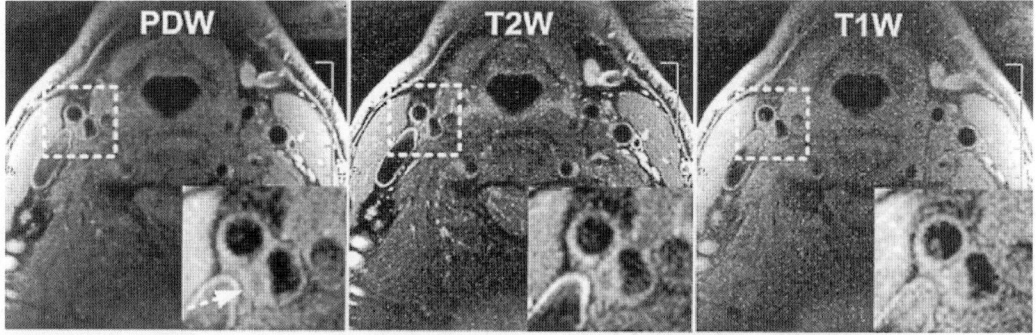

Figure 5–5. Multi-sequence TSE MR images acquired of an atherosclerotic plaque found in the right internal carotid artery (arrow). Insets correspond to close-ups of boxed regions. Note the different image appearances and contrasts achieved. PDW, T2W, and T1W correspond to proton density-weighted, T2-weighted, and T1-weighted TSE, respectively.

weighted imaging (T2W) TSE, and (3) T_1-weighted imaging (T1W) TSE. Images of a carotid plaque acquired with these three image contrasts are shown in (Figure 5-5). The relative appearance of plaque components (relative to adjacent muscle tissue) obtained with these three imaging sequences is outlined in (Table 5-1).[7,33] In summary, calcium appears very dark during PDW, T2W, and T1W TSE imaging due to its low water proton concentration. T2W TSE imaging is particularly useful for delineating the collagenous/fibrous tissue, which appears hyperintense, from the lipid core, which appears hypointense.[10,34,35] T1W TSE is particularly useful for locating the lipid core, which appears hyperintense, and acute (< one week old) and recent (< one month old) intraplaque hemorrhage, which have been reported to appear hyperintense.[33] As suggested by Hatsukami et al.,[36] 3-D TOF bright-blood imaging may also be performed in conjunction with TSE imaging to visualize the fibrous cap, which appears hypointense.

MRI contrast agents have also been used to improve depiction of atherosclerotic arterial wall. Work by Aoki et al.[37] in patients reported the presence of a hyperintense rim in the carotid arteries after contrast injection, claiming the ability to directly visualize the vascularity of the arterial wall. Recent work in human carotid plaques with contrast enhanced MR imaging has reported postcontrast enhancement of fibrocellular

TABLE 5-1. PLAQUE CHARACTERIZATION WITH MR

Relative MR Signal Intensity

	T1 W	P D W	T2 W
Calcium	hypointense	very hypointense	very hypointense
Lipid	very hyperintense	hyperintense	hyperintense
Fibrous	isointense to slightly hyperintense	isointense to slightly hyperintense	isointense to slightly hyperintense
Thrombus†	variable	variable	variable
Hemorrhage†	variable	variable	variable

*Relative to adjacent muscle tissue

†Variable signal intensity may be due to thrombus/hemorrhage age

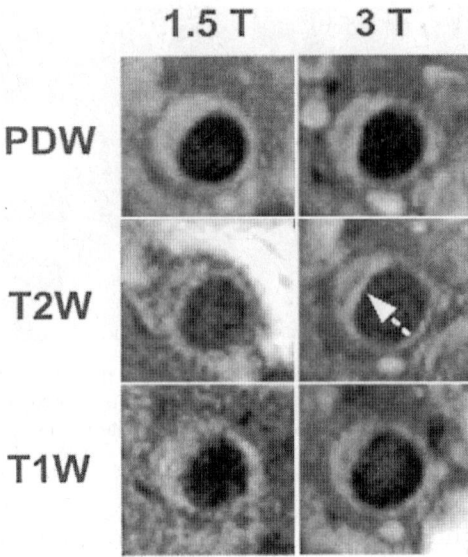

Figure 5–6. PDW, T2W, and T1W TSE images acquired at 1.5 T and 3 T. Atherosclerotic thickening of the common carotid artery is clearly visible at both field strengths. Note the improved image quality and SNR at 3 T. During T2W imaging, the layered composition of the plaque is clearly visible (arrow). According to the criteria of Table 1, the plaque appears to consist of a bright fibrous cap overlying a lipid core.

tissue,[38] the ability to identify regions of neovascularization within fibrous tissue,[39] and the ability to quantify microvessel area within plaque.[40]

FUTURE DIRECTIONS

MR imaging of atherosclerotic plaque is an active area of research. Methods to improve imaging efficiency, SNR, and sensitivity and specificity to plaque composition are currently under investigation.

One area of active research is plaque imaging on 3 T clinical scanners, rather than 1.5 T. Three Tesla plaque imaging should theoretically double image SNR over 1.5 T imaging, and may improve image contrast so as to more accurately characterize plaque composition. Preliminary 3 T vessel wall imaging studies have shown very good image quality, and significant gains in SNR over 1.5 T imaging.[41-43] A direct comparison of carotid artery images acquired at 1.5 T and 3.0 T using multispectral MRI is shown in (Figure 5-6).

Use of atherosclerotic plaque targeting MRI contrast agents is another area of active research. Plaque targeting agents may improve imaging sensitivity for detecting plaque and may eventually facilitate rapid assessment of plaque burden in the body. Ultrasmall superparamagnetic iron oxide particle (USPIOs)-based contrast agents detectible with MRI have been shown to accumulate via macrophagic phagocytosis in atherosclerotic plaques.[44-45] Gadofluorine, a gadolinium-based MRI contrast agent, has been found to selectively enhance atherosclerotic arterial wall during MR imaging.[46-47]

As described in this chapter, MRI is a powerful imaging modality for noninvasive assessment of atherosclerosis. MRI has the ability to locate atherosclerotic plaques, assess plaque morphology, and characterize plaque composition. With continued research, further advances in the field of MR plaque imaging are to be expected.

REFERENCES

1. American Heart Association. Heart Disease and Stroke Statistics–2005 Update. Dallas; 2005.
2. Glagov S, Weisenberg E, Zarins CK, et al. Compensatory enlargement of human atherosclerotic coronary arteries. *N Engl J Med*. 1987;316:1371–1375.
3. Glagov S, Zarins C, Giddens DP, et al. Hemodynamics and atherosclerosis. Insights and perspectives gained from studies of human arteries. *Arch Pathol Lab Med*. 1988;112: 1018–1031.
4. Stiel GM, Stiel LS, Schofer J, et al. Impact of compensatory enlargement of atherosclerotic coronary arteries on angiographic assessment of coronary artery disease. *Circulation*. 1989; 80:1603–1609.
5. Falk E, Shah PK, Fuster V. Coronary Plaque Disruption. *Circulation*. 1995;92:657–671.
6. Stary HC, Chandler AB, Dinsmore RE, et al. A Definition of Advanced Types of Atherosclerotic Lesions and a Histological Classification of Atherosclerosis: A Report From the Committee on Vascular Lesions of the Council on Arteriosclerosis, American Heart Association. *Circulation*. 1995;92:1355–1374.
7. Fayad ZA, Fuster V. Clinical imaging of the high-risk or vulnerable atherosclerotic plaque. *Circ Res*. 2001;89:305–316.
8. McConnell MV, Aikawa M, Maier SE, et al. MRI of rabbit atherosclerosis in response to dietary cholesterol lowering. *Arterioscler Thromb Vasc Biol*. 1999;19:1956–1959.
9. Yonemura A, Momiyama Y, Fayad ZA, et al. Effect of lipid-lowering therapy with atorvastatin on atherosclerotic aortic plaques detected by noninvasive magnetic resonance imaging. *J Am Coll Cardiol*. 2005;45:733–742.
10. Toussaint JF, LaMuraglia GM, Southern JF, et al. Magnetic resonance images lipid, fibrous, calcified, hemorrhagic, and thrombotic components of human atherosclerosis in vivo. *Circulation*. 1996;94:932–938.
11. Gold GE, Pauly JM, Glover GH, et al. Characterization of atherosclerosis with a 1.5-T imaging system. *J Magn Reson Imaging*. 1993;3:399–407.
12. Yuan C, Tsuruda JS, Beach KN, et al. Techniques for high-resolution MR imaging of atherosclerotic plaque. *J Magn Reson Imaging*. 1994;4:43–49.
13. Yuan C, Murakami JW, Hayes CE, et al. Phased-array magnetic resonance imaging of the carotid artery bifurcation: preliminary results in healthy volunteers and a patient with atherosclerotic disease. *J Magn Reson Imaging*. 1995;5:561–565.
14. Edelman RR, Chien D, Kim D. Fast selective black blood MR imaging. *Radiology*. 1991;181: 655–660.
15. Steinman DA, Rutt BK. On the nature and reduction of plaque-mimicking flow artifacts in black blood MRI of the carotid bifurcation. *Magn Reson Med*. 1998;39:635–641.
16. Yuan C, Beach KW, Smith LH, Jr., et al. Measurement of atherosclerotic carotid plaque size in vivo using high resolution magnetic resonance imaging. *Circulation*. 1998;98:2666–2671.
17. Simonetti OP, Finn JP, White RD, et al. "Black blood" T2-weighted inversion-recovery MR imaging of the heart. *Radiology*. 1996;199:49–57.
18. Felmlee JP, Ehman RL. Spatial presaturation: a method for suppressing flow artifacts and improving depiction of vascular anatomy in MR imaging. *Radiology*. 1987;164:559–564.
19. Parker DL, Goodrich KC, Masiker M, et al. Improved efficiency in double-inversion fast spin-echo imaging. *Magn Reson Med*. 2002;47:1017–1021.
20. Yarnykh VL, Yuan C. Multislice double inversion-recovery black-blood imaging with simultaneous slice reinversion. *J Magn Reson Imaging*. 2003;17:478–483.
21. Ku DN, Giddens DP. Pulsatile flow in a model carotid bifurcation. *Arteriosclerosis*. 1983;3:31–39.
22. Wildy KS, Yuan C, Tsuruda JS, et al. Atherosclerosis of the carotid artery: evaluation by magnetic resonance angiography. *J Magn Reson Imaging*. 1996;6:726–732.
23. Zhang S, Hatsukami TS, Polissar NL, et al. Comparison of carotid vessel wall area measurements using three different contrast-weighted black blood MR imaging techniques. *Magn Reson Imaging*. 2001;19:795–802.

24. Davies MJ, Thomas AC. Plaque fissuring—the cause of acute myocardial infarction, sudden ischaemic death, and crescendo angina. *Br Heart J*. 1985;53:363–373.

25. Ambrose JA, Tannenbaum MA, Alexopoulos D, et al. Angiographic progression of coronary artery disease and the development of myocardial infarction. *J Am Coll Cardiol*. 1988;12:56–62.

26. Fuster V. Lewis A. Conner Memorial Lecture. Mechanisms leading to myocardial infarction: insights from studies of vascular biology. *Circulation*. 1994;90:2126–2146.

27. Little WC, Constantinescu M, Applegate RJ, et al. Can coronary angiography predict the site of a subsequent myocardial infarction in patients with mild-to-moderate coronary artery disease? *Circulation* 1988;78:1157–1166.

28. Yuan C, Mitsumori LM, Ferguson MS, et al. In vivo accuracy of multispectral magnetic resonance imaging for identifying lipid-rich necrotic cores and intraplaque hemorrhage in advanced human carotid plaques. *Circulation*. 2001;104:2051–2056.

29. Yuan C, Mitsumori LM, Beach KW, et al. Carotid atherosclerotic plaque: noninvasive MR characterization and identification of vulnerable lesions. *Radiology*. 2001;221:285–299.

30. Mitsumori LM, Hatsukami TS, Ferguson MS, et al. In vivo accuracy of multisequence MR imaging for identifying unstable fibrous caps in advanced human carotid plaques. *J Magn Reson Imaging*. 2003;17:410–420.

31. Cappendijk VC, Cleutjens KB, Kessels AG, et al. Assessment of human atherosclerotic carotid plaque components with multisequence MR imaging: initial experience. *Radiology*. 2005; 234:487–492.

32. Cai JM, Hatsukami TS, Ferguson MS, et al. Classification of human carotid atherosclerotic lesions with in vivo multicontrast magnetic resonance imaging. *Circulation*. 2002;106: 1368–1373.

33. Kampschulte A, Ferguson MS, Kerwin WS, et al. Differentiation of intraplaque versus juxtaluminal hemorrhage/thrombus in advanced human carotid atherosclerotic lesions by in vivo magnetic resonance imaging. *Circulation*. 2004;110:3239–3244.

34. Toussaint JF, Southern JF, Fuster V, et al. T2-weighted contrast for NMR characterization of human atherosclerosis. *Arterioscler Thromb Vasc Biol*. 1995;15:1533–1542.

35. Winn WB, Schmiedl UP, Reichenbach DD, et al. Detection and characterization of atherosclerotic fibrous caps with T2-weighted MR. AJNR *Am J Neuroradiol*. 1998;19:129–134.

36. Hatsukami TS, Ross R, Polissar NL, et al. Visualization of fibrous cap thickness and rupture in human atherosclerotic carotid plaque in vivo with high-resolution magnetic resonance imaging. *Circulation*. 2000;102:959–964.

37. Aoki S, Aoki K, Ohsawa S, et al. Dynamic MR imaging of the carotid wall. *J Magn Reson Imaging*. 1999;9:420–427.

38. Wasserman BA, Smith WI, Trout HH, 3rd, et al. Carotid artery atherosclerosis: in vivo morphologic characterization with gadolinium-enhanced double-oblique MR imaging initial results. *Radiology*. 2002;223:566–573.

39. Yuan C, Kerwin WS, Ferguson MS, et al. Contrast-enhanced high resolution MRI for atherosclerotic carotid artery tissue characterization. *J Magn Reson Imaging*. 2002;15:62–67.

40. Kerwin W, Hooker A, Spilker M, et al. Quantitative magnetic resonance imaging analysis of neovasculature volume in carotid atherosclerotic plaque. *Circulation*. 2003;107:851–856.

41. Botnar RM, Stuber M, Lamerichs R, et al. Initial experiences with in vivo right coronary artery human MR vessel wall imaging at 3 tesla. *J Cardiovasc Magn Reson*. 2003;5:589–594.

42. Koktzoglou I, Simonetti O, Li D. Coronary artery wall imaging: initial experience at 3 Tesla. *J Magn Reson Imaging*. 2005;21:128–132.

43. Koktzoglou I, Chung Y-C, Mani V, et al. Multi-Slice Carotid Imaging with Regional Saturation and Rapid Extended Coverage: Comparison at 1.5T and 3.0T. In: *Proceedings of the 13th Annual Meeting of ISMRM*, Miami Beach, 2005. p. 1745.

44. Ruehm SG, Corot C, Vogt P, et al. Magnetic resonance imaging of atherosclerotic plaque with ultrasmall superparamagnetic particles of iron oxide in hyperlipidemic rabbits. *Circulation*. 2001;103:415–422.

45. Kooi ME, Cappendijk VC, Cleutjens KB, et al. Accumulation of ultrasmall superparamagnetic particles of iron oxide in human atherosclerotic plaques can be detected by in vivo magnetic resonance imaging. *Circulation* 2003;107:2453–2458.
46. Barkhausen J, Ebert W, Heyer C, et al. Detection of atherosclerotic plaque with Gadofluorine-enhanced magnetic resonance imaging. *Circulation*. 2003;108:605–609.
47. Sirol M, Itskovich VV, Mani V, et al. Lipid-rich atherosclerotic plaques detected by gadofluorine-enhanced in vivo magnetic resonance imaging. *Circulation*. 2004;109:2890–2896.

6

Tips on Coding for Endovascular Procedures

Sean P. Roddy, MD

INTRODUCTION

Vascular surgeons provide comprehensive treatments to the patient with atherosclerosis through medical management, endovascular therapy, and open surgery. Though patient care and quality outcomes are of highest importance, the process by which care is rendered must continuously be evaluated in order to optimize billing, coding, and, ultimately, reimbursement. Patient assessment, operative intervention, and diagnostic evaluation can all be described with a diagnosis and a procedure. A claim is generated when a diagnosis code is paired to a procedure code, and up to three modifiers are added. That claim is then submitted to an insurance carrier for payment, usually electronically. The correctness of the coding involved leads to timely reimbursement by the insurance carrier as well as minimizes the possibility of "insurance fraud." The probability that a rejected claim will ever be paid to the physician decreases significantly each time a claim is denied for any reason. Therefore, all efforts should be centered on generating a "clean" claim that is without error, is medically appropriate, and describes the intervention correctly. This chapter will describe endovascular treatments in the arterial system and is therefore only a guideline for the physician since each insurance payer has their own rules and regulations. Please consult your local carriers for specific details on claim submission.

DIAGNOSIS CODING

The International Classification of Diseases was created by the World Health Organization (WHO) in 1948. The 9th Edition (ICD-9) was published in 1977 in an effort to track disease processes worldwide. In the United States, the National Center for Health Statistics altered this manual and therefore "Clinical Modification" was added to the title. The concept for an organized categorization evolved from the "London Bills of Mortality" which described the reasons for death in England during the 1600's. In 1937, this model was renamed the International List of Causes of Death for use across the globe. In 1948, the WHO created the

International Classification of Diseases tracking mortality and, for the first time, morbidity. The current edition is updated annually, effective October 1st each year, and divided into two sections. The first section is a numerical list of diseases presented as code numbers in a tabular form and the second section is an alphabetical index of the disease entries with corresponding diagnostic code numbers. Each ICD-9 code is comprised of a three, four, or five digit number. There is increasing specificity as more digits are added. A common error is the use of a probable, suspected, or "rule out" diagnosis. A patient has the diagnosis of epigastric abdominal pain and not mesenteric ischemia while in the emergency room. Only after angiography or laparotomy, if significant ischemia is identified, does the patient officially have the diagnosis of acute mesenteric ischemia. If the patient has another etiology for the pain identified in the workup or through exploratory surgery, that diagnosis should be included in claims to the insurer. It is also important to use the most clinically appropriate description listed in the ICD-9 manual for a patient's given condition whenever possible. That said, there are instances where several diagnoses will all be medically suitable.

PROCEDURAL CODING

Procedure billing is taken from codes summarized in the Current Procedural Terminology (CPT) manual which is currently in its 4th edition. This book is created, maintained, and copyrighted by the American Medical Association (AMA) who updates it annually, effective January 1st each year. It is used by physicians, researchers, and managed care as a systematic listing of all procedures that are currently performed by health care providers. CPT descriptors are always five digits and broken down into standard codes and add-on codes. Standard codes are those that can be submitted by themselves. Add-on codes cannot and must be accompanied by other specific code(s) as well. An example of an add-on code is CPT 35683 (autogenous composite, three or more segments of vein from two or more locations). This code provides value for the added difficulty in performing a spliced vein leg bypass surgery compared to a single piece of vein harvested from the ipsilateral extremity. Therefore, payment for CPT code 35683 would also require one of the nine standard lower extremity revascularization codes be submitted as well.

CPT codes for professional fee billing are designated as either Category I or Category III. Category I codes are the typical five digit number codes with which most people are familiar. On the other hand, Category III codes are four digits followed by a "T". These are referred to as temporary or emerging technology codes. They usually describe the use of a device not approved by the Federal Drug Administration or an investigational procedure. Most Category III codes are not reimbursed by insurers unless converted at some point to a Category I code but are in place to help with data collection by Medicare, private insurers, and other interest groups. An example is CPT code 0078T which describes endovascular repair of an abdominal aortic aneurysm using a fenestrated modular bifurcated prosthesis. Category III codes are limited in duration with a maximum of 5 years. The CPT code 0078T is due to expire on December 31, 2010 unless it is converted at some point to a Category I code.

More than one procedure on the same date, same session, or within a global period may require use of a modifier. Modifiers are always two digit numbers that can be appended to a claim. They describe circumstances which allow for full or partial payment in situations that would otherwise be denied as "global" or inclusive to another procedure. Additionally, there is an organization whose sole purpose is to ensure multiple codes, when billed together, are appropriate. That entity is the National Correct Coding Initiative (or CCI) who reviews CPT codes quarterly to decide what can and cannot be billed together routinely based on billing patterns and trends. For example, the -59 modifier can be used to notate distinct procedural services or an exception to the CCI. The modifiers are listed both in the front of the CPT manual each year as well as their own section in the Appendix.

Two specific modifiers important in billing radiologic codes include the -TC (or technical component) modifier and the -26 (or professional component) modifier. When the equipment is owned by a practice in an office setting, that practice would bill with no modifier. Billing for both the technical and professional fees associated with a radiologic study is termed "billing global". If a test is performed in the hospital where the hospital owns the equipment, a physician would bill for the professional fee only using a -26 modifier. This signifies that the physician is performing and interpreting the test but does not own the equipment, the disposables, or the facility and does not employ the staff required to perform the procedure.

It is also important to understand that when more than one CPT code is billed on the same session, the code designated the highest degree of work is paid in its entirety. All subsequent non-radiologic codes are paid at 50% of their assigned work value. This decrease is termed the "multiple procedure discount". Imaging codes (i.e., codes that begin with the number 7) or vascular laboratory codes are not subject to this discount. Additionally, add-on codes are exempt from this fee reduction.

CPT codes are usually grouped into three general categories as outlined in Table 6–1. These include evaluation and management (E&M) codes, surgical procedure codes, and radiologic codes. Evaluation and management codes are typically patient and practitioner interaction such as office visits, consultations, and hospital evaluations. Patient encounter billing is a separate topic and will not be discussed further in this chapter. Surgical procedure codes involve the work and care around the time of an operation. This is best described by a "global surgical package". This package includes all pre-operative care, intra-procedural care, and post-operative care for a given time period. In most instances, that global period extends from the day before surgery

---

TABLE 6-1. CPT-4 CODING CATEGORIES

Evaluation and Management (E&M)

Open surgical Procedures

   90-day global codes

   10-day global codes

   0-day global codes

Endovascular procedures

   Catheter manipulation

   Imaging

   Intervention

     Embolization

     Percutaneous transluminal angioplasty (PTA)

     Endovascular stent placement

     Atherectomy

     Thrombolysis infusions

     Transcatheter foreign body retrieval

     Endograft aneurysm repair

to 90 days after the procedure. Minor surgery, however, may have a zero day global period (just the actual date of the procedure) or a ten day global period associated with it that extends from the day of surgery to 10 days after the procedure. Global packages also include discussion with the patient about the procedure, alternatives, risks, benefits and consent issues, and documentation of preoperative notes. All radiologic codes in CPT are further classified in one of three categories: catheter manipulations, imaging studies, and interventions. Endovascular billing uses all three and is termed "component coding". Catheter manipulations occur when vessels are traversed and selected most commonly via a femoral or brachial artery puncture. Imaging includes the interpretation of angiography in various vascular beds. Interventions include things such as embolization, angioplasty, stent placement, atherectomy, thrombolysis, intravascular foreign body retrieval, or endograft deployment. In the coding world, there are five interventional systems. These include arterial, venous, lymphatic, portal, and pulmonary. The remainder of this chapter will be dedicated to endovascular treatments on the arterial side.

CATHETER MANIPULATION

Catheterization coding requires description in an operative record of the arterial entry site, vessels traversed within the body, and final resting point for the end of the catheter at the time of imaging. Any movement of the catheter should be noted including the subsequent imaging and/or intervention. An important topic in endovascular coding is selective and non-selective catheterization with regards to a vascular family. Non-selective implies that the puncture vessel itself is used for imaging or a catheter is advanced along the cannulated artery retrograde into the aorta. It does not matter whether the access site is the brachial artery or the femoral artery. If a catheter is advanced from either extremity vessel into the aorta, a non-selective aortic catheterization has occurred. There are instances when introduction of a catheter into the aorta is simple and quick. There will also be circumstances where vessel tortuosity and/or stenosis may required multiple wire and catheter exchanges. In the coding world, both situations are described by the same CPT code, 36200.

Selective catheterization occurs when cannulation of a vessel is performed at an arterial branch point off a non-selected vessel. The network of vessels that originate from this arterial branch point is also designated a "vascular family". In most circumstances, this will be a named vessel coming off the aorta itself. The initial artery traversed off the aorta is termed a first order branch. As further branching occurs within that family, the arteries are designated second order and third order. There is work involved manipulating the catheter to access the desired vessel. Branch point negotiation beyond third order is not recognized in component coding. When selective catheterizations occur below the diaphragm, CPT codes 36245, 36246, and 36247 describe first, second, and third order catheterizations, respectively. When selective catheters are placed within vascular families above the diaphragm, CPT codes 36215, 36216, and 36217 again describe first, second, and third order catheterizations, respectively. Every vascular family that is selected during an angiogram for imaging and/or intervention purposes will generate a separate and distinct catheter CPT code. Also, the same vessel can be different based on the puncture site or anatomic variation (e.g., normal versus bovine aortic arch anatomy). Therefore, when describing catheter manipulations in an operative report, it is important to note all branch entry points in a given exam for billing purposes. This was set up to describe the quantity of physician work dedicated to placing a catheter into a given artery. Advancing a catheter further into a vessel has a different amount of work associated with it compared to pulling that catheter back into the aorta and placing the catheter in a separate and distinct vessel. If the catheter is brought back into a non-selective position and a separate vascular family is catheterized, this will necessitate an additional catheter code. For example, a left common femoral artery puncture generates the non-selective CPT catheterization code 36140 which describes retrograde femoral artery access. If the catheter is advanced into the aorta, the non-selective catheterization code 36200 would be recorded and nullify the 36140 code. The 36200 code contains the work described within the 36140 code as well as the additional work required to negotiate the iliac anatomy and advance the catheter into the aorta. Similarly, if the left renal artery is cannulated as a first order catheterization, the code 36245 would take the place of the 36200 code; 36245 contains the relative value associated with the work required to not only get the catheter into the aorta but also to select the left renal artery. If this catheter is pulled back into the aorta and then placed in the right renal artery which is an entirely different vascular family, a separate and distinct 36245 code would be appropriate. Bilateral renal artery selective catheterization would allow for billing the CPT code 36245 twice. If a catheter is further advanced within a given vascular family, branch points will require navigation. A selective catheterization of the celiac artery would be termed "first order" similar to the renal artery cannulation described above and billed at 36245. However, if the catheter is advanced into the common hepatic artery past the left gastric and splenic artery branch points, the catheter is now in a "second order" vessel. Second order catheterization below the diaphragm is CPT code 36246 and includes the work of 36245 plus the work to enter the second order vessel. Further advancement of the catheter into the proper hepatic artery past the gastroduodenal artery branch point is a "third order" catheterization. Third order catheterization is billed as a 36247 and, following the previous examples, voids and replaces the prior 36246 code.

If one enters a vascular family and proceeds to second or third order catheterization, there are times when the catheter is pulled back within that family (but not back into the aorta) and a separate second or third order branch is selected for further angiography. An example is selective catheterization through the innominate artery into the right common carotid artery for carotid imaging. This is a second order catheterization above the diaphragm (36216). The catheter is pulled back into the innominate artery and then into the right subclavian artery for further imaging. Placement of the catheter into the right subclavian artery is a "subsequent second or third order" catheterization and is billed with the CPT add-on code 36218. Similarly, if this occurred below the diaphragm, 36248 would be used.

IMAGING

Imaging includes image intensifier manipulation, table positioning, contrast injection, and interpretation of the angiography in a specific vascular bed. All hospital based imaging necessitates use of the -26 modifier to designate only the professional component of the imaging CPT code. As a general rule, when a catheter is repositioned and imaging occurs, another code is generated. Some imaging requires a selective catheter placement. Therefore, non-selective catheterizations such as 36200 could never be used at the same time as any of these imaging codes. Examples include external carotid, renal, visceral, spinal, adrenal, and pelvic arteriography as listed in Table 6–2. Coding these imaging with a non-selective catheterization would be a red flag to insurance carriers for inappropriate billing practices.

To start, the basic exam is coded first followed by subsequent exams. Abdominal aortography (75625) and bilateral lower extremity arterial runoff (75716) are standard basic imaging codes for vascular surgeons. However, some subsequent exams include the basic exam. An example for this includes a renal artery selective arteriogram. Both the unilateral (75722) and bilateral (75724) renal arteriogram codes include selective renal angiography as well as flush aortography. Therefore, a basic abdominal aortogram (75625) would never be coded at the same time as a selective renal arteriogram (75722) since the renal study includes the work for interpreting the aortogram as well as the selective renal images. Visceral angiography (75726) is similar and also includes a flush aortogram.

In previous years, many practices did a diagnostic angiogram and identified a lesion that could be treated with an endovascular therapy. Anywhere from one day to several days later, the same angiogram was repeated at the time of percutaneous intervention. This allowed for payment on the angiography twice for the same clinical condition. To discourage this practice and to ensure that Medicare would only pay once for angiography, version 10.3 of the National Correct Coding Initiative created an edit on October 1, 2004 in the policy manual that bundled imaging with intervention except if the -59 modifier was added to the imaging CPT code. Therefore, one must dictate into the operative report if no prior angiography was done in a given clinical situation which then allows addition of the -59 modifier to the imaging codes for reimbursement.

ENDOVASCULAR INTERVENTION

The last component of endovascular billing is the concept of interventions. These include embolization, transluminal angioplasty, stent placement, atherectomy, thrombolysis, transcatheter foreign body retrieval, or endograft deployment. Most of these procedures are described through two CPT codes: one code which begins with a three and another code that begins with a seven. The latter code is the radiology supervision and interpretation code submitted with a -26 modifier to signify professional fee billing.

TABLE 6-2. ARTERIAL IMAGING CPT CODES REQUIRING SELECTIVE CATHETERIZATION

CPT code	Description
75660	Unilateral external carotid angiography
75662	Bilateral external carotid angiography
75722	Unilateral renal angiography
75724	Bilateral renal angiography
75726	Visceral angiography
75731	Unilateral adrenal angiography
75733	Bilateral adrenal angiography
75736	Pelvic angiography

Multiple interventions are often performed on the same vessel in the same session. The American Medical Association CPT correct coding guidelines would allow for reporting all the endovascular techniques required to percutaneously treat an occluded vessel provided each was done with appropriate intent. There was a change in Medicare policy effective October 1, 2007 as described in Version 13.3 of the National Correct Coding Initiative Policy Manual for Medicare Services. Previously, one could perform an angioplasty and have an inadequate result such that a stent was required. Both the angioplasty and stent were billed. The angioplasty required appending a -59 modifier in the claim to certify an attempt with a balloon was pursued but the result was inadequate requiring stent salvage. With the above outlined alteration, the Center for Medicare and Medicaid Services officially reimbursed only for the final endovascular procedure which was considered successful. Therefore, a patient could have an atherectomy that required angioplasty with subsequent stenting. Only the stenting procedure would be reimbursable. This is in line with the overall Medicare policy that unsuccessful procedures are not reportable. An appeal was submitted by the Society for Vascular Surgery and the Society for Interventional Radiology. In response, Medicare and the NCCI rescinded the new policy retroactive to the October 1, 2007 creation date. The CPT Editorial panel thereafter created a workgroup composed of representatives from the American College of Cardiology, the Society for Cardiac Angiography and Interventions, the American College of Radiology, the Society of Interventional Radiology, and the Society for Vascular Surgery. Coding for lower extremity arterial endovascular interventions is now being revised by this collection of physicians for tentative publication in the 2011 CPT manual.

INTERVENTIONAL CODING DESCRIPTIONS

Percutaneous transluminal angioplasty (PTA) involves inflation of a balloon within a stenotic or occluded vessel. The procedure is coded per vessel treated and grouped into "renal or other visceral", "aortic", "iliac", "femoral-popliteal", "brachiocephalic trunk or branches", "tibioperoneal trunk and branches", and "venous" for coding purposes. An additional radiology supervision and interpretation code is added for each vessel (CPT 75962-75968, 75978) treated. The first peripheral artery PTA includes use of 75962 while all subsequent peripheral vessels treated with PTA allow for the add-on code 75964. Similarly, the initial renal and visceral PTA permits billing 75966 while all subsequent renal or visceral PTA require the add-on code 75968. If several inflations are performed at varying locations along a given vessel, only one intervention can be submitted for reimbursement. There is one set of codes that describe open angioplasty (CPT 35450-35460) and another set that cover a percutaneous approach (CPT 35470-35476) to the same vessel. It is important to differentiate between the two. For example, iliac PTA done at the time of a leg bypass through a contralateral percutaneous groin puncture would be billed differently than an iliac PTA approached retrograde through the exposed ("open") common femoral artery. A hard copy image of the inflation must be preserved for documentation purposes in all cases.

Atherectomy follows the same rules as PTA. There are similar groupings as listed above (except there is no venous category) and a likewise division between open (CPT 35480-35485) and percutaneous (35490-35495) approaches. The radiology supervision and interpretation codes (75992-75996) mirror PTA for each vessel subject to plaque excision.

Endovascular stent placement is based on a different convention. There are actually only four stent codes for all vessels (excluding carotid and vertebral arteries). CPT code 37205 describes percutaneous deployment of the first stent while 37206 is an add-on code used to describe each additional *vessel* treated. Similarly, CPT code 37207 and the add-on code 37208 are used in the open setting. All four codes require use of the same radiology supervision and interpretation code (75960). If four vessels are treated with stents through percutaneous access, four 75960 codes, three 37206 codes, and one 37205 code can be submitted for reimbursement. It is important to remember that stents are coded per vessel and not per stent. There is no difference in superficial femoral artery or renal artery stent placement as far as billing is concerned for deployment of the device. The ICD-9 diagnosis will differ on the claim but the stent CPT coding is identical. Also, if three individual stents are placed in the superficial femoral artery, component coding guidelines would treat the intervention as if only one stent was placed for that endovascular therapy. However, CPT Assistant (an update published by the AMA) states that lesions in the superficial femoral artery that are distinct from those in the popliteal artery are separately reportable. Also, when both an external iliac artery and an ipsilateral common femoral artery stenosis are treated, each therapy is reportable provided the lesions are not contiguous.

Only the carotid and vertebral artery have different codes for stenting. Cervical carotid artery stenting with (37215) or without (37216) distal protection is special in that this represents a divergence from component coding. The work associated with catheter placement, selective imaging of the carotid arteries, placement of the stent, and use of a protection device are all bundled into one code. The inclusion of multiple procedures in one CPT code is termed bundling. Arch angiography which is typically performed before selective carotid catheterization is not bundled into these codes and may be reported separately. A similar situation exists with regard to intrathoracic carotid and extrathoracic vertebral artery stenting. Bundling for this intervention is described by CPT code 0075T, a Category III code, for the initial vessel and 0076T, an add-on code, for each subsequent vessel treated at the same session.

Embolization (37204, 75894) implies percutaneous placement of a thrombogenic material through a selective catheter in an attempt to occlude an aneurysm, arteriovenous malformation, or bleeding site. Glue and coils are typical agents employed in the process. Additionally, most embolization procedures are followed by contrast angiography to evaluate the adequacy of the thrombosis. This follow-up study is reportable (75898) for each operative field treated. In 2007, a bundled CPT code (37210) was introduced to describe all work associated with uterine fibroid embolization. This includes all catheters, imaging, and techniques for vessel occlusion. There is no associated radiology supervision and interpretation code. As is usually the case, creation of an all-encompassing procedure unfortunately lowered the total relative value of this intervention compared to the prior component coding descriptions.

Thrombolysis is the administration of a clot desolving agent through a catheter which may open a clotted artery or vein. It is important to note that there is a difference between injection and infusion in the CPT manual. The CPT codes for thrombolysis (37201, 75896) necessitate an actual prolonged infusion by pump of the agent in an area outside the angiography suite. Instilling a thrombolytic drug through a catheter as a bolus by hand is termed "injection" and therefore not reimbursable. Thrombolysis is usually administered in a hospital setting and a follow-up study is performed to evaluate the effectiveness of the treatment. Follow-up angiography when the patient returns to the angiography suite through an existing catheter is coded 75898. It is inappropriate to rebill the thrombolytic codes as they are only for the initiation of therapy and not for continued use on subsequent dates of service. Additionally, the infusion catheter may be exchanged to continue thrombolysis and reposition the catheter for optimal drug delivery. The removal and replacement of this catheter is described by CPT codes 37209 and 75900.

Primary arterial mechanical thrombectomy (37184) includes both clot disruption by an endoluminal device and instilling thrombolytic agent while in the angiography area. This code is reported per vessel. Each additional vessel treated in the same setting on the same date of service can be described by the add-on CPT code 37185. This is in direct contrast to secondary arterial mechanical thrombectomy (37186) for salvage after an embolic event is identified from arterial manipulation, PTA, or stent deployment. This add-on CPT code describes the work associated with extracting debris from a distal vessel by all endovascular methods. Primary means the patient went to the angiography for the purpose of mechanical thrombectomy and secondary implies salvage after an untoward event has occurred.

Both thoracic (TEVAR) and infrarenal (EVAR) aortic aneurysm repair by endograft follow similar conventions. In a stepwise fashion, report the main device deployment first. This is based on the type of endograft implanted. EVAR is reported based on the main body graft configuration: aorta to aorta tube graft (34800), modular with one docking limb (34802), modular with two docking limbs (34803), bifurcated unibody graft (34804), or aorto-uniiliac graft (34805). The radiology supervision and interpretation code for all of the above listed EVAR possibilities include 75952. Placement of the initial docking limb(s) is bundled into the main body code. When a modular bifurcated graft is transformed into an aorta-uniiliac prosthesis with either a formal graft converter or an aortic cuff placed proximally, the two devices are collectively reported with CPT code 34805. Additional extensions both proximally and distally per vessel treated are reported separately. The first extension is described by CPT codes 34825 and 75953. Each additional vessel treated by endograft extension is represented by 34826 and 75953. The radiology supervision and interpretation CPT code 75953 is the same for the first as well as the subsequent extensions such that subsequent submissions would require the use of a 59 modifier to identify that the replication of an identical code is not an accidental duplicate bill. TEVAR reporting is somewhat different. The initial graft placement is predicated on coverage of the left subclavian artery. If the graft occludes the orifice of the left subclavian artery, CPT codes 33880 and 75956 are appropriate. If the graft is placed caudad to that artery, CPT codes 33881 and 75957 are correct. Any additional distal endograft extensions at the time of the initial TEVAR are not separately reportable. However, proximal endograft extensions done at the time of initial TEVAR are appropriate. The first proximal extension is described by 33883 and 75958. Any additional proximal extensions are codes with 33884 and 75958. If a proximal extension(s) causes coverage of the left subclavian artery, the 33881, 33883, and 33884 as well as their radiology supervision and interpretation codes are voided and are replaced by 33880 with 75956. Distal extensions are only reportable when done at a separate setting from the initial graft placement. Codes 33886 and 75959 describe placement of as many distal TEVAR extensions necessary at a date subsequent to the main body deployment.

Next, the arterial catheter placements are considered. Most patients will have two non-selective catheters (36200 x 2): one in each femoral artery that extends into the aorta. If selective catheterization is performed, appropriate component coding rules apply. Any open arterial exposure is described. Usually femoral artery exposure and simple repair is coded with 34812 but complex primary repair (35226), prosthetic patch angioplasty (35286), and common femoral endarterectomy (35371) may supersede an exposure code. CPT code 34820 denotes iliac artery exposure as necessary and 34833 conveys iliac artery exposure with the additional creation of a prosthetic graft conduit to assist in sheath insertion when small or heavily diseased external iliac arteries are encountered. When a brachial artery exposure (and repair) is warranted, CPT code 34834 is appropriate. All radiological supervision and interpretation is then summarized. Any separately reportable services are then added such as stenting or PTA outside of the endograft landing zone (e.g., left renal stent placement), embolization of arteries that do not contain an endograft (e.g., internal iliac artery or inferior mesenteric artery), or deployment of an aneurysm pressure sensor (34806). Cross femoral bypass with prosthetic conduit at the time of EVAR is described by the add-on code 34813. With regards to TEVAR, left arm revascularization may be required. Open subclavian to carotid artery transposition at the time of TEVAR is coded 33889. Carotid to subclavian artery bypass with prosthetic, an alternative to transposition, is reported with the traditional coding, 35606. If the left subclavian and the left common carotid artery are both occluded and a carotid to carotid artery bypass with prosthetic is placed in a retropharyngeal tunnel, a specially designed CPT code for use at the time of TEVAR is appropriate (33891).

ADDITIONAL BILLING ISSUES

Central to all reimbursement in a physician practice is some type of billing, scheduling, and registration information technology system. These software packages must be user friendly for support staff and organize the large volume of demographic data required in claim submission. They also allow for reasonable office schedule templates and maximal use of clinic time. Many systems have interfaces with most insurance companies including Medicare, United Healthcare, Aetna, and Blue Cross/Blue Shield that provide immediate eligibility verification. They also employ scrubbing programs that identify global periods, medical necessity policies, and National Correct Coding Initiative edits. Use of these computer models promotes efficiency in patient check-in/scheduling, higher clean claim creation rates, and improved throughput for charge entry. Electronic medical records (EMR) in both the office and the vascular lab are also beneficial on many levels. Physicians can have access to them after hours which can help in immediate patient care issues. EMR can include all the necessary information for billing at a given encounter level and allow for templating with future follow-up visits as well. There are immediate fax options which may improve communication in a timely fashion with referring MD's and therefore may increase referrals.

The largest income source in a vascular surgery practice is typically reimbursement for procedures performed. There must be a system of checks and balances in regard to this procedure billing. Procedures (both open and endovascular) should be tracked from booking to charge entry. Having all procedure reports faxed to one central number for review to ensure none are misplaced is an added failsafe mechanism. Missing even one procedure per month can lead to thousands of lost cash revenue per year for a practice.

Review rejection reports for trends on a routine basis. Insurers will periodically upgrade the scrubbing software and this may lead to denial of claims that were previously paid. Only by systematic evaluation can changes be identified and remedied. Be aware of medical necessity edits or local coverage determinations (LCD's). These may limit payments on procedures such as vascular lab studies, debridements, or Unna boot placement.

SUMMARY

Vascular surgery open coding and endovascular component coding are complex and difficult. Physicians must be involved in this process. Operative notes and angiography reports are also "billing receipts ". Treat them as such and include an appropriate diagnosis for medical necessity, a list of all imaging, catheterizations, and interventions for endovascular work, and individual procedures for open surgery. The physician must have a general understanding of what is billed in a given procedure so he or she can dictate a description that is clear and not disputable for each CPT code involved. Computer software eases the burden significantly.

REFERENCES

2008 Physicians' Professional ICD-9-CM International; Classification of Diseases Volumes 1&2. Salt Lake City: The Medical Management Institute, 2007.

Current Procedural Terminology cpt 2008 Professional Edition. Chicago: American Medical Association, 2007.

The National Correct Coding Sourcebook Version 13.3. Salt Lake City: The Medical Management Institute, 2007.

The National Correct Coding Sourcebook Version 10.3. Salt Lake City: The Medical Management Institute, 2004.

Surgery: Cardiovascular System, 35474 (Q&A). CPT Assistant. August 2006;16:8, p. 10.

Bonus Feature: Surgery: Cardiovascular System. CPT Assistant. December 2007;17:12.

The 2008 SIR Interventional Radiology Coding CD. Fairfax. Society of Interventional Radiology, 2008.

SECTION **II**

Carotid Stenting for Carotid Stenosis

7

Guidelines for Training and Credentialing in Carotid Artery Stenting

Russell C. Lam, M.D. and
K. Craig Kent, M.D., F.A.C.S.

Carotid angioplasty and stenting (CAS) is a minimally invasive treatment option for cerebrovascular occlusive disease. Although patients with acceptable risk should continue to be referred for carotid endarterectomy (CEA), the recently published SAPHIRE trial has raised the possibility that CAS might be an equivalent alternative to CEA in high surgical risk patients.[1] Moreover, the role of CAS in low-risk patients is now being investigated in a number of ongoing clinical trials. It is clear to those who treat carotid artery disease, whether by surgery or by endovascular means, that excellent outcomes are related to technical expertise and experience. With all new technology, there is a learning curve. There is the need to disseminate a new procedure from the few who were participants in its development to the large number of practitioners who treat patients for which the procedure was designed. It is necessary to define optimal outcomes, determine the best venue for training, and choose criteria for optimal training, as well as to determine the volume necessary to maintain skills. For carotid artery stenting, these tasks have been particularly challenging. The following chapter will focus on the current guidelines that are in place for training and credentialing in CAS.

It is necessary to begin by reaffirming that credentialing of physicians is a local process, the sole responsibility of hospitals and their credentialing committees. Consequently, there will likely not be uniformity in the requirements for credentialing for any procedure. Hospital A may set the bar at 25 carotid stents before an interventionalist is credentialed to independently perform carotid stenting, whereas hospital B, across the street, may set the threshold at 15. Hospitals, however, often do rely on published guidelines when determining credentialing requirements. These guidelines are often produced by either relevant societies or consensus groups composed of individuals with clinical expertise.

One of the challenges in producing uniform credentialing criteria is the fact that physicians that perform CAS have arisen from many different specialties including vascular surgery, cardiology, interventional radiology, neurosurgery, neuroradiology, and neurology. The background and experiences of individuals from each of these specialties is different, thus one could presume that the training paradigm that is required to learn CAS might vary among specialists. For example, a vascular surgeon might have a great deal of knowledge about pathophysiology, natural history, and anatomy of carotid artery disease, but have less experience with catheterization of the cerebral circulation. Alternatively, a neuroradiologist may have significant experience with carotid and cerebral angiography but little exposure to extracranial carotid atherosclerotic disease. The value of physicians from different backgrounds and with diverse specialty training becoming involved with CAS is that each brings a variety of strengths, experiences, and skills to the table .

Currently, there are several publications that have addressed the issue of CAS credentialing. The elements of training for CAS that are recommended in all three publications include the need for clinicians to attain clinical and cognitive skills related to the treatment of carotid artery disease as well as technical skills related to CAS. Three multispecialty consensus recommendations are available for review. The first report was published in 2003 by Barr et al.[2] and represents the views of a collaborative panel from the American Society of Interventional and Therapeutic Neuroradiology, the American Society of Neuroradiology, and the Society of interventional Radiology. In this document, it is recommended that interventionalists attain a thorough knowledge of cerebrovascular anatomy as well as an understanding of the hemodynamics, physiology, and pathophysiology of cerebrovascular occlusive disease. The clinical manifestations and natural history of cerebrovascular disease must also be understood, as well as the risks and benefits of CAS and treatment alternatives such as CE or medical management. The practitioner should be familiar with antiplatelet and anticoagulation therapy, and the clinical neurological examination and radiation physics and safety. It is expected that the clinician will be able to recognize complications of CAS including intracranial complications, and have the knowledge and skills to treat these complications. The authors of this document go on to state that these requirements may be met by obtaining formal residency/fellowship training in neuroendovascular surgery or interventional neuroradiology. Alternatively, these requirements can be met through a postgraduate experience that should include, for physicians with no prior catheter experience, 200 diagnostic cervicocerebral angiograms with acceptable indications and outcomes. For physicians with experience sufficient to meet the AHA requirement for peripheral intervention, at least 100 diagnostic cervicocerebral angiograms are required. In addition, physicians must possess experience with arterial stents, having performed either 25 noncarotid stent procedures and a minimum of four successful CAS cases, or 10 consecutive CAS procedures with acceptable results as principal operator.[2]

In 2004, a consensus statement by Connors et al. representing the American Academy of Neurology, the American Association of Neurological Surgeons, the American Society of Interventional and Therapeutic Neuroradiology, the Congress of Neurological Surgeons, the AANS/CNS Cerebrovascular Section, and the Society of Interventional Radiology[3] readdressed the issue of training and credentialing in diagnostic cervicocerebral angiography, carotid stenting, and cerebrovascular intervention. Similar to the previous published guidelines by Barr et al. the new consensus statement recognizes the need for interventionalists to acquire the cognitive and technical skills necessary to achieved competence in CAS. It is asserted in this document that there should be formal training for a minimum of six months in radiology, neuroradiology, neurosurgery, neurology, or vascular neurology. The goal of this training would be to allow the clinician to acquire an adequate depth of cognitive knowledge of the brain and its associated pathophysiological vascular processes. In addition, it is recommended that there be the performance of a minimum of 100 diagnostic cervicocerebral angiograms before initiating training in CAS. This prerequisite of 100 diagnostic cervicocerebral angiograms prior to CAS is based on the doctrine that extensive knowledge of the brain and the ability to correctly interpret a cervicocerebral angiogram is the foundation for the technical performance of cervicocerebral angiography and interventions such as CAS. Unlike the guidelines established previously by Barr et al. the new consensus statement did not establish a minimum requirement for arterial stenting or CAS.[3]

In 2005, a clinical competence statement was published by Rosenfield et al.[4] representing the views of the Society for Vascular Surgery, the Society for Cardiovascular Angiography and Intervention, and the Society for Vascular Medicine and Biology. Also expressed in this manuscript was the need for interventionalists to acquire the cognitive, technical, and clinical skills required for CAS. The training of physicians to perform CAS can be achieved by one of two pathways. The first pathway is through an accredited postgraduate residency or fellowship program in vascular surgery, interventional cardiology, or interventional radiology. For physicians already in practice, credentialing in peripheral interventions would be mandatory prior to learning carotid intervention. Physicians would also be required to develop a comprehensive understanding of the pathophysiology of carotid artery disease and stroke. They would also need to learn the risk factors, epidemiology, natural history, the clinical manifestations, associated pathology, angiographic anatomy, and therapeutic alternatives and selection criteria for interventions in patients with extracranial carotid artery disease. In addition to these cognitive requirements, the clinician needs to perform a minimum of 30 diagnostic cervicocerebral angiograms with at least half as primary operator and 25 carotid stent procedures with at least half as primary operator. Angiograms and stents may be performed in the same patients, provided that the interventionalist has experience with a minimum of 15 diagnostic angiograms before performing the first stent as a primary operator. Other technical elements considered fundamental to training in CAS include high levels of expertise with antiplatelet and periprocedural anticoagulation, and the ability to recognize and manage intraprocedural complications. Lastly, it is expected that the clinician will be sufficiently knowledgeable to be able to manage patients clinically before, during, and in follow-up postintervention.[4] Table 7-1 summarizes the cognitive and technical requirements for CAS from the respective documents.

TABLE 7-1. COMPARISON OF COGNITIVE AND TECHNICAL REQUIREMENTS FOR CAS

Authors, Year	Formal Cognitive Training	Diagnostic Cervicocerebral Angiogram	CAS
Barr et al., 2003[2]	Not required	200	4
Connors et al., 2005[3]	6 months in radiology, neuroradiology, neurology, or neurosurgery residency/fellowship	100	*Not specified
Rosenfield et al., 2005[4]	Not required	30	25

*Although not specified in this report, the authors did endorsed the principles and standards described by Barr et al. in 2003.[2]

There appears to be general agreement within all three documents that interventionalists who perform CAS should have a thorough understanding of the pathophysiology, natural history, and proper management of carotid artery disease. For those individuals who acquire CAS skills as part of a formal training program, it is anticipated that these training programs will have appropriate curriculum that will provide this knowledge. However, for practicing physicians seeking training in CAS, the mechanism for the acquisition of this knowledge seems more elusive. Vascular surgeons who are in practice will already have familiarity with the management of carotid artery disease. The challenge is for other specialists who do not currently treat carotid artery stenosis to gain the necessary cognitive skills to successfully manage these patients.

Analysis of these three documents reveals considerable controversy over the prescription for CAS training. The recent report by Connors et al. mandates formal training through postgraduate residency or fellowship in radiology, neuroradiology, neurosurgery, neurology, or vascular neurology as a prerequisite for performing CAS. Whether training in interventional cardiology or vascular surgery could be an additional pathway to credentialing in CAS was not mentioned. A favorable interpretation of this document would be its purpose was to describe credentialing for neurologists, interventional radiologists, neurointerventionalists, and neurosurgeons. This interpretation seems reasonable since, as previously discussed, the requirements for credentialing may and should be different for clinicians from varying backgrounds. It is safe to assume that the intent of this document was not to exclude vascular surgeons and cardiologists who are appropriately trained in the performance of CAS.

The most significant difference among these documents resides in the number of cerebral angiograms and carotid sents required for credentialing. The Barr and Connors manuscripts set a threshold of 100 cerebral angiograms for experienced interventionalists, and the Rosenfield manuscript sets this bar at 30.[2-4] Moreover, the Barr manuscript sets the threshold for carotid stents at four, if there is pervious experience with stenting. Alternatively, the Rosenfield document sets this threshold at 25 with 13 as primary operator. As is obvious, the difference in numbers is quite substantial. All interventionalists who have performed carotid stenting would agree that prior expertise in cervical angiography is a prerequisite of CAS. The debate is focused on how extensive this experience needs to be. There is little data to support either number. However, enrollment as an interventionalist in CREST did not require a prerequisite number of cerebral angiograms, only a prerequisite number of carotid stents. Yet the outcomes of interventionalists in CREST are at least equivalent if not superior to those of any other CAS trials.[5,6] Moreover, a prerequisite of 100 cerebral angiograms has not been a standard for enrollment as a CAS investigator in any of the clinical trials that to date have set the standards for outcome in carotid stenting. There is a downside to requiring extensive experience with cerebral angiography prior to CAS. Establishing such a high threshold may encourage unnecessary angiographic procedures in an era when the diagnosis and treatment for carotid occlusive disease is increasingly made using noninvasive techniques such as duplex ultrasound, MRA, and CTA. While there is no data supporting the necessity of a large number of diagnostic cervicocerebral angiograms for the safe and effective performance of CAS, there are published reports from clinical trials demonstrating improved patient outcome with increasing operator experience with CAS.[5-9] In CREST, the stroke rate with CAS was lower among those interventionalists who had performed at least 15 procedures prior to randomization.[9]

Another issue not addressed in these documents is the number of carotid stents that need to be performed following initial training to allow maintenance of skills. In recent years, it has been demonstrated for a variety of vascular procedures—including carotid endarterectomy—that yearly volume correlates in a positive manner with outcome. These threshold numbers are difficult to determine and the required volume for maintenance of skills in CAS is clearly not known. Nevertheless, the ultimate goal of credentialing is to produce interventionalists who can provide optimal outcomes for their patients. Thus, monitoring of outcomes and maintenance of skills is as important as the initial credentialing process.

Currently, the demand for CAS training far exceeds the programs through which training is available. In many institutions, there are an insufficient number of cases available to train current fellows, let alone practicing physicians, who wish to retrain in CAS. This dearth of training opportunities is related to 1) the small number of individuals who are currently proficient in carotid stenting and capable of training, and 2) the current restriction of carotid stenting for high-risk symptomatic patients or clinical trials. There are, however, a number of CAS training programs currently offered by academic institutions, societies, and industry. These programs vary considerably depending on the sponsor and the venue. There are FDA-mandated courses sponsored by industry where the emphasis is on acquiring familiarity with specific devices. These courses are not designed to train physicians to perform CAS nor are they meant to be used by physicians for hospital credentialing. These industry-sponsored courses usually begin with precourse Web-based instruction in CAS and cerebral anatomy. Courses then include didactic teaching, case discussion, simulator training, product education, and in-hospital proctoring.[10] More substantial exposure to CAS is usually gained by preceptorships or minifellowships performed at high-volume centers. An alternative mechanism is the propagation of CAS techniques from one individual to others within the same group. However, the number of centers where CAS is performed in high volume is limited, and thus, the opportunities for training.

There are several possible solutions to the limited opportunity for training. One approach would be to continue with current paradigms using the existing credentialing guidelines outlined in this chapter as the standard. Eventually, the problem will be solved. As and if the indications for CAS increase, there will be more procedures performed and the opportunity for training will increase. The concern with this approach is that if the indications for CAS abruptly change, there may not be a sufficient number of experienced interventionalists to meet the demand.

A second alternative would be, as more data become available, to alter the training requirements for CAS. There is some belief that for experienced interventionists, the required number of CAS procedures may be in the range of 15 rather than 25. Given the diversity of the background of clinicians seeking training in CAS, it would not be surprising that the training requirements might vary with an individual's prior training and experience. While there will never be a training requirement at which patient safety is universally guaranteed, among those clinicians applying as interventionalists in CREST, the stroke rate was least amongst those who had performed 15 cases or more, suggesting that 15 may be a more appropriate threshold.[6] In a recently published roundtable discussion, experience in peripheral angioplasty and stenting—including the performance of iliac, superficial femoral, tibial, and renal artery interventions—was considered an excellent prerequisite for performance of CAS.[11] Credentialing committees might take into consideration the trainee's baseline level of experience in dealing with carotid occlusive disease and catheter-based intervention in considering an individual's application for CAS privileges.

While there is no substitute for hands-on experience, the use of simulation in conjunction with formal mentorship could play an important role in training for CAS. Endovascular simulators have been shown in a randomized trial to enhance the assimilation of catheter skills. It has not been proven whether simulation is beneficial to the advanced interventionalist learning CAS; however, there are reasons to believe that this might be the case. Simulators allow investigators to rehearse the stepwise progression of a CAS procedure. Simulation can also familiarize clinicians with the catheters, guidewires, sheaths, protection devices, and stents necessary to perform catheter-carotid intervention. In addition, simulators can be used to demonstrate arch and cervicocerebral anatomy; challenging variations in anatomy can be modeled through simulation.[12] The use of simulators have been shown to decrease operative and fluoroscopy time necessary to complete CAS, as well as to enhance the operator's comfort with device usage.[13-15] Thus far, simulation is being used only as an adjunct in CAS training programs, but there is the belief that simulation training has the potential to reduce the required number of cases necessary for CAS credentialing. This hypothesis awaits validation.

In summary, CAS has become an integral part of the treatment of patients with carotid artery occlusive disease, and it is anticipated that the role of CAS relative to carotid endarterectomy will increase as techniques improve and as validating studies become available. Thus, all interventionalists, including surgeons, who desire to participate in the care and treatment of these patients, must obtain training in CAS. Vascular surgeons who perform carotid endarterectomy already have the cognitive and clinical skills necessary to care for these patients. The most appropriate mechanism for a surgeon to achieve expertise in CAS is to first develop advanced catheter and guidewire skills, then acquire specific training in CAS. Although credentialing requirements may vary with each hospital, the desired goal would be to perform as part of a mentored program a minimum of 30 cerebral angiograms and 25 carotid stents. Although a significant focus has been placed on initial credentialing, the most important assessment of competence is through the measurement of outcomes. No matter what treatment is employed in patients with carotid occlusive disease, the perioperative risk of stroke needs to remain low.

REFERENCES

1. Yadav JS, Wholey MH, Kuntz RE, et al; Stenting and Angioplasty with Protection in Patients at High Risk for Endarterectomy Investigators. Protected carotid-artery stenting versus endarterectomy in high-risk patients. *N Engl J Med*. 2004;351(15):1493–1501.
2. Barr JD, Connors JJ 3rd, Sacks D, Wojak JC, et al; American Society of Interventional and Therapeutic Neuroradiology; American Society of Neuroradiology; Society of Interventional Radiology. Quality improvement guidelines for the performance of cervical carotid angioplasty and stent placement. *J Vasc Interv Radiol*. 2003;14(9 Pt 2):S321–335.
3. Connors JJ 3rd, Sacks D, Furlan AJ, et al; NeuroVascular Coalition Writing Group; American Academy of Neurology; American Association of Neurological Surgeons; American Society of Interventional and Therapeutic Radiology; American Society of Neuroradiology; Congress of Neurological Surgeons; AANS/CNS Cerebrovascular Section; Society of Interventional Radiology. Training, competency, and credentialing standards for

diagnostic cervicocerebral angiography, carotid stenting, and cerebrovascular intervention: a joint statement from the American Academy of Neurology, American Association of Neurological Surgeons, American Society of Interventional and Therapeutic Radiology, American Society of Neuroradiology, Congress of Neurological Surgeons, AANS/CNS Cerebrovascular Section, and Society of Interventional Radiology. *Radiology*. 2005;234(1): 26–34. Epub 2004 Nov 4.

4. Rosenfield KM; SCAI/SVMB/SVS Writing Committee. Clinical competence statement on carotid stenting: training and credentialing for carotid stenting—multispecialty consensus recommendations. *J Vasc Surg*. 2005 Jan;41(1):160–168.

5. Hobson RW 2nd, Howard VJ, Roubin GS, et al.; CREST. Credentialing of surgeons as interventionalists for carotid artery stenting: experience from the lead-in phase of CREST. *J Vasc Surg*. 2004 Nov;40(5):952–957.

6. Roubin GS, New G, Iyer SS. Immediate and late clinical outcomes of carotid artery stenting in patients with symptomatic and asymptomatic carotid artery stenosis: a 5-year prospective analysis. *Circulation*. 2001;103:532–537.

7. Henry M, Amor M, Massoa I, et al. Angioplasty and stenting of the extracranial carotid arteries, *J Endovasc Surg*. 1998;5:293–304.

8. White CJ, Gomez CR, Iyer SS, et al Carotid stent placement for extracranial carotid artery disease: current state of the art. *Catheter Cardiovasc Interv*. 2000;5:339–346.

9. Al-Mubarak N, Roubin GS, Hobson RW, et al. Credentialing of stent operators for the Carotid Revascularization Endarterectomy vs Stenting Trial (CREST). *Stroke*. 2000;31:292.

10. Yadav JS, Roubin GS, Iyer S, et al. Elective stenting of the extracranial carotid arteries, *Circulation*. 1997;95:376–381.

11. Katzen BT, Ohki T, Gray WA, et al. CAS accreditation roundtable. *Endovasc Today*. 2004;3: 47–60.

12. Schneider PA. Optimal training strategies for carotid stenting. *Semin Vasc Surg*. 2005;18(2): 69–74.

13. Dayal R, Faries PL, Lin SC, et al. Computer simulation as a component of catheter-based training. *J Vasc Surg*. 2004;40(6):1112–1117

14. Patel AD, Gallagher AG, Nicholson WJ, Cates CU. Learning curves and reliability measures for virtual reality simulation in the performance assessment of carotid angiography. *J Am Coll Cardiol*. 2006;47(9):1796–802. Epub 2006 Apr 17.

15. McChesney C. CAS training programs. *Endovascular Today*. 2004;Nov:20–22.

8

Assessing Competence in the Components of Vascular Surgery

Anton N. Sidawy, M.D., M.P.H., John J. Ricotta, M.D., Robert S. Rhodes, M.D.

In the last few years, many external and internal factors have influenced the practice of medicine in general and surgery in particular. One prominent such factor has been increased public demand for quality and accountability. Interest in physician accountability increased especially after the publication of the Institute of Medicine report, "To Err is Human," which estimated that 98,000 lives are lost annually in hospitals around the United States due to medical errors.[1] To reduce the incidence of such errors, this report recommended that patients be involved in their own care. It also called for improving data collection, analysis, and reporting in the hopes of improving patients' safety. The Institute of Medicine report caused a ripple effect in the health care industry that culminated in many health care organizations changing how physicians are taught, monitored, certified, and credentialed. This chapter will detail those changes that relate to board certification in vascular surgery, and discuss their relationship to the assessment of competence and their application in granting hospital privileges.

WHAT IS COMPETENCE?

As applied to the practice of medicine, competence has been both difficult to define and to measure. For instance, the traditional requirements for certification by member boards of the American Board of Medical Specialties (e.g., certification in Vascular Surgery through the American Board of Surgery) require satisfactory completion of an accredited residency training program. Certification in vascular surgery also requires that the program director attest to the professionalism, technical skills, and communication skills of the applicant, as well as the satisfactory completion of both a written multiple-choice and an oral examination. Yet these seemingly stringent requirements only measure physicians' qualifications and not what they actually do in practice. Knowledge is the basis of understanding and clinical judgment but does not

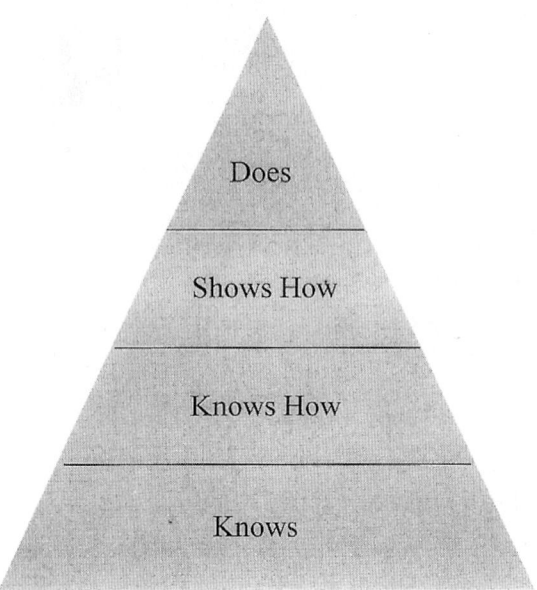

Figure 8-1. Miller's pyramid.

automatically translate into actual practice. This distinction is reflected by Miller's pyramid (Figure 8–1).[2] The current requirements for certification reflect the lower two levels of the pyramid whereas patients and the public are most interested in the top level. The fact that knowledge (*Knows*) may not always be applied in practice (*Does*) is exemplified by the difference between the percentage of surgeons that correctly respond to questions about the timing of prophylactic antibiotics and the percentage that actually appropriately administer them in a timely fashion. Whereas nearly 90% of surgeons respond correctly to questions about such timing, Figure 8–2 indicates that

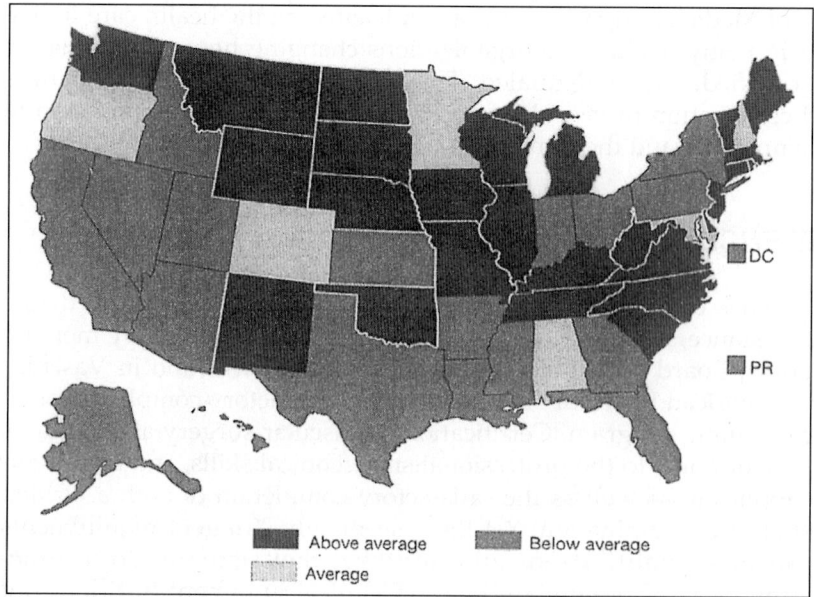

Figure 8-2. State variation in appropriate timing of prophylactic antibiotics, 2005[1]

TABLE 8-1. THE STAGES OF COMPETENCE [DREYFUS]

Novice	Learns context-free elementary rules.
Advanced Beginner	Begins to appreciate situational features.
Competent	Able to identify and focus on specific goals.
	Able to extract meaningful information from a seemingly overwhelming amount of data.
	Decision-making remains a conscious behavior.
Proficient	Intuitive behavior begins to replace consciously reasoned responses.
Expert	Both the evaluation of situations and the decisions for action become increasingly intuitive.

the timely administration of these antibiotics actually occurs considerably less frequently.[3] The national average was 75.2% with a range from 54.6% to 89.8%, a 36% differential among states.

A second concern related to the definition of competence tends to be the thought that competence is a duality (i.e., if one is not competent they are incompetent). A more appropriate view is that competence is a continuum.[4] The postulated stages of competence and their definitions are shown in Table 8–1. It has been suggested that completion of residency training should reflect, at a minimum, the *Competent* stage and that further increases in competence occur with experience in practice. This model underscores the concept that the development of surgical competence involves intuitive intellectual skills as well as technical skills. Dreyfus' concept of competence parallels the performance levels described by Rasmussen[5] in that progressive competence in the Dreyfus model corresponds with skill-based performance (versus knowledge-based and rule-based performance) in the Rasmussen model.

To address the issues of defining and measuring competence, the Accreditation Council for Graduate Medical Education (ACGME) and the American Board of Medical Specialties (ABMS) identified six competencies characteristic of good physicians (Table 8–2). Yet the choice of the term competencies emphasizes the difficulties of defining competence as a single attribute. Even these six competencies may not be all inclusive; thus, these specific behaviors are necessary but may not be sufficient for a competent physician. The ACGME has sought to incorporate assessments of these

TABLE 8-2. THE SIX ACGME AND ABMS COMPETENCIES AND THEIR SCOPE

Competency	Scope
Medical Knowledge	Evolving biomedical, clinical, and cognate sciences, and the application of this knowledge to patient care.
Patient Care	Compassionate, appropriate, and effective treatment of health problems and promotion of health.
Interpersonal and Communication Skills	Effective information exchange and teaming with patients, their families, and other health professionals.
Professionalism	A commitment to professional responsibilities, adherence to ethical principles, and sensitivity to a diverse patient population.
Practice-based Learning and Improvement	Evaluation of one's own patient care and outcomes, assimilation of scientific evidence, and targeted improvement efforts.
Systems-based Practice	An awareness of and responsiveness to the systems and environments that affect the delivery of health care, and the ability to best coordinate those systems to provide optimal care.

competencies into residency training, but their actual assessment, other than traditional tests of medical knowledge, has been an elusive goal. Similarly, the important concepts of the Dreyfus and Rasmussen models currently lack sufficient criteria to be readily measurable.

MAINTENANCE OF CERTIFICATION

This process has been implemented by the ABMS and its member boards to ensure documentation of ongoing postgraduation efforts of practicing surgeons to maintain competence acquired during the initial training period. Diplomates who certify or recertify after June 1, 2005, will automatically be entered into this process. To assess ongoing competencies, the ABMS member boards divided them into four components of a process called Maintenance of Certification (MOC) (Table 8–3). While MOC uses some measures that are already part of traditional recertification, this process differs from traditional recertification in two substantive ways. The first is that MOC is intended to emphasize a more continuous process as opposed to the episodic—most commonly every 10 years—nature of traditional recertification. The second difference is the addition of Part 4, Evaluation of Performance in Practice, a change that places greater emphasis on the top level of Miller's pyramid.

Completion of Parts 1 and 2 of MOC will be required every three years. For certification in Vascular Surgery, specific documentation of hospital privileges and clinical assessment (Part 1) in Vascular Surgery will be required. For Part 2, 50% of CME credits will be required in areas specific to Vascular Surgery and 100% of the self-assessment requirement will be in Vascular Surgery. Individuals who hold multiple certificates (e.g., vascular surgery and surgery) will be allowed to count their Parts 1 and 2 efforts in vascular surgery toward their surgery certification.

Part 3 of MOC, the secure written examination, will continue to be offered in years 8 to 10 of the recertification cycle. Each certificate will require successful completion of a separate secure written examination. It is important to recognize that entrance to the secure examination (Part 3) will not be possible unless the candidate has successfully completed the other requirements of MOC (i.e., Parts 1, 2, and 4) at the time the recertification examination is processed. This means at least two cycles of Parts 1 and 2 and one cycle of Part 4.

Part 4 of the MOC process is new and involves evaluation of practice performance. Its goal is to demonstrate that the diplomate is continuously evaluating and improving his or her practice performance. The challenge of Part 4 of MOC is to identify appropriate criteria that reflect such performance. The previous example of the timing of

---

TABLE 8-3. THE COMPONENTS OF MAINTENANCE OF CERTIFICATION (MOC)

Part 1—Professional Standing through maintenance of an unrestricted medical license, hospital privileges, and satisfactory references.

Part 2—Lifelong Learning through continuing education and periodic self-assessment.

Part 3—Cognitive Expertise based on performance on a secure examination.

Part 4—Evaluation of Performance in Practice through tools such as outcome measures and quality improvement programs, and the evaluation of behaviors such as communication and professionalism.

antibiotics is one such criterion but to date, relatively few other criteria of surgical performance have emerged. The specific requirements for Part 4 MOC have not been completely developed at the present time. However, essential to this process is participation in efforts to assess and improve practice. Examples include participation in databases and programs such as NSQIP, SCIP, and registries such as the SVS carotid database, the AVF venous registry, regional databases, and the ACS Web portal. While independent audited registries appear to be the Holy Grail of outcome measures, this approach is fraught with difficulties. Problems include the substantial cost for establishing and maintaining such registries, the number of data points necessary to ensure statistical validity, and issues of risk adjustment. Development of more specific methods to use for Part 4 MOC is in evolution.

CASE REQUIREMENTS FOR RESIDENCY TRAINING

The procedural experiences required for accreditation of residency training in vascular surgery are established by the Residency Review Committee for Surgery (RRC-S) of the ACGME. The goal of these requirements is to ensure technical proficiency and sufficient experience with operative decision-making so that such decisions can develop in accord with the Dreyfus criteria of competence. Ideally, these requirements should be based on validated criteria but such criteria only appear to exist in a relatively limited way. The existing criteria tend to be of four types: supervisor assessments, learning curve analyses of a large number of trainees/procedures (e.g., CUSUM analyses),[6-7] the ability to recognize errors,[8] and trainees' opinion of the number of procedures needed to acquire confidence.[9]

Given the relative lack of validated criteria, the RRC-S requirements for procedural experience are to a large extent historical, and as a consequence, have shortcomings. These shortcomings relate to both the acquisition of technical skills as well as operative decision-making. Many of the RRC-S criteria were established years ago and have not been routinely updated. The RRC-S did establish *defined minimums* (i.e., minimum numbers of procedures within broad categories of related procedures), but these minimums are often based on the 10th percentile of experience among all programs rather than any demonstrable relationship between number of cases and the acquisition of proficiency. Moreover, these minimums are based on an unproven assumption that transference of skills occurs from one procedure to another within a specific procedure category. Even though some procedures within a defined category might require unique decision-making and/or technical skills, it is possible to satisfy the RRC-S category requirements without experience with these procedures. The role of specific case volumes is of particular concern given the emerging data on the relationship between surgeon volume and outcomes. If one couples the fact that the threshold volumes for the best outcomes often considerably exceed actual resident experience with the fact the volume-outcome relationships are based on surgeons who already completed their training, it should be clear that there is a desperate need to establish evidence-based experience criteria for residency training. Until such criteria are developed, the assessment of both technical prowess and intra-operative decision skills will rest on the opinions of supervising surgical faculty. The observation that surgery residents' self-assessment continues to show relatively high numbers of residents who feel only somewhat prepared for practice suggests this process is imperfect.[10]

CASE REQUIREMENTS FOR HOSPITAL PRIVILEGING FOR VASCULAR SURGERY TRAINEES

Since satisfactory completion of an ACGME-accredited residency may not ensure proficiency in all aspects of a specialty, particularly in its more complex or infrequent procedures, external panels often attempt to establish guidelines for hospital privileges. In the case of vascular surgery, a committee from the Clinical Practice Council of the Society for Vascular Surgery (CPC-SVS) updated the guidelines for hospital privileges in vascular and endovascular surgery.[11] This committee based its guidelines on multiple sources that included the requirements of the RRC-S, the recommendations of the Inter-societal Commission for Accreditation of Vascular Laboratories (ICAVL), and previously established guidelines also published by a committee of the SVS. The guidelines referred to in this chapter are primarily drawn from the work of this committee and its publication.[11]

Open Surgery

The foundation for case numbers established for residency training by the RRC-S is discussed above. Given the emergence of endovascular technologies and the recent establishment of two years as the minimum duration of a residency, training, and the case numbers for trainees and programs have been recently updated (Table 8–4).[11]

Endovascular Interventions

Guidelines regarding the number of catheter-based interventions have been previously published.[12] Graduating vascular surgery residents are expected to have acquired sufficient training to perform catheter-based vascular interventions. These minimum numbers of endovascular procedures for training, established by the RRC-Surgery, are included in Table 8–4. Diagnostic catheterizations should be balanced among the various vascular beds[12] and at least half should be selective catheterizations. Three-quarters of the total diagnostic and therapeutic interventions should be arterial and 25% venous.[13] These specific requirements were placed to ensure the endovascular experience of the resident is based mainly on arterial and venous interventions, and that

---

TABLE 8-4. MINIMUM RRC-S REQUIRED CASE NUMBERS; MINIMUM 250 MAJOR VASCULAR RECONSTRUCTIVE CASES DURING RESIDENCY TRAINING

Open Procedures

- 30 abdominal vascular operations
- 25 cerebrovascular procedures
- 45 peripheral reconstructions
- 10 complex procedures

Endovascular Interventions

- 100 endovascular diagnostic catheterizations
- 80 endovascular therapeutic interventions
- 20 EVAR[A]

*This required EVAR number of 20 has been recently increased from five cases previously determined by RRC to be the minimum number; this increase reflects the increasing trend in the use of EVAR in the treatment of abdominal aortic aneurysm repair.

interventions on hemodialysis fistulas, grafts, and catheters do not constitute the majority of the resident's experience.

Special Requirements for Endovascular Credentialing Guidelines for Vascular Surgery Trainees.   Experience in specific areas that requires special skills such as TEVAR and CAS during residency training have been established.

1. *TEVAR:* For thoracic endovascular aortic repair (TEVAR), recent guidelines have been published and include full basic endovascular privileges in addition to an experience of at least 25 EVARs (12 as primary operator).[14] The term "full basic endovascular privileges" was defined by guidelines established by publications of either the American Heart Association guidelines or multispecialty guidelines.[13] In addition, vascular residents performing TEVAR should be familiar with the peri-operative management of aortic surgical patients. Although the surgeon does not have to have preexisting open thoracoabdominal privileges to perform TEVAR,[14] he or she should have experience performing adjunctive procedures for TEVARs including iliac conduits, femoral artery exposures and repairs, and carotid-subclavian bypasses, surgical skills that a graduating vascular surgery trainee should have.

2. *CAS:* Credentialing guidelines for carotid stenting have been endorsed by major vascular societies interested in the management of carotid artery disease, including the SVS as well as radiology and cardiology societies (Society for Vascular Medicine and Biology; Society for Cardiovascular Angiography and Intervention).[15] In addition to specifying minimal knowledge and clinical skills, this document recommends "a minimum of 30 diagnostic cervico-cerebral angiograms, with half as the primary operator, and a minimum of 25 carotid stent procedures, with half as the primary operator."[14] This document also stated that the number of diagnostic and therapeutic procedures does not need to be satisfied using separate encounters; rather, diagnostic and stenting procedures may both be counted toward their specified numbers if performed during the same procedure.

Noninvasive Vascular Laboratory Diagnosis

In order to interpret vascular laboratory studies, a graduating vascular resident must meet certain basic requirements to include knowledge of the vascular anatomy and physiology, as well as ultrasound physics and evidence of CME activity specific to noninvasive vascular diagnostics. Recent graduates of postgraduate ACGME-approved training programs where interpretation of vascular laboratory studies was an integral component of the training program are initially exempt from the CME requirement for three years following completion of their ACGME approved training program.

As suggested by the Inter-societal Commission for Accreditation of Vascular Laboratories (ICAVL), a minimum number of supervised interpreted studies during postgraduate training are required for individuals wishing to apply for privileges in interpretation of specific individual areas of the vascular laboratory. These minimum numbers are included in Table 8–5.[11]

Individuals may seek privileges only in those areas in which they have sufficient qualifications and training rather than in all areas of vascular laboratory testing. The

TABLE 8-5.

100 Peripheral Arterial Physiologic Tests
100 Peripheral Arterial Duplex Scanning
100 Peripheral Venous Duplex Scanning
100 Carotid Duplex Scanning
100 Transcranial Duplex/Doppler scanning
75 Visceral Vascular Duplex Scanning

American Registry of Diagnostic Medical Sonographers (ARDMS) provides two types of certification:

1. Registered Physician in Vascular Interpretation (RPVI)
2. Registered Vascular Technologist (RVT)

Graduating vascular residents are encouraged to obtain certification in either examination. Both the RVT and the RPVI are obtained by passing examinations administered by the ARDMS.

Medical Management of Vascular Disease and its Complications

Training in medical management of peripheral vascular disease is considered an important part of a vascular residency. Vascular residents should have a thorough understanding of vascular disease risk factors and their management in addition to knowledge in the management of nonsurgical vascular diseases such as nonatherosclerotic vascular disease, management of venous thromboembolism (VTE), chronic venous insufficiency, and lymphedema.[16] Vascular residents are also expected to be closely involved in the management of vascular surgical patients in intensive care settings.

TRAINING REQUIREMENTS FOR NEW PROCEDURES FOR ALREADY CREDENTIALED SURGEONS

The explosion in medical knowledge and technology has greatly accelerated the rate of change in medical practice. As a result, the knowledge acquired and procedures learned during residency training are likely to remain current for only a fraction of one's practice career. This is particularly true with endovascular therapies. As a consequence, standards are needed to ensure proficiency in new technologies acquired after traditional graduate medical education. Vascular surgeons are expected to acquire proficiency in new and evolving procedures, which should include evidence of participation in CME courses relevant to the topic. However, some new devices can be used without special certification by physicians trained in endovascular interventions. Whether a mentor is required or not will depend on the complexity of the procedure and will need to be determined on a case by case basis. A recent example of procedures that required special training are TEVAR[14] and CAS.[15]

DISCUSSION

Public demands for transparency has resulted in the publication, by many private or governmental organizations, of provider or hospital-specific risk adjusted or nonadjusted clinical outcomes.[17,18] This increased emphasis on surgical outcomes has lead various organizations involved in graduate and postgraduate medical training to devise new methods to evaluate the competence of medical providers, and most of all, surgeons. Surgical practice presents an especially complex challenge since it does not only include maintenance and improvement in cognitive knowledge, but also technical skills. In particular, vascular surgical practice presents a new set of challenges since it has recently undergone a major shift in adopting endovascular therapy in the management of vascular disease as an equal alongside open surgery, and more and more as a primary management tool, two completely different domains with dissimilar technical skills. In fact, the across-the-board adoption of endovascular therapy in the management of vascular disease has had, and continues to have, its own set of challenges. It has taken a long time and considerable effort to educate established vascular surgeons in endovascular tools, which has been done very successfully by the vascular surgery community. Now, after endovascular means have matured, the challenge has recently been the ability to teach trainees in vascular residencies and fellowships open vascular surgery as the number of these procedures is decreasing. Furthermore, many discussions currently revolve around the scope of practice of the vascular surgeon. Although when one thinks about the scope of practice in surgical specialties, one thinks about the actual surgical treatment of the disease, arguably, the scope should span prevention, diagnosis to include imaging, medical management, surgical and endovascular treatment, perioperative management to include critical care, and long-term surveillance of vascular procedures. Although it has been argued that the advantage for the patient who is being cared for by a vascular surgeon is the ability of the vascular surgeon to choose the best means to treat established disease, whether the best approach is open surgical or endovascular, a more complete vascular practice that provides maximum benefit to the patient is one that includes all the elements of practice detailed above. It may be rather difficult for a vascular surgeon to be proficient and competent in all these elements; in such situations, various members in a practice can primarily practice in one element over others. This "super specialization" has not matured yet, but it can be observed in some very busy, large practices where some members continue to perform mainly open surgery while other typically younger members of the practice perform more endovascular therapy. Furthermore, some members of a practice may limit themselves to venous disease management while others' practice emphasizes arterial disease management. If this trend continues to evolve, organized vascular surgery is going to face the question of whether modular competence assessment and certification in vascular surgery is the appropriate way to go.

Last, in considering the complexities of defining and measuring competence and its application to credentialing, it is important to remember that the above guidelines are exactly that: guidelines. The American Board of Surgery does not involve itself in local credentialing issues because in many cases, each institution or organization needs to set standards based on its particular culture and needs. Nonetheless, the Board feels that such standards should increasingly recognize training, experience, and outcomes relative to one's peers.

REFERENCES

1. Kohn LT, Corrigan J, Donaldson MS (eds): *To Err Is Human: Building a Safer Health System. Committee on Quality of Health Care in American, Institute of Medicine.* Washington, DC: National Academy Press, 2000.
2. Miller GE. The assessment of clinical skills/competence/performance. *Acad Med.* 1990;65 (9 Suppl):S63–S67.
3. http://www.ahrq.gov/qual/nhqr07/Chap3.htm. Accessed September 16, 2008
4. Dreyfus HL, Dreyfus SE. From Socrates to Expert Systems: The Limits and Dangers of Calculative Rationality [monograph on the Internet]. Berkeley, CA. 2004. Available from: http://socrates.berkeley.edu/~hdreyfus/html/paper_socrates.html.
5. Rasmussen J, Jensen A. Mental procedures in real-life tasks: A case study of electronic trouble shooting. *Ergonomics.* 1974;17:293–307.
6. Forbes TL, DeRose G, Kribs Sw, Harris KA. Cumulative sum failure analysis of the learning curve with endovascular abdominal aortic aneurysm repair. *J Vasc Surg.* 2004;39:102–108.
7. Forbes TL, Chu MWA, Lawlor DK, DeRose G, Harris KA. Learning curve analysis of thoracic endovascular repair in relation to credentialing guidelines. *J Vasc Surg.* 2007;46: 218–222.
8. Bann S, Datta V, Darzi A. Surgical skill is predicted by the ability to detect errors. *Am J Surg.* 2005;189:412-415.
9. Park A, Kavic SM, Lee TH, Heniford BT. Minimally invasive surgery: The evolution of fellowship. *Surgery.* 2007;142:505–513.
10. Blumenthal D, Gokhake M, Campbell EG, Weissman JS. Preparedness for clinical practice: Reports of graduating residents at academic health centers. *JAMA.* 2001;286:1027-1034.
11. Calligaro KD, Toursarkissian B, Clagett GP, Towne J, Hodgson K, Moneta G, Sidawy AN, Cronenwett JL. Guidelines for Hospital Privileges in Vascular and Endovascular Surgery: Recommendations of the Society for Vascular Surgery. *J Vasc Surg.* 2008,47:1-5.
12. ACC/ACP/SCAI/SVMB/SVS Clinical Competence Statement on Vascular medicine and Catheter-Based Peripheral Vascular Interventions. A report of the American College of Cardiology/American Heart Association/American College of Physicians Task Force on Clinical Competence (ACC/ACP/SCAI/SVMB/SVS Writing Committee to Develop a Clinical Competence Statement on Peripheral Vascular Disease. *J.A.C.C.* 2004;44(4):941-957.
13. White RA, Hodgson KJ, Ahn SS, et al. Endovascular interventions training and credentialing for Vascular Surgeons. *J Vasc Surg.* 1999; 29:177-186.
14. Clinical competence statement on thoracic endovascular aortic repair (TEVAR)- multispecialty consensus recommendations. A report of the SVS/SIR/SCAI/SVMB Writing Committee to Develop a Clinical Competence Standard for TEVAR. *J Vasc.Surg.* 2006;43(4): 858-862.
15. Clinical competence statement on carotid stenting: training and credentialing for carotid stenting. Multispecialty consensus recommendations. A report of the SCAI/SVMB/SVS writing committee to develop a clinical competence statement on carotid interventions. *J Vasc Surg.* 41(1):160–168.
16. Plummer D, Macsata R, Sidawy AN. Training in vascular medicine for vascular surgeons: what is it? And how will we accomplish it? *Semin Vasc Surg.* 2006;12:200–2004.
17. http://www.leapfroggroup.org/. Accessed August 22, 2008.
18. http://www.healthgrades.com/. Accessed August 22, 2008.

9

Preprocedure Imaging to Facilitate Carotid Artery Stenting

Richard J. Powell, M.D.

Carotid endarterectomy (CEA) has been a standard treatment for selected patients with symptomatic and asymptomatic carotid occlusive disease at risk for stroke. This has been the most extensively studied vascular surgical procedure with over six thousand patients having been enrolled in randomized trials to compare carotid endarterectomy to best medical management.[1-4] The outcomes of these studies for both symptomatic and asymptomatic patients are outlined in Tables 9–1 and 9–2. Historically, preopera-

TABLE 9-1. POOLED ANALYSIS OF RANDOMIZED TRIALS FOR SYMPTOMAT PATIENTS TREATED WITH CEA NASCET, ECST, VA (6,092 PATIENTS)

Risk Reduction of 30-day Stroke and Death versus Medical Management

Stenosis	Absolute	Relative	P<
<30%	+2.2%	+23%	.05
30–49%	–3.2%	–18%	ns
50–69%	–4.6%	–25%	.04
70–99%	–16%	–61%	.0001

TABLE 9-2. OUTCOMES OF CAROTID ENDARTERECTOMY IN ASYMPTOMATIC PATIENTS

	Total	ACAS	ACST
Piatients	4,782	1.662	3,120
Op CVA, death	2.8%	2.3%	3.1%
Surgica—5 yr*	6.0%	5.1%	6.4%
Medical—5 yr*	11.5%	11.0%	11.8%
Absoute RR	5.5%	5.9%	5.4%
Realtive RR	48%	54%	46%

ACST: Benefit for men and women <age 75, any stenosis >60% (ACAS; JAMA 1995)

*30-day death, stroke, ipsilat late stroke (ACST; Lancet 2004)

tive evaluation of the patient with carotid occlusive disease prior to CEA included thoracic arch and cerebral arteriography. The use of preoperative arteriography was associated with a stroke rate as high as 1%. More recent studies have shown that diffusion weighted infarcts on MRI, though usually asymptomatic, are common after cerebral arteriography, though the incidence can be decreased through the use of heparinization and air filters. Because of the concern of stroke associated with arteriography, most surgeons have moved away from using this invasive diagnostic test prior to CEA, and now use some type of noninvasive vascular testing. Duplex ultrasonogaphy remains the most commonly utilized diagnostic study to confirm the presence of a significant internal carotid artery stenosis. Additional studies utilized to determine the need for CEA depend largely on the local expertise available but may include magnetic resonance arteriography (MRA) or computed tomographic arteriography (CTA) evaluation to confirm the findings of duplex. Frequently, duplex ultrasound is the sole diagnostic study that many surgeons use prior to carotid endarterectomy, especially in asymptomatic patients. Symptomatic patients who have suffered a stroke should in most cases undergo some form of brain imaging such as a computed tomography or magnetic resonance imaging scan to determine if there is a cerebral infarct, and if an infarct is present, to assess size and the presence of parenchymal hemorrhage.

Carotid stent placement to treat extracranial carotid occlusive disease has slowly developed as a viable option to CEA in *selected* patients.[3-9] However, early enthusiasm for the procedure as a potential replacement therapy for CEA has now been tempered by recent randomized trials that been associated with relatively high stroke rates in the CAS treated patients.[8,10-13] Criticisms of these trials have focused on the limited experience of the CAS interventionists. To date, most interventionists utilize duplex arterial ultrasound as a screening tool to define the severity of carotid stenosis and then proceed to arteriography.

Many decisions regarding whether or not to proceed with carotid stenting are based on the arteriographic evaluation at the time of CAS. This may not be an optimal approach as the potential for the interventionist to push ahead despite the presence of difficult anatomy is significant. Since at this point in the procedure arterial access has been gained and "there is already a catheter in the arch," the allure to proceed with CAS and "see how it goes" is difficult to overcome. This concern is supported by the recent EVA-3S Trial that has shown worse outcomes for CAS versus CEA on an intention to treat basis. In this trial, in which preprocedure imaging to define anatomy was not performed, the stroke and death rate at 30 days was 9.6% in the CAS group and 3.8% in the CEA group.[10] The technical failure rate for CAS was 5%. The SPACE trial showed a trend toward improved 30-day stroke or death per protocol outcomes in CEA (stroke and death rate 5.7%), patients versus CAS (stroke and death rate 7.3%).[13] In this trial, the technical failure rate for CAS was 3%. When these trials are compared to the CARESS Trial, in which surgeon preference allowed patients to be placed into either the CAS or CEA group, it becomes clear that selecting therapy based on individualized physician assessment of the patient results in better outcomes.[3] In this trial, the 30-day stroke and death rate for the CAS group was a low 2.1%. Likewise, the Dartmouth experience in which preoperative CTA was used to screen potential CAS patients for unsuitable anatomy had a 2.7% 30-day stroke and death rate for patients undergoing CAS, and this includes the initial CAS patients that would be considered part of the learning curve.[14] Thus, preprocedural knowledge of the thoracic aortic arch, common carotid, and internal carotid artery may assist interventionists in avoiding patients at high risk for CAS.

Much effort has been placed on defining the high-risk CEA patient, but data are lacking to define the high-risk CAS patient. Determining what high-risk CAS criteria are will help make CAS a safer procedure and define the patient population in which it is best utilized.

Currently, factors considered high risk for CAS include patients greater than 80 years of age. Abundant registry data, the lead-in data from CREST, and randomized controlled trials have shown that asymptomatic patients greater than 80 years old have at least a two-fold higher risk of stroke and that in symptomatic patients greater than 80 years old, this may increase to as high as three-fold.[11,15-16] Additional factors that increase patient risk for CAS include the presence of "tortuous" anatomy. What defines tortuous anatomy, however, is largely left up to the discretion of the interventionist. General recommendations have included avoiding the type three arch (Figure 9–1); however, this admonition is not routinely followed by many interventionists. Certainly, as the investigators gain experience with CAS, they can better define who should not have this procedure based on anatomy. However, the learning curve for CAS is extensive, requiring anywhere from 50 to 150 procedures before stroke and death rates are minimized. In order to identify high-risk anatomy for CAS prior to performing arteriography, we have used CTA with three-dimensional reconstruction (3-D-CTA, M2S, Medical Media Systems, Lebanon, NH) to assess arch and carotid artery morphology, tortuosity, and intracranial anatomy prior to arteriography.

Patients who are considered for CAS undergo 3D-CTA of the arch, carotids, and circle of Willis. This information has proven helpful in many respects with regards to planning CAS. In a series of 57 patients who had preprocedure CTA prior to planned CAS, this changed the interventional plan in a third of cases. Patients with a tortuous aortic arch or a large arch atherosclerotic burden as shown in Figure 9–2 underwent CEA or best medical management. Those patients who had hostile neck due

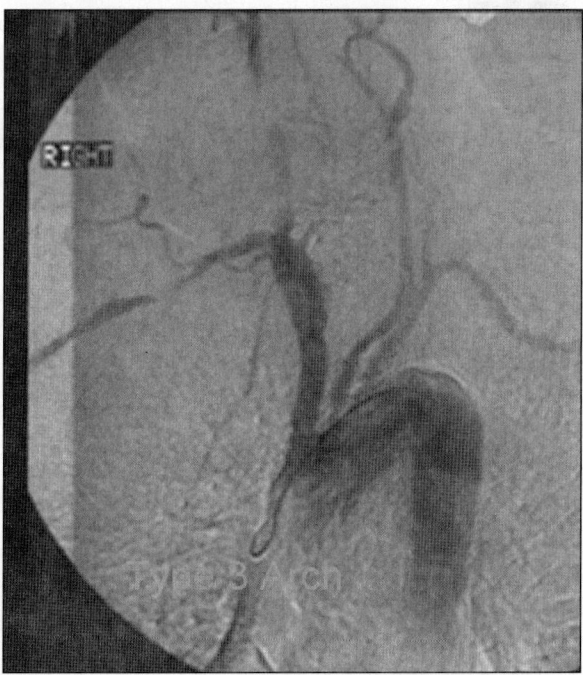

Figure 9-1. Example of Type 3 aortic arch. This degree of tortuosity would increase risk of CAS through transfemoral approach. Transcervical CAS or CEA would be appropriate interventional options.

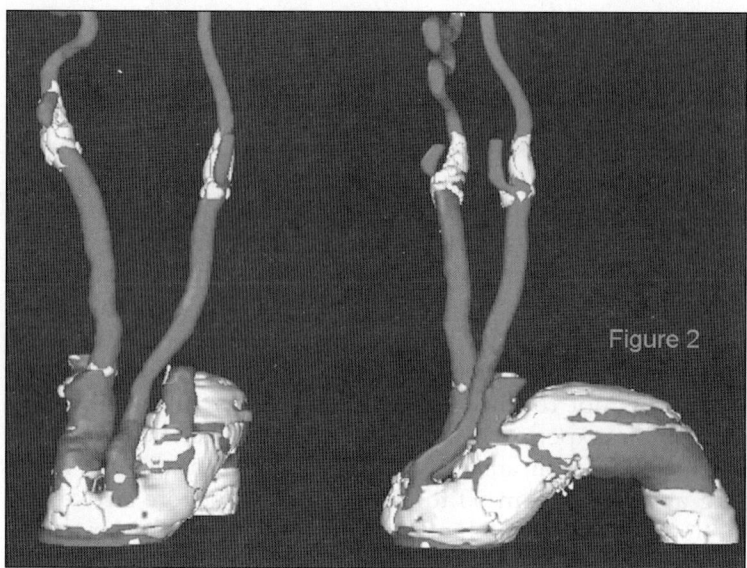

Figure 9-2. 3-D-CTA shows severity of arch tortuosity as well as atherosclerotic disease burden. Plaque is shown in grey and calcification shown in white.

to radiation or previous carotid endarterectomy, in addition to severe aortic arch disease, had the carotid stent procedure performed through a small cervical incision under local anesthesia. A relative contraindication to transcervical CAS is if the carotid bifurcation is low in the neck or the lesion extends proximally into the common carotid artery near the region of the clavicle. The location of the carotid bifurcation and extent of the lesion can be indentified by superimposing the saggital reconstruction of the 3-D-CTA onto the three dimensional model as shown in Figure 9–3.

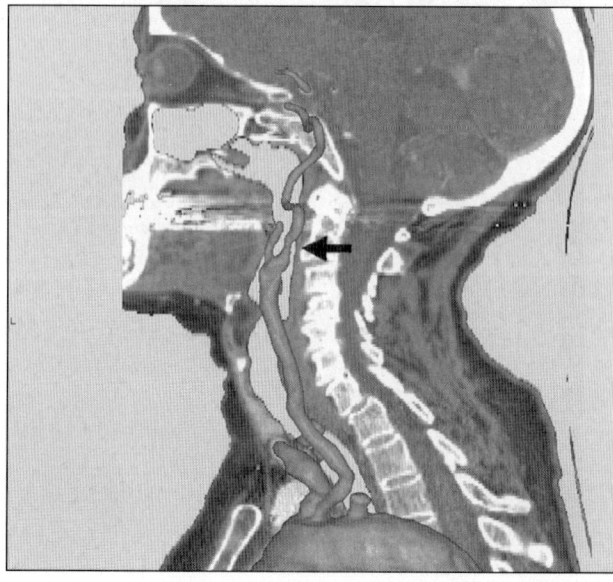

Figure 9-3. Saggital reconstruction superimposed on 3-D model allows for identification of carotid bifurcation (black arrow) relative to vertebral bodies. This will allow identification of high carotid lesions prior to CEA and prohibitively low carotid bifurcations prior to transcervical CAS.

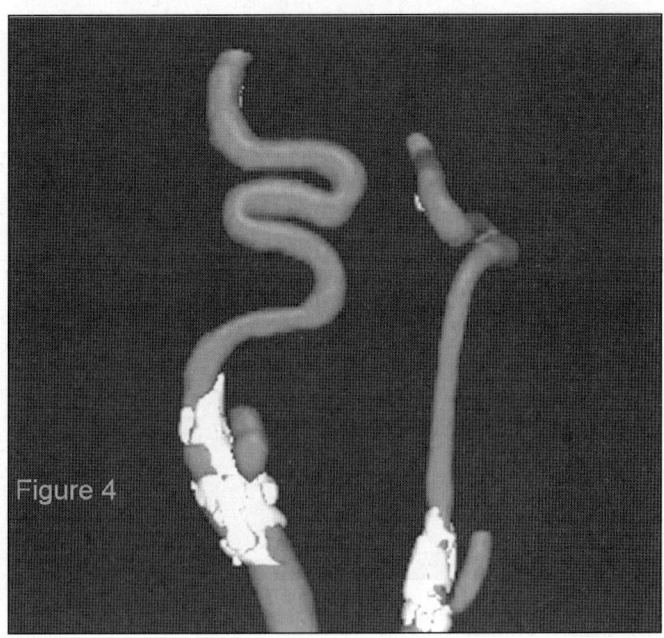

Figure 9-4. 3-D-CTA shows severity of ICA tortuosity. ·

Patients with severely tortuous internal carotid arteries as shown in Figure 9–4 would either undergo CEA or optimal medical management, and forgo CAS altogether. Similarly, the degree of calcification can also be accurately assessed. This is not possible with arteriography. Heavy circumferential calcification is a relative contraindication to CAS, and these patients are often best treated by CEA or medical therapy (Figure 9–5).

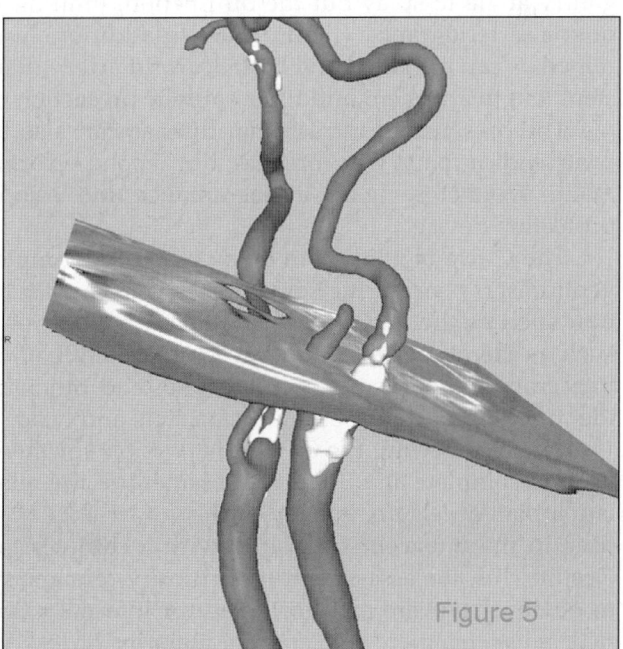

Figure 9-5. Axial slice of CTA superimposed onto 3-D model. Severity of internal carotid artery calcification can be evaluated (black arrow).

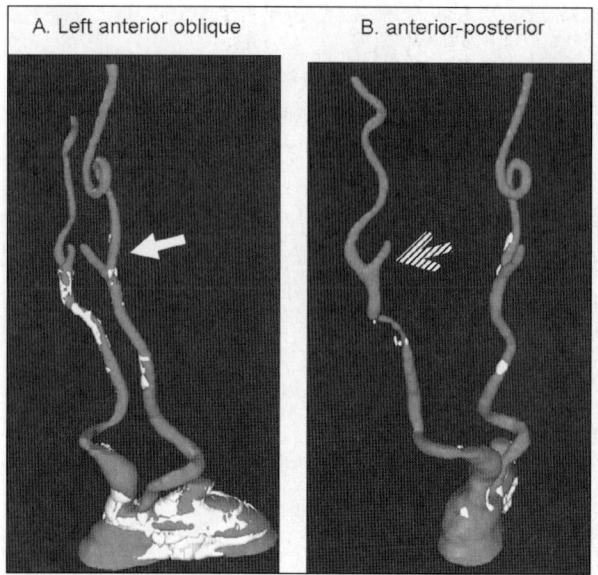

Figure 9-6. Preprocedure planning can be facilitated by 3-D-CTA. **(A)** Left carotid bifurcation best viewed by left anterior oblique (LAO) projection (arrow). **(B)** Right carotid bifurcation best viewed by anterior-posterior (AP) projection (arrow).

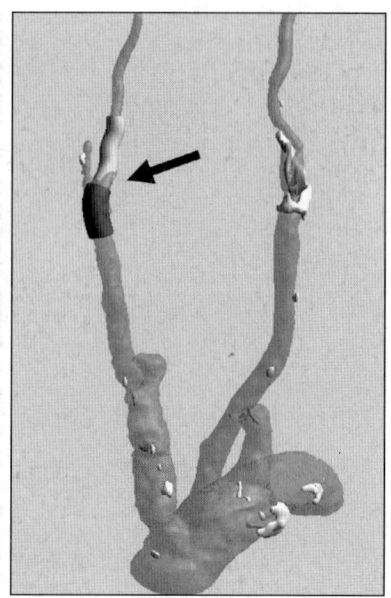

Figure 9-7. Preprocedure imaging can facilitate determination of stent length and choice of stent and embolic protection diameter. "Virtual stent" placed (black arrow) to assess for vessel wall approximation.

In addition to determining if a patient is a candidate for CAS, the 3-D-CTA also helps with procedural planning. The 3-D model can be used to determine the best gantry angle to splay out the bifurcation, limiting the need for multiple arteriograms or spin arteriography (Figure 9–6). In addition, lesion length can be accurately determined as can proximal and distal carotid artery diameter. This will help with selecting stent length and stent and filter embolic protection device diameter (Figure 9–7).

The presence of intracranial disease can also be assessed. This is typically not a contraindication to CAS or CEA, but when performing CAS, ideally, it would be optimal to avoid crossing any intracranial carotid lesion with the distal wire of the embolic protection device.

The Circle of Willis can be assessed for completeness. This is helpful if the interventionist is considering some occlusive form of internal carotid artery embolic protection such as the PercuSurge occlusion balloon or the carotid flow reversal systems such as the neuroprotection system (NPS, W.L. Gore, Flagstaff, AZ). The presence of intracranial aneurysms, occult stroke, and other intracranial pathology may also be identified on CT/CTA of the chest, neck, and head.

When reviewing the CTA, it is possible for the interventionist to perform this on a PC and complete an in-depth assessment of the relevant vascular anatomy and formulate a plan at leisure, not under the constraints of reviewing the anatomy for the first time in the interventional suite with a catheter in the aortic arch or carotid artery. Despite this, the assessment of tortuosity remains subjective. Prohibitive anatomy due to obviously severe arch tortuosity or internal carotid artery tortuosity can be identified; however, there remains the majority of less severe cases that the interventionist

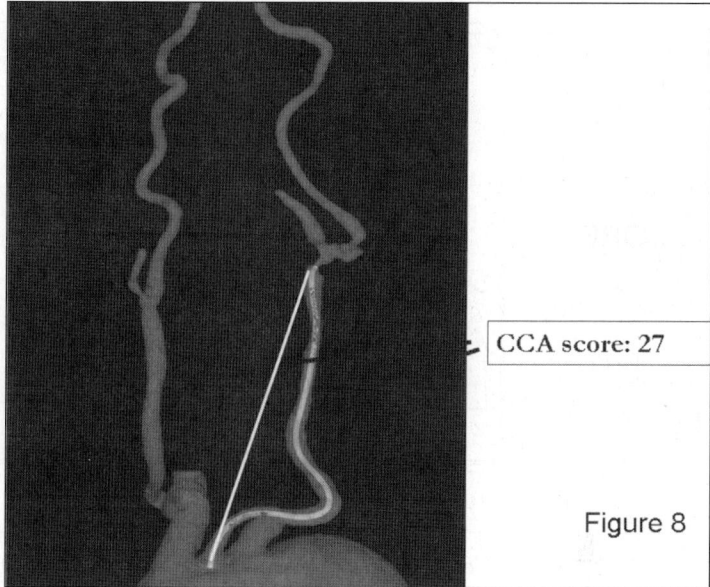

Figure 9-8. Vessel tortuosity measurement. Score measured as centerline length divided by straightline length x 100. The larger the number, the more tortuous.

must assess. Operator experience is very important during the evaluation to determine if one should push ahead with CAS in the face of difficult arch or carotid anatomy. In order to assist with this decision-making, we have analyzed the degree of aortic arch and carotid artery tortuosity of patients who underwent successful transfemoral stent placement, and compared this to the tortuosity of patients who either were refused CAS or had an unsuccessful attempt at CAS. Tortuosity index was measured by comparing the vessel straightline to the centerline as shown in Figure 9–8. We found that the total CCA/ICA tortuosity index predicted success (Figure 9–9). As show in

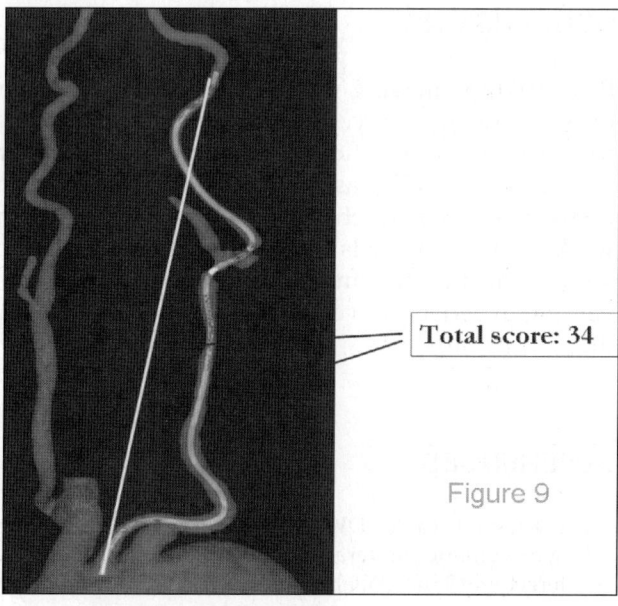

Figure 9-9. The total carotid artery tortuosity determined by adding the internal carotid and common carotid artery scores. This was the most predictive of CAS technical failure.

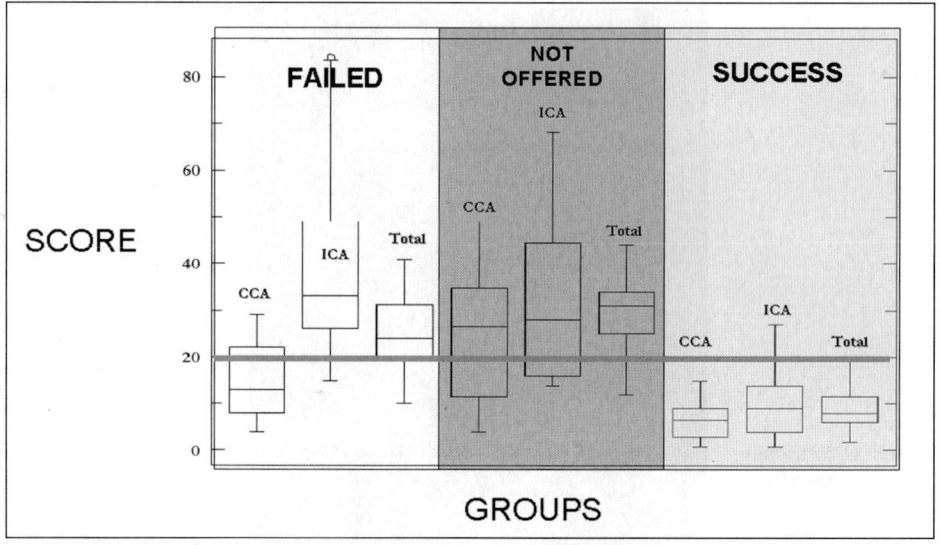

Figure 9-10. Tortuosity score for patients who had failed attempt at CAS, those who were refused CAS after review of 3-D-CTA, and patients who underwent successful transfemoral CAS. Total score p<.001 Successful versus other groups.

Figure 9–10, no patient with a total carotid artery tortuosity score of greater than 20 had a successful transfemoral CAS procedure performed. This measure of carotid artery tortuosity may not be of help to interventionists with extensive CAS experience; however, this may be useful for less experienced or low-volume interventionists and may also be useful as a screening tool in order to select appropriate patients for CAS in clinical trials.

CONCLUSIONS

Preprocedure imaging with 3-D-CTA helps the operator avoid high-risk CAS patients prior to arteriography. This imaging modality allows the interventionist to tailor the treatment to the specific vascular anatomy. In patients who are identified as good CAS candidates, 3-D-CTA assists in planning the CAS procedure by allowing the interventionist to know beforehand which gantry angles and devices will be required. Future work in this area needs to be performed to further define various degrees of tortuosity and/or calcification, and develop risk stratification models to help interventionists of varying experience levels assess the risk of CAS based on preoperative assessment of the vascular anatomy.

REFERENCES

1. Barnett HJ, Taylor DW, Eliasziw M, et al. Benefit of carotid endarterectomy in patients with symptomatic moderate or severe stenosis. North American Symptomatic Carotid Endarterectomy Trial Collaborators. *N Engl J Med.* 1998;339:1415–1425.

2. European Carotid Surgery Trialists' Collaborative Group. Randomised trial of endarterectomy for recently symptomatic carotid stenosis: final results of the MRC European Carotid Surgery Trial (ECST). *Lancet*. 1998;351:1379–1387.

3. Goodney, PP, Schermerhorn ML,and Powell, RJ. Current status of carotid artery stenting. *J Vasc Surg*. Feb 2006;43(2):406–411.

4. Rothwell PM, Eliasziw M, Gutnikov SA, et al. Analysis of pooled data from the randomised controlled trials of endarterectomy for symptomatic carotid stenosis. *Lancet* 2003;361: 107–116.

5. Ederle J, Featherstone RL, Brown MM. Percutaneous transluminal angioplasty and stenting for carotid artery stenosis. *Cochrane Database Syst Rev*. 2007;3:CD000515.

6. Gray WA, Yadav JS, Verta P, et al. The CAPTURE registry: results of carotid stenting with embolic protection in the post approval setting. *Catheter Cardiovasc Interv*. 2007;69:341–48.

7. Gurm HS, Yadav JS, Fayad P, et al. Long-term results of carotid stenting versus endarterectomy in high-risk patients. *N Engl J Med*. 2008;358:1572–1579.

8. Mas JL, Chatellier G, Beyssen B, et al. Endarterectomy versus stenting in patients with symptomatic severe carotid stenosis. *N Engl J Med*. 2006;355:1660–71.

9. Yadav JS, Wholey MH, Kuntz RE, et al. Protected carotid-artery stenting versus endarterectomy in high-risk patients. *N Engl J Med*. 2004;351:1493–1501.

10. Eckstein HH, Ringleb PA, Allenberg J-R, et al. Stent-protected angioplasty versus carotid endarterectomy for symptomatic stenoses (SPACE): two-year results. *Lancet* Neurol. 2008;7:893–902.

11. Hobson RW, Howard VJ, Roubin GS, et al. Carotid artery stenting is associated with increased complications in octogenarians: 30-day stroke and death rates in the CREST lead-in phase. *J Vasc Surg*. 2004;40:1106–1111.

12. Mas JL, Chatellier G, Beyssen B. Carotid angioplasty and stenting with and without cerebral protection: clinical alert from the Endarterectomy versus angioplasty in patients with symptomatic severe carotid stenosis (EVA-3S) trial. *Stroke* 2004;35:e18–20.

13. Ringleb PA, Allenberg J, Bruckmann H, et al. 30-day results from the SPACE trial of stent-protected angioplasty versus carotid endarterectomy in symptomatic patients: a randomised noninferiority trial. *Lancet*. 2006;368:1239–1247.

14. Powell RJ, Schermerhorn ML, Nolan B, Lenz J, Rzuidlo E, Fillinger F, Walsh D, Wyers M, Zwolak R, Cronenwett JL. Early results of carotid stent placement for treatment of extracranial carotid bifurcation occlusive disease. *J Vasc Surg*. Jun 2004;39(6):1193–1199.

15. Kastrup A, Groschel K, Schulz JB, Nagele T, Ernemann U. Clinical predictors of transient ischemic attack, stroke, or death within 30 days of carotid angioplasty and stenting. *Stroke* 2005; 36: 787–791.

16. Yuo TH, Goodney PP, Powell RJ, and Cronenwett JL. Medical "high risk" designation is not associated with survival after carotid artery stenting. *J Vasc Surg*. January 2008;

10

Evaluation of Cerebrovascular Anatomy During Carotid Bifurcation Stenting

Douglas W. Massop, M.D.

The procedure of stent-assisted angioplasty with embolic protection is gaining increasing support, based on well-controlled randomized trials and databases. A clear understanding of the access anatomy at the aortoiliac level and of the aortic arch is essential to gaining access for the sheaths and delivery systems for these devices.[1] Further, this understanding provides a basic fund of knowledge regarding the cerebrovascular anatomy involving these cases to assist in the procedural planning as well as the intraprocedural and postprocedural evaluation of these patients.

ANGIOGRAPHIC TECHNIQUE

The routine angiographic assessment involves understanding of both the cervical and cerebral vascular anatomy, as well as a clear understanding of the angiographic views and injection techniques to evaluate this.[2] The minimum evaluation involves ipsilateral injection of each carotid system with biplane views of each of these injections. Methods of selective catheterization of the common carotid arteries are well described in numerous texts.[3]

Optimal injection rates and volumes need to be adjusted to the patient's anatomy. The standard initial injection into the common carotid artery for visualization of the anterior cerebral circulation should be 8 cc of nonionic isoosmolar contrast at 6 cc/sec. The rate and volume of injections can be influenced by the anatomy encountered. For instance, if there is combined high-grade disease of both the external and internal carotid, flow through the common carotid will be slower and injection rate probably should be slowed to 4 or 5 cc/sec. Injection rates faster than this will only reflux contrast back to the aortic arch. The volume of injection can be adjusted in instances where there is a contralateral occlusion and this particular vessel is supplying a larger vascular bed with patent communicating arteries. In this instance, the injection rate

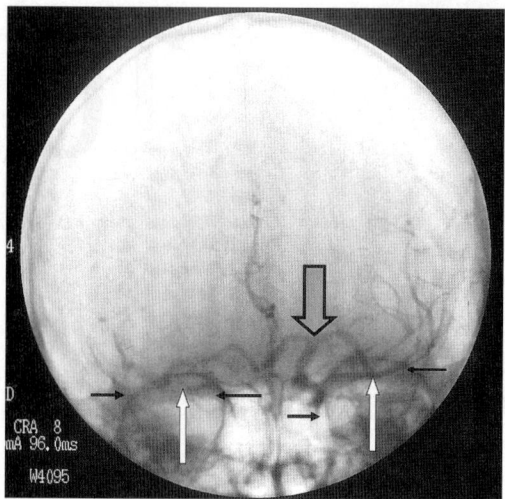 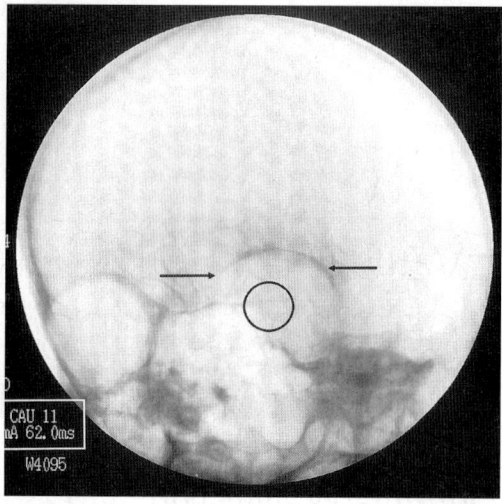

Figure 10-1. Anterior-posterior view of cerebral angiogram, 8 degrees cranial angulation, black arrow = rim of boney orbit, white arrow = superior ridge of sphenoid bone, bold grey arrow = bifurcation of intracranial internal carotid artery.

Figure 10-2. Transorbital oblique view (LAO 20, caudal 11), black arrow = rim of boney orbit, circle = foramen of optic nerve.

may be increased to 7 or 8 cc/sec with total volumes of 10–14 cc, depending on the individual anatomy to be imaged.

The cerebral views involve first a straight lateral of the head where the external auditory canals are aligned with the head facing in a neutral anatomic position. The anterior view involves cranial angulation of the image intensifier so as to line up the superior orbital rims with the superior ridge of the sphenoid bone (Figure 10–1). This projects the vessels above the large amount of bone in this area and minimizes artifactual distortions of the vessels themselves. Frequently, this involves cranial angulation anywhere from 8–20 degrees, depending on the nature of the patient's skull anatomy and position on the angiographic table. Optional views that can be encountered include a transorbital oblique that frequently involves ipsilateral oblique angulation of 10–25 degrees to align the bony orbit itself with the foramen of the optic nerve (Figure 10–2). This improves visualization of the communicating segment of the internal carotid as well as the anterior communicating arteries and the branching pattern of the middle cerebral artery (Figure 10–3). This is particularly helpful when there is suspicion for an intracranial aneurysm. Several other views have been described.[4] Familiar knowledge of these three cranial images is basic for visualizing the anterior circulation of the brain.

CEREBRAL VASCULAR ANATOMY

The normal anatomy of the intracranial anterior circulation requires an understanding of the intracranial internal carotid, the anterior cerebral artery, the anterior communicating artery, and the middle cerebral artery, as well as the takeoff of the posterior communicating arteries and/or fetal posterior cerebral arteries.

The intracranial internal carotid enters the skull at its foramen and goes through the petrous portion of the sphenoid bone, then gently curving to the lacerum segment

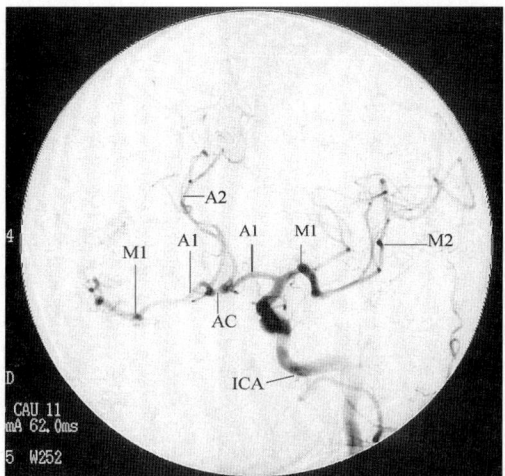

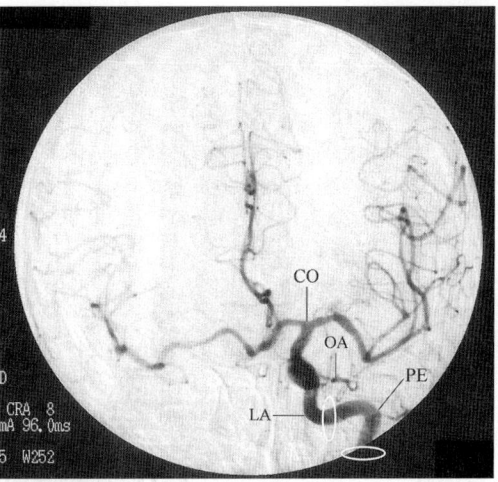

Figure 10-3. Transorbital oblique angiogram, left (LAO 20, caudal 11), ICA = left internal carotid artery, AC = anterior communicating artery, A1 and A2 = segments of anterior cerebral artery, M1 and M2 = segments of middle cerebral artery.

Figure 10-4. Anterior-posterior view of cerebral angiogram, segments of the intracranial internal carotid artery: PE = petrous, LA = lacerum, CO = communicating; OA = ophthalmic artery; circles = exo- and endo-foramina of the sphenoid bone.

and then the cavernous, ophthalmic, and communicating segments follow (Figures 10–4 and 10–5). It is important to understand the relationship of this artery to the base of the skull as it is frequently quite fragile, and positioning of the cerebral protection devices during carotid stenting requires the operator to be aware of the possibility of dissection by passing stiff delivery systems near the base of the skull. The branches of the intracranial internal carotid are described and illustrated in Figures 10–6 and 10–7).

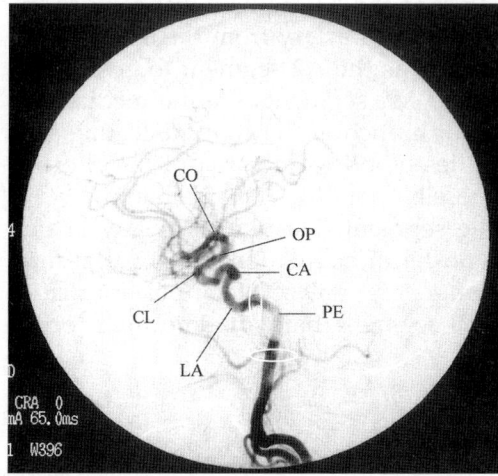

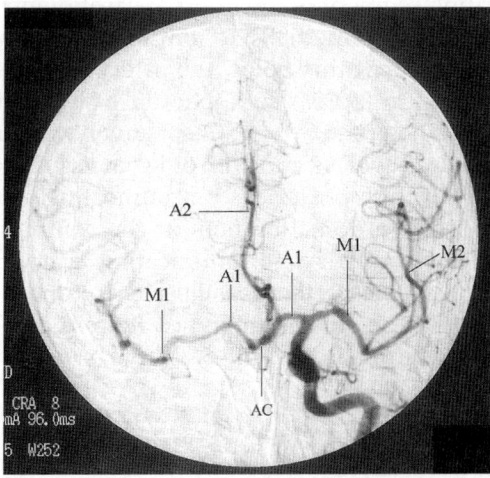

Figure 10-5. Lateral view of cerebral angiogram, segments of the intracranial internal carotid artery: PE = petrous, LA = lacerum, CA = cavernous, CL = clinoid, OP = ophthalmic, CO = communicating; circles = exo- and endo-foramina of the sphenoid bone.

Figure 10-6. Anterior-posterior view of cerebral angiogram, intracranial branches: AC = anterior communicating, A1 and A2 = segments of the anterior cerebral artery, M1 and M2 = segments of the middle cerebral artery.

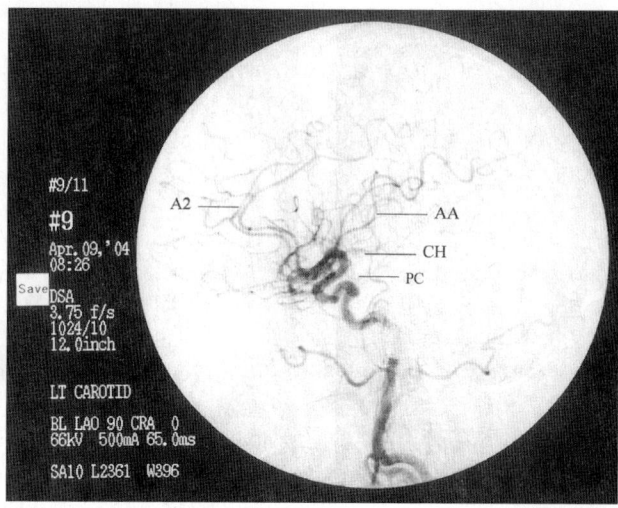

Figure 10-7. Lateral view of cerebral angiogram, intracranial branches: PC = posterior communicating, CH = choroidal artery, AA = angular artery, A2 = segment of anterior cerebral artery.

The middle cerebral artery arises as a lateral branch of the communicating segment of the internal carotid and frequently bifurcates in the M1 segment. This bifurcation point is a frequent site of intracranial aneurysms. The vertical portion of the middle cerebral is called the M2 segment, and the recurring segment at the insula is the M3 segment. The cortical branches are called the M4 segment of the middle cerebral artery. The most posterior branch of the middle cerebral artery coursing out the Sylvian fissure is called the angular artery.

The anterior cerebral artery also arises as an anteromedial branch of the communicating segment of the internal carotid and gives rise to the A1 segment that courses anteriorly and medially to join the anterior communicating artery from the opposite A1 segment. At this point, the artery ascends vertically as the A2 segment to give blood supply to the frontal lobe. Off of both the A1 and M1 segments are the medial and lenticulostriate arteries respectively. An important branch of the communicating segment as well is the choroidal artery that supplies blood to the area of the choroid plexus. The posterior communicating artery (possible fetal posterior cerebral artery) arises as a dorsal branch off the communicating segment. This varies greatly in size and typically is a communicating artery to the posterior circulation. However, it may exclude the vertebrobasilar system and be a completely replaced fetal posterior cerebral artery. This occurs when there is an absent P1 segment that would normally occur at the bifurcation of the basilar artery.

VARIATIONS

Significant variations in the communication of these vessels occur in the head. The so-called normal interconnection of the vessels is called the circle of Willis. This circle is actually a nine-sided polygon made up of the anterior communicating artery which then connects on each side with the A1 segment of the anterior cerebral artery, the communicating segment of the internal carotid artery, the posterior communicating artery, and the P1 segment of the posterior cerebral artery. The complete circle of Willis is seen in only approximately 45% of cases. The most significant variations of clinical importance include an absent or a significantly hypoplastic A1 segment on one or both sides. The other significant variation is an absent or hypoplastic posterior communicating artery on one or both sides.

The middle cerebral artery can be an isolated terminal branch of the internal carotid artery. This variation occurs when the A1 segment and the posterior communicating segment on the same side are absent or significantly hypoplastic. Therefore, occlusion or embolization of the internal carotid artery during cervical intervention will probably result in an extensive cerebrovascular accident.

The other significant variation that is important to understand is the so-called anterior-posterior communications that can occur on a congenital basis. This frequently involves hypoplasia or absence of the cervical portion of a vertebral artery. There is then a congenital interposition of vessel from some portion of the internal carotid to the vertebrobasilar system. These can occur in ascending level of communication described as the proatlantal, hypoglossal, trigeminal, otic, and more normally the posterior communicating artery. These variations are important when considering carotid bifurcation disease that presents in an unusual manner, possibly with posterior circulation symptoms. This also is important when delivering endovascular devices up near the cervical portion of the internal carotid, as these variations do occur in 1–2% of patients.

The operator performing carotid stenting also needs an understanding of intracranial aneurysms.[5] The risk of an intracranial aneurysm in the general population is 1–2%. Ninety percent of aneurysms occur in the anterior circulation with 10% occurring in the posterior circulation. The most common sites of aneurysms in the anterior circulation are at the level of the takeoff of the anterior communicating artery in 35% of patients, the bifurcation of the M1 segment in 30% of cases, and the origin of the posterior communicating artery in another 25% of cases. The posterior circulation aneurysms most frequently occur at the bifurcation of the basilar artery and can account for up to 10% of cases. There is also some frequency of aneurysms at the takeoff of the cerebellar arteries off the basilar artery.

It is important to realize that intracranial aneurysms, if discovered, should be treated on their own merit with referral to a neurosurgeon for consideration of repair.[6] The other important fact is that if one intracranial aneurysm is discovered, a thorough search of all intracranial vessels is necessary as multiple aneurysms occur in 20% of patients.

The periprocedural evaluation of the anatomy as described is important for a number of reasons. The preinterventional evaluation establishes a baseline of the patient's anatomy, and if complications should occur during the procedure, a clear understanding of which vessels possibly have undergone embolization, spasm, or thrombosis can be determined. The angiographic evaluation is to clearly understand the arterial, parenchymal, and venous phases of the angiogram. Large thromboembolic obstructions will produce loss of flow in a region seen in the arterial phase whereas smaller parenchymal level embolizations will produce a standing column of contrast in a particular parenchymal branch as washout occurs through all the other major arteries on the injection. This can guide neurointerventional rescue to perform catheter-directed thrombolysis in a particular area.

Several anatomic and neuroanatomic references are available to discuss this further for the interested reader. A highly recommended reference is Diagnostic Cerebral Angiography by Ann Osborn, currently in its 2nd edition and published by Lippincott.

REFERENCES

1. Osborn AG. *Introduction to cerebral angiography.* Philadelphia, PA; Harper & Row: 1980.
2. Latchaw RE. The use of nonionic contrast agents in neuroangiography. A review of the literature and recommendations for clinical use. *Invest Radiol.* 1993;28(suppl 5):55-59.
3. Morris P. *Practical neuroangiography.* Baltimore, MD; P Williams & Wikens: 1997.
4. Osborn AG. *Diagnostic cerebral angiography.* Philadelphia, PA; Lippincott; 1999.
5. Atkinson JL et al. Angiographic frequency of anterior circulation aneurysms. *J Neurosurg.* 1989;70:551-555.
6. Bederson JB et al. Recommendations for the management of patients with un-ruptured intracranial aneurysms. *Stroke.* 2000;31:2742-2750.

SECTION **III**

Techniques in Carotid Angioplasty and Stenting

11

Techniques for
Carotid Artery Stenting

Mark K. Eskandari, M.D.

While the actual limits of carotid angioplasty and stenting (CAS) have yet to be defined, this minimally invasive approach remains a viable treatment option for some patients with occlusive cervical carotid artery disease. As with many percutaneous interventions, a transfemoral approach is most widely used; however, access from the arm or directly from the carotid artery has been described with acceptable results. In this chapter, the techniques and nuances of each approach will be outlined along with a description of some of their corresponding pitfalls.

TRANSFEMORAL APPROACH

In the majority of CAS cases, a standard percutaneous transfemoral approach is employed. This technique allows for easy access to a large caliber vessel away from the head and neck region. At times, anatomic anomalies or tortuosity make this approach more difficult, at which point an alternative access vessel can be chosen.

Access

Achieving appropriate femoral access cannot be overemphasized. Insertion of the arterial sheath in the short segment of common femoral artery below the inguinal ligament and above the femoral bifurcation allows for hemostasis of the puncture site at the conclusion of the procedure by way of manual compression anteriorly, directly over the femoral head, which lies posteriorly. Alternatively, an arterial closure device can be safely utilized in this segment of artery. Punctures at or below the femoral bifurcation (i.e., superficial femoral or profunda femoris artery) frequently result in a hematoma, pseudoaneurysm, arteriovenous fistula, and/or arterial thrombosis.[1] Obtaining hemostasis after arterial access above the inguinal ligament, usually angiographically denoted by the origins of the inferior epigastric and lateral circumflex arteries, is difficult since the artery courses cephalad to the femoral head at this point and lies within the pelvis. Manual compression in this circumstance frequently is inadequate and results in a retroperitoneal hematoma, while suture-mediated closure devices have been shown to entrap the inguinal ligament and lead to either a delayed retroperitoneal hematoma or pseudoaneurysm once the patient begins to ambulate. Adjuncts to assist in obtaining appropriate femoral access include initial access with a micropuncture kit (22-gauge needle and 4-Fr system) and/or ultrasound guided arterial access. Confirmation of access is best viewed angiographically in an ipsilateral 20–30° oblique projection, which clearly shows the origins of the superficial and deep femoral arteries.

Arch and Carotid Imaging

Once femoral access is obtained, a standard arch aortogram in a 30–40° left anterior oblique angle (LAO) is performed. This view will provide several important pieces of information: 1) arch type (origin of the great vessels relative to the apex of the arch); 2) identification of supra-aortic trunk origin disease; 3) anatomic anomalies; 4) patency of the common, internal, and external carotid arteries; and 5) extent of arterial calcification. Moreover, tortuosity of the innominate and carotid arteries can be appreciated. Once it has been determined that the anatomy is conducive to proceed with CAS, the target common carotid artery (CCA) is selectively engaged with a 4- or 5-Fr diagnostic catheter. Typically, a simple curved catheter is first chosen (i.e., vertebral, DAV, JB-1, or headhunter) while reserving more complex curved catheters (i.e., Simmons or Vitek) for tortuous anatomy. The latter is more commonly employed when cannulation of the left CCA is required in a patient with a bovine arch configuration. Catheterization of the right CCA can sometimes be problematic, particularly in a LAO view. In these circumstances, a right anterior oblique (RAO) projection will provide a clearer view of the origins of the right subclavian and common carotid arteries (Figure 11–1). In general, systemic heparin is administered prior to selective catheterization of the carotid arteries. After the catheter is well positioned within the intended CCA, identification of the extent of carotid bifurcation disease is assessed. The severity of stenosis is based on the NASCET measurements.[2] The need for intracranial imaging is more physician preference than a requirement; however, appropriate imaging would include at least two intracranial views: 1) anterior-posterior and 2) lateral.

Sheath or Guiding Catheter Placement

CAS has been facilitated by advances in sheaths and catheters that are placed within the CCA and provide a stable access platform to deliver the necessary components for a successful intervention. The two broad options are either a sheath or guiding catheter. Advantages of a long sheath (90–100 cm) are the ability to place it securely within the distal CCA just proximal to the carotid bifurcation and the smaller arterial puncture (6-Fr). On the other hand, guiding catheters are designed in a variety of angled configurations allowing for easy manipulation into the target CCA, but require larger arterial access (8-Fr). My personal preference is the Shuttle sheath (Cook Inc., Bloomington, IN) for the majority of cases, but I rely on the guiding catheters for proximal CCA lesions or very tortuous anatomy when the external carotid artery (ECA) is either occluded or severely narrowed (Figure 11–2).

After the diagnostic catheter has been placed within the CCA, a stiff 0.035-inch wire is advanced into the ECA. Once this is in position, the diagnostic catheter is removed,

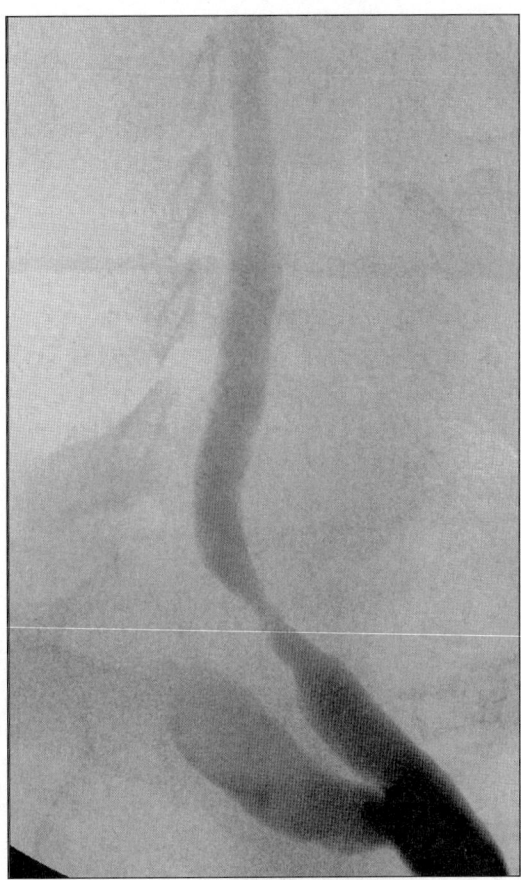

Figure 11-1. Right anterior oblique angle angiogram of the right subclavian and common carotid arteries. Note stenosis in the proximal right common carotid artery and the ability to visualize the origins of the two vessels in this projection.

and the sheath and introducer are advanced over the wire into the distal CCA. Care should be taken to pay close attention to the tip of the stiff wire to ensure that it does not perforate or otherwise traumatize a branch of the ECA. Hematoma formation and airway compromise can be a devastating complication. Sometimes for an angulated CCA, a stiff wire will not successfully pass into the ECA. In these circumstances, the use of a 0.035-inch angled glidewire or stiff angled glidewire will facilitate passage of the diagnostic catheter into the ECA, which will then allow for introduction of stiff wire into the ECA. An alternative option is to use a "telescoping" technique whereby the diagnostic catheter is passed through the sheath that is positioned in the proximal descending thoracic aorta. After the CCA is engaged with the diagnostic catheter and the wire, which are positioned in the mid portion of the CCA, the sheath is advanced over the wire and catheter into the CCA. The Shuttle Select system by Cook, Inc. has a unified system to accommodate this approach.

TRANSBRACHIAL APPROACH

A transbrachial approach is less frequently used, but may be a good alternative in situations were femoral access is not feasible or aortic arch vessel angulation is too severe.[3]

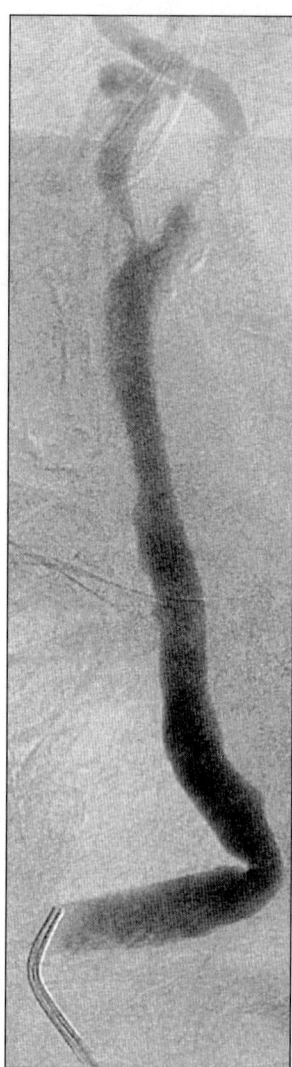

Figure 11-2. Left carotid angiogram showing severe tortuosity of the proximal left common carotid artery and a severe stenosis of the origin of the left external carotid artery.

Access can be from either side, but obviously a right-sided approach to the left CCA (or vice versa) increases the risk of bilateral hemispheric embolic events by crossing the origin of both CCAs.

Access

The critical strategies to successful brachial access for CAS are ultrasound assessment of the caliber of the artery and ultrasound-guided micropuncture access. Unlike the femoral artery, two unique factors an interventionalist has to contend with in the brachial artery are spasm and the risk of nerve impairment from a brachial sheath hematoma. Spasm is typically relieved with the intra-arterial administration of nitroglycerine (100 micrograms) via the sheath. The occurrence of a brachial sheath hematoma requires a high index of suspicion since the majority of cases do not present with an obvious large hematoma at the puncture site, but rather with manifestations of nerve impairment in the median nerve distribution. If new onset parathesias within the median nerve distribution are acknowledged by the patient, it is strongly recommended that the patient undergo an immediate exploration of the brachial artery puncture site and relief of the sheath hematoma in order to avoid permanent neurologic impairment. The majority of brachial access sites are managed postprocedure with manual compression alone, but on occasion, closure devices have been attempted.

Arch and Carotid Imaging

Imaging of the arch and carotid arteries is performed similar to the transfemoral approach, and simple curved diagnostic catheters are preferred over complex curved catheters when using a brachial approach to selectively cannulate the CCA.

Sheath or Guiding Catheter Placement

Similarly, sheath and guiding catheter placement is done as it is when using a transfemoral approach using a stiff 0.035-inch wire placed within the ECA as support to advance the long sheath or guiding catheter. Unlike the transfemoral access, systemic heparin is usually administered early and shortened dwell times of the sheaths in the brachial artery become critically important since these devices are commonly completely occlusive to distal forearm flow.

TRANSCERVICAL APPROACH

Recently, the use of a transcervical approach has been employed in circumstances when femoral or brachial access is prohibitive or for patients with very tortuous aortic arch anatomy.[4] Options included a purely percutaneous approach or open cutdown on the CCA.

Access

While a completely percutaneous approach has been attempt by a brave few, most opt for a small cutdown on the CCA at the base of the neck. The obvious difficulty with an entirely percutaneous approach is the risk of a substantial neck hematoma causing airway compromise. The open approach to the CCA allows for direct visualization of the puncture site and direct suture repair at the conclusion of the procedure. As is acknowledged in traditional carotid surgery, care must be taken not to injury the vagus nerve, particularly as a result of a clamp or traction injury to avoid vocal cord paralysis. Moreover, this approach can be performed under local, regional, or general anesthesia.

Arch and Carotid Imaging

Unlike the transfemoral or transbrachial approaches described above, imaging of the aortic arch is not mandatory since the target CCA is directly cannulated. Placement of a short sheath within the CCA allows for complete extracranial and intracranial imaging of the ipsilateral carotid circulation.

Sheath Placement

Typically, in this approach, the use of short devices (catheters and wires) is best because of the shorter working distance. A short 6-Fr sheath placed securely within the CCA will suffice for the majority of cases.

EMBOLIC PROTECTION DEVICES

While embolic protection devices (EPDs) are widely used during CAS and appear to reduce the risk of periprocedural stroke, no randomized level 1 data is available to support this concept.[5] Nevertheless, it is advocated to use an EPD for CAS whenever feasible. There exist three general categories of EPDs: 1) distal balloon occlusion; 2) distal filter; and 3) proximal balloon occlusion.[6] Each device has limitations and anatomic constraints; however, only distal filters have on-label approval for use during CAS, which will be the focus of this section.[7]

Distal Filter EPD Delivery

This category of EPD requires delivery of a constrained filter element across the stenotic target lesion and into the distal normal ICA. An obvious concern is the risk of distal embolization when attempting to deliver the filter element through the atherosclerotic lesion. A primary requirement of an EPD is the ability to safely deliver it to the distal ICA. It is generally recommended that if the constrained filter element does not pass because of the severity of stenosis, it may be best to abort the CAS procedure rather that dilate the lesion with a small balloon without distal protection to facilitate passage of the device. If the EPD does not advance beyond the lesion because of angulation of the vessel, the use of a "buddy wire" to straighten the vessel may be employed using a stiffer 0.014-inch wire (Figure 11–3).

Another requirement when using an EPD is the ability to place the filter element in a portion of the distal ICA that is relatively straight and distal from the intended distal extent of the stent. This anatomic limitation should be taken into consideration when choosing which brand of filter EPD to use. The "landing zone", or length of the deployed element from end to end, is variable between manufacturers, and a shorter device may be more applicable when the straight segment of the distal ICA is relatively short. One of the limitations of filter elements is the inability to assess circumferential basket-vessel wall apposition. Gaps between the filter element and the vessel wall may be regions where debris is not captured and can embolize into the distal intracranial circulation.[8] It is known that this problem occurs more frequently when the filter is placed in regions of sharp angulation of the ICA.

Pitfalls of Filter EPDs

Rare complications of filter EPDs have been reported including filter detachment, filter entanglement with the stent, and iatrogenic ICA dissection, but the more common occurrences are ICA spasm, filter thrombosis, and inability to retrieve the filter. One of the primary problems with distal EPD devices when working over long distances—femoral approach to the carotid artery—is minimizing movement of the filter during the CAS procedure. Newer filter delivery systems have addressed this to a certain degree by having the filter "free floating" on a specific wire in the ICA such as the

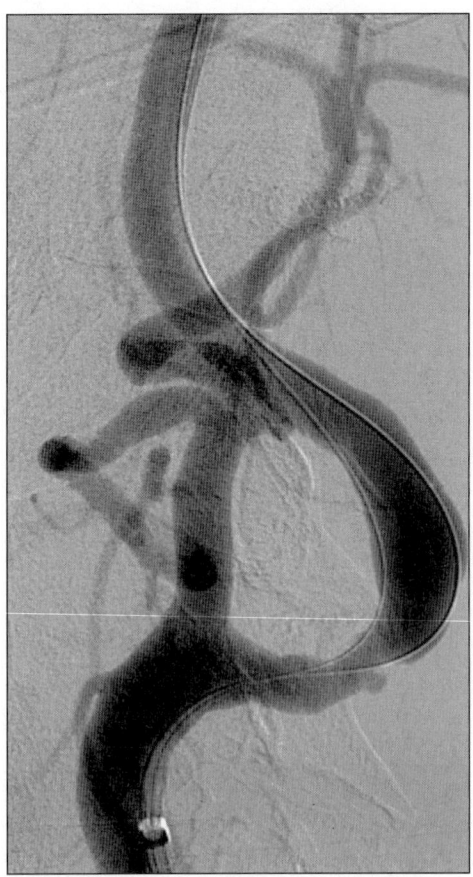

Figure 11-3. Use of the "buddy wire" technique to straighten out the carotid bifurcation and allow for delivery of the EPD. Note the two 0.014-inch wires crossing the internal carotid artery lesion.

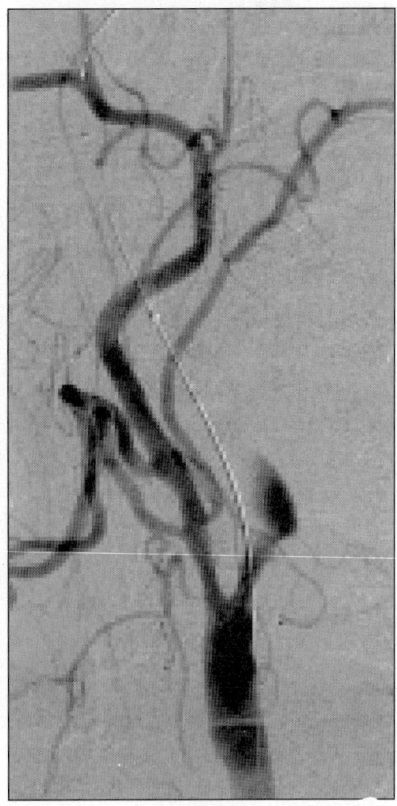

Figure 11-4. A carotid angiogram after an initial angioplasty of the internal carotid artery lesion showing flow arrest at the level of the EPD.

Emboshield system (Abbott Vascular, Santa Rosa, CA). Nevertheless, motion of the filter in the distal ICA can induce varying degrees of vasospasm that may be severe enough to halt flow through the collapsed filter element (Figure 11–4). Fortunately, this can be easily remedied with an intra-arterial administration of nitroglycerin (100 micrograms) (Figure 11–5). In rare circumstances, it can only be relieved by removing the filter, but it is important to differentiate spasm from thrombosis of the filter.

Determining the causation for flow arrest at the level of the filter element can be challenging and anxiety provoking. Generally, it is either due to intense vasospasm or filter thrombosis. While the former typically improves with nitroglycerine, the latter may require additional maneuvers. A first step is to re-dose systemic anticoagulation—heparin or angiomax—and re-check the activated clotting time to ensure that it is greater than 250 seconds. Next, try intra-arterial nitroglycerine. If these simple steps do not improve the flow, an attempt to aspirate captured debris from inside the filter basket should be made. Available devices to achieve this are the Pronto system (Vascular Solutions, Minneapolis, MN) and the Export catheter (Medtronic, Sunnyvale, CA). After aspirating from the filter down into the CCA with several passes and removal of

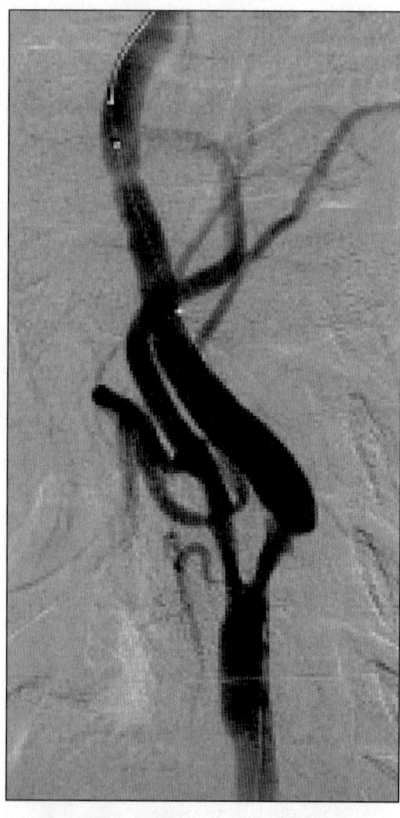

Figure 11-5. Carotid angiogram after the intra-arterial administration of nitroglycerin to alleviate the severe vasospasm induced by the indwelling EPD. Adequate antegrade flow has now been restored through the EPD and distal internal carotid artery.

at least 50 cc of blood, flow should be re-assessed. If there is still no improvement, intra-arterial tissue plasminogen activator (TPA) can be given. Once adequate flow is restored or if all else fails, the filter should then be removed. Luckily, this is an infrequent phenomenon.

Last, inability to retrieve the filter element can occur due to vessel tortuosity or "fish scaling" of an open cell stent. All current filter EPD design systems use a specific catheter to collapse and retrieve the filter basket at the conclusion of the procedure. Some use a catheter with a shapeable tip whereas others use a tapered tip to allow easy passage through the stented segment. It is important to watch the tip as is passes through the stent to ensure that it does not catch a stent strut and deform the stent or pull down the filter basket. If the catheter does not pass unimpeded, torquing the catheter to alter the tip angle, having the patient turn his or her head, or advancing the sheath within the stented segment will usually allow the catheter to negotiate through angulated anatomy (Figures 11–6A and 11–6B).

BALLOON ANGIOPLASTY

While CAS is often referred to as carotid *angioplasty* and stenting, in fact it is rarely the case that angioplasty alone is sufficient to treat the target lesion. However, angioplasty is part of the procedure for carotid stenting and commonly involves two inflations. The first is after the EPD has been deployed and usually is performed with a short 3.0 or 4.0

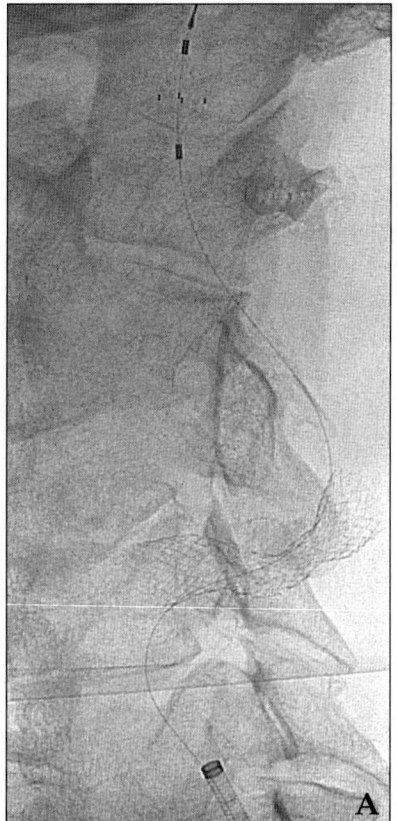 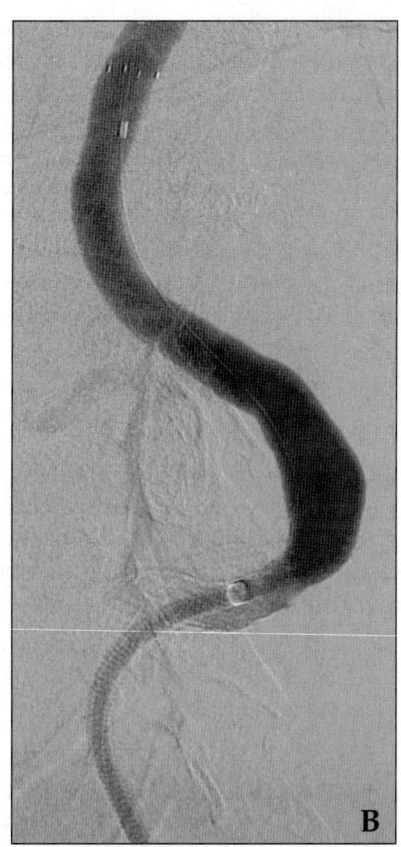

Figure 11-6. Severe angulation of the carotid bifurcation. **(A)** X-ray image showing the position of the stent and the distal filter element. **(B)** Advancement of the sheath over the wire and retrieval catheter were necessary to allow for capture of the EPD.

millimeter (diameter) x 20 millimeter (length) balloon inflated to nominal pressure. This balloon angioplasty to the target lesion is performed to allow for easy passage of the stent delivery system across the atherosclerotic plaque. Some data has shown that systemic administration of atropine (0.4–1.0 mg) given intravenously prior to balloon angioplasty of the carotid will minimize the effects on the baroreceptors and the clinic manifestation of profound bradycardia or asystole.[9] The second angioplasty is performed after the stent has been deployed in the carotid and is typically done with a 5.0 millimeter (diameter) x 20 millimeter (length) balloon to resolve any residual stenosis.

STENTS

Current approved self-expanding stents for the carotid artery are either open or closed cell designs. The cell design confers scaffolding and flexibility to the stent such that a closed cell stent is generally more rigid than an open cell stent, but because the stent struts are all interconnected, "fish-scaling"—or stent strut protusion into the lumen— does not occur. Stents also are designed in taper and nontapered configurations, with the goal of the former being better accommodation to the natural carotid bifurcation.

Whether specific stent design systems confer an impact on clinical outcomes remains controversial today, but some speculate that closed cell stents may be associated with a lower periprocedural stroke risk in symptomatic patients treated with CAS.[10]

Other important points in regards to stent deployment for CAS: 1) a residual stenosis of 10–20% is not significant and is best left alone rather than overdilating the vessel; 2) remember that the lesion is longer than what is seen angiographically, so use a longer stent (30 or 40 millimeter lengths are most commonly used); 3) stenting across the origin of the ECA is very common and will not alter flow into the ECA in the vast majority of cases;[11] and 4) when using a nontapered stent, size the stent according to the CCA so that the stent is not undersized and free floating in the CCA.

CONCLUSION

CAS requires a unique set of skills and proficiency in using an array of devices (sheaths/guiding catheters, balloons, stents, and EPDs). A stepwise approach to CAS, as with other important vascular beds, allows treating physicians to avoid recognized complications. Successful outcomes can be expected with good patient selection, advanced endoluminal training, and a solid understanding of the limitations of current CAS systems.

REFERENCES

1. Eliasziw M, Smith RF, Singh N, Holdsworth DW, Fox AJ, Barnett HJ. Further comments on the measurement of carotid stenosis from angiograms. North American Symptomatic Carotid Endarterectomy Trial (NASCET) Group. *Stroke*. Dec 1994;25(12):2445–2449.
2. Beneficial effect of carotid endarterectomy in symptomatic patients with high-grade carotid stenosis. North American Symptomatic Carotid Endarterectomy Trial Collaborators. *N Engl J Med*. Aug 15 1991;325(7):445–453.
3. Al-Mubarak N, Vitek JJ, Iyer SS, New G, Roubin GS. Carotid stenting with distal-balloon protection via the transbrachial approach. *J Endovasc Ther*. Dec 2001;8(6):571–575.
4. Criado E, Fontcuberta J, Orgaz A, Flores A, Doblas M. Transcervical carotid stenting with carotid artery flow reversal: 3-year follow-up of 103 stents. *J Vasc Surg*. Nov 2007;46(5): 864–869.
5. Barbato JE, Dillavou E, Horowitz MB, et al. A randomized trial of carotid artery stenting with and without cerebral protection. *J Vasc Surg*. Apr 2008;47(4):760–765.
6. Eskandari MK. Design and development of mechanical embolic protection devices. *Expert Rev Med Devices*. May 2006;3(3):387–393.
7. Eskandari MK, Najjar SF, Matsumura JS, Kibbe MR, Morasch MD. Technical limitations of carotid filter embolic protection devices. *Ann Vasc Surg*. Jul 2007;21(4):403–407.
8. Siewiorek GM, Eskandari MK, Finol EA. The Angioguard embolic protection device. *Expert Rev Med Devices*. May 2008;5(3):287–296.
9. Cayne NS, Faries PL, Trocciola SM, et al. Carotid angioplasty and stent-induced bradycardia and hypotension: Impact of prophylactic atropine administration and prior carotid endarterectomy. *J Vasc Surg*. Jun 2005;41(6):956–961.
10. Bosiers M, de Donato G, Deloose K, et al. Does free cell area influence the outcome in carotid artery stenting? *Eur J Vasc Endovasc Surg*. Feb 2007;33(2):135–141; discussion 142–133.
11. Woo EY, Karmacharya J, Velazquez OC, Carpenter JP, Skelly CL, Fairman RM. Differential effects of carotid artery stenting versus carotid endarterectomy on external carotid artery patency. *J Endovasc Ther*. Apr 2007;14(2):208–213.

12

Cerebral Protection Devices During Carotid Stenting

Juan C. Parodi, M.D., F.A.C.S. Hon.,
Federico E. Parodi, M.D.,
and Michel A. Bartoli, M.D.

Carotid Stenting is becoming an alternative to surgery for selected patients with carotid stenosis. Carotid endarterectomy is an established treatment that has proven to be efficacious and safe; there are, however, subgroups of patients who would benefit from a less invasive procedure such as carotid artery stenting (CAS). According to the randomized, prospective SAPPHIRE trial, CAS has less morbidity than surgery when high-risk patients are treated. Acute myocardial infarction, stroke, and death resulted in 5.8% of the cases in the CAS arm, while surgery produced 12.8% of such adverse events.

The main limitation of CAS is cerebral embolization, which was called the Achilles' heel of CAS (Figure 12–1). Secondary problems are access and restenosis although the latter does not seems to be a significant one. Using Transcranial Doppler (TCD) monitoring, it becomes evident that High Intensity Transitory Signals (HITS) are produced by particles traveling in the insonated artery, usually the middle cerebral artery (MCA). Transitory signals, however, also can be produced by artifacts and by air bubbles in addition to the ones produced by solid particles. If two transducers are used in tandem, it is possible to differentiate artifacts from particles, and among the particles, the solid ones and the air bubbles. Embolic signals occur throughout all the different stages of CAS (Figure 12–2). In addition, three in vitro studies using carotid endarterectomy specimens, showed that embolization is universal during CAS.[1-3]

Jacques Theron suggested in the mid-eighties the possibility of using an occlusion balloon in the internal carotid artery (ICA) to stop the flow and prevent cerebral embolization during CAS. Aspiration of the isolated segment of the ICA before reestablishing flow resulted in retrieval of multiple fragments of plaque or thrombus.

In the present chapter, we will describe the different stages in our experience on CAS, which started doing CAS without protection. Following stages came along when different cerebral protection devices (CPD) became available.

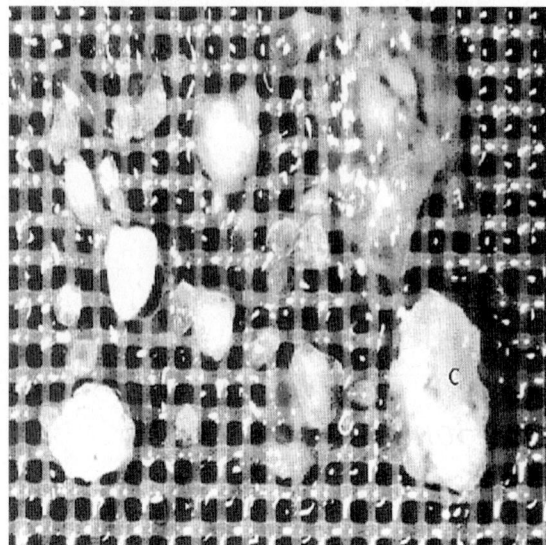

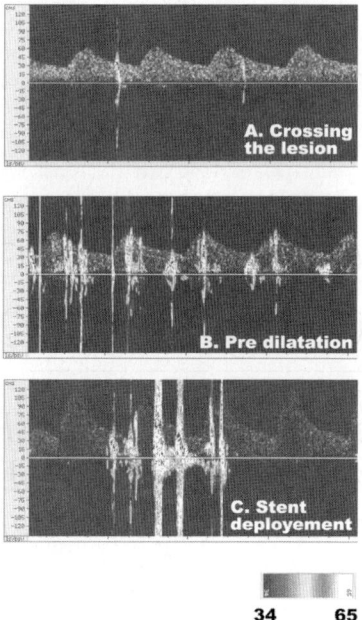

34   65

Figure 12-1. Particles of different characteristics obtained performing stent assisted carotid angioplasty in vitro. Specimens of carotid endarterectomies were used. Adapted from: Ohki T, et al. Efficacy of a filter device in the prevention of embolic events during carotid angioplasty and stenting: An ex vivo analysis. *J Vasc Surg.* 1999;30(6): 1034-1044.

Figure 12-2. Transcranial Doppler monitoring of the middle cerebral artery during carotid stenting without cerebral protection. HITS were evident in all stages of the procedure.

CAS WITHOUT CEREBRAL PROTECTION

Our initial experience was done in patients with carotid restenosis after surgery. Using TCD monitoring routinely, we learned that HITS occurred in all cases although clinical consequences of the HITS were not evident in all of them. In this initial experience before starting to use CPD, TIAs and minor strokes were seen in a small number of patients as was reported in 2000.[4] From the beginning, coronary systems were utilized to minimize trauma to the vessels. Alarmed by the HITS and some clinical adverse events, we moved to the first protection device that became available, the Percusurge system (Guardwire, Medtronic, Santa Rosa, California) (Figure 12-3) .

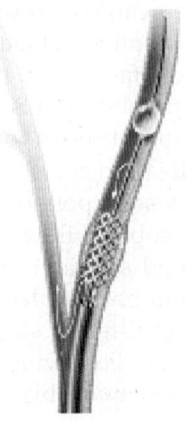

Figure 12-3. Percusurge in position. Aspiration is applied before deflating the balloon.

BALLOON OCCLUSION OF THE ICA

Following Theron's advice, a hypotube with a balloon at the tip was advanced inside the ICA across the lesion and the balloon was then inflated in the distal ICA, balloon predilatation of the lesion, followed by stenting and balloon dilatation of the stent was performed under the protection of the balloon. After careful aspiration of the area, the balloon was deflated and removed (Figure 12–4). We were part of the CAFÉ trial directed by Patrick Whitlow, which was published recently in *Stroke*.[5] Results of the initial cases were uniformly good although HITS were detected throughout the procedure insonating the ipsilateral MCA (Figure 12–5A). The group in Lennox Hill in New York also described those findings.[6]

What were the Drawbacks of the Procedure?

1. Crossing the lesion produced a shower of particles detected by the transducer of the TCD positioned over the MCA in most of our patients (Figure 12–6). As mentioned before, HITS continued throughout the procedure. After deflating the balloon, the number of emboli increased temporarily, suggesting that trapped particles stayed attached to the balloon or on its side, and were released when the balloon was deflated (Figure 12–5B). HITS over the MCA while the balloon was inflated were originated by particles coming from the stented area and traveling through communications between external carotid artery (ECA) and branches of the ICA. Communications between the ECA and the vertebral artery are sometimes seen and represent an additional risk to posterior circulation embolization. Transitory or permanent amaurosis after CAS using the Percusurge device was reported in France (Amor M., Personal communication). In a reported series, we found lining thrombus in 24% of the carotid plaques removed during carotid endarterectomy.[7] The group in Stanford reported the presence of thrombus in more than 49% of highly stenotic plaques (>75%).[8] It became clear that just crossing the lesion could produce an ischemic stroke. Ohki, in one of his publications, reported that 12% of the total number of particles generated during stenting using distal protection devices was originated crossing the stenosis.[9]

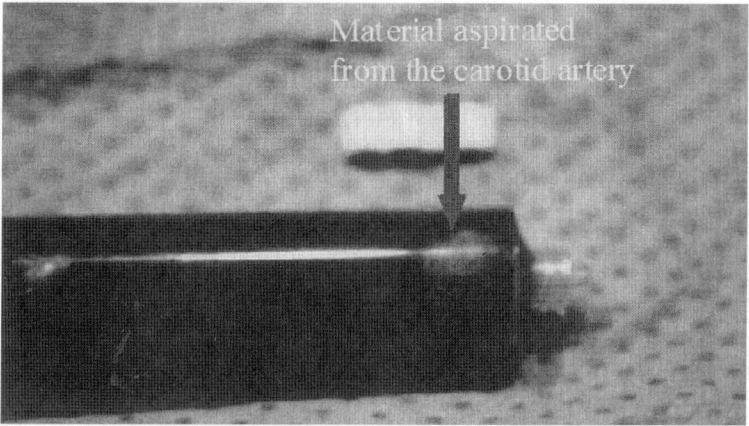

Figure 12-4. Material aspirated using the Percusurge as protection device.

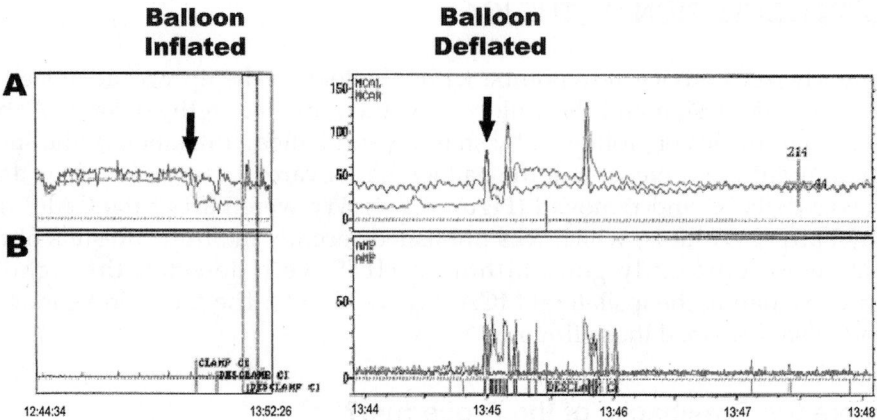

Figure 12-5. Transcranial Doppler monitoring of both Middle Cerebral Artery (MCA) during carotid stenting using the Percusurge device. Upper section: The red (lightger) line represents flow velocity in the ipsilateral MCA, note drop in velocity during balloon inflation in the Internal carotid Artery (ICA), green (darker) line: contralateral MCA with no variations. Lower section: Presence of HITS is noticed throughout the procedure. Shower of particles after balloon deflation in spite of intense aspiration of the stump.

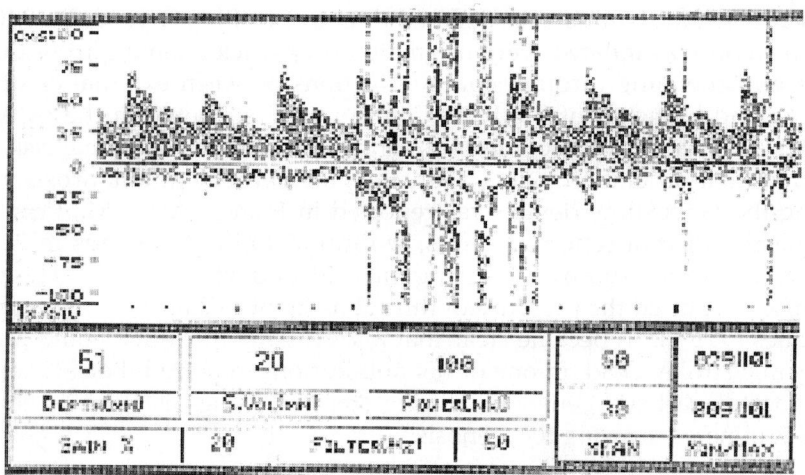

Figure 12-6. Shower of emboli reaching the MCA crossing the lesion

2. Spasm and damage to the friable intima of the distal ICA were seen with certain frequency with the use of the Percusurge. The hypotube used as guidewire constitutes one piece with the balloon; thus, when the wire is moved, the movement is transmitted to the balloon. Rubbing the intima produces denudation of endothelial cells and eventually can produce a dissection of the artery. Spasm is often seen at the level of balloon inflation. Long-term consequences of trauma to the artery and endothelial denudation are still ignored.
3. Intolerance to balloon inflation occurs in a small proportion of patients. It is often related to the development of hypotension. Lack of communicating arteries could be a contraindication for the use of occlusion devices although intolerance to balloon inflation, in our experience, never ended in a permanent neurological deficit. As with carotid endarterectomy, ischemic complications most of the time are related to emboli.

4. Impossibility to cross the lesion or to advance the balloon in the ICA sometimes requires balloon predilatation of the lesion and the use of a "buddy" wire. Both procedures entail increased risk of embolization.[10]
5. A distinct concern also arose in relation to the impossibility of aspirating large particles because of the small lumen of the aspirating catheter. It is obvious that particles larger than the lumen of the catheter will remain free in the lumen of the artery. Following the use of filters in the next stage, we learned that they captured particles larger than 300 microns, which cannot be aspirated by the catheter.

FILTERS

The above-mentioned findings using distal balloon occlusion prompted us to start using filters for cerebral protection (Figures 12–7, 12–8, and 12–9). The Angioguard filter (Cordis, Warren, NJ) was the initial one we used. Clinical results were very impressive although analysis of information also produced concerning data. Most of the filters contained material at the end of the procedure, sometimes particles of large size.

The following are the comments we can make about filters based on our and others experience.

1. Filters can embolize crossing the lesion of the carotid artery. Profile of the filters is larger (2.9 to 3.6 Fr) than the Percusurge. Need for predilatation is seen in significant number of patients. Coggia reported that crossing the lesion with a filter produced 50,000 particles as average.[2] In the SAPPHIRE trial, even using the Angioguard filter, stroke resulted in more than 4.4% of the patients and in the ARCHeR trial, the incidence of stroke was 5.3% using the AccuNet filter (Guidant, Indianapolis, IN).
2. Filters are often rigid and not easily tracked mainly in tortuous arteries.

Figure 12-7. Illustration of the Accunet filter.

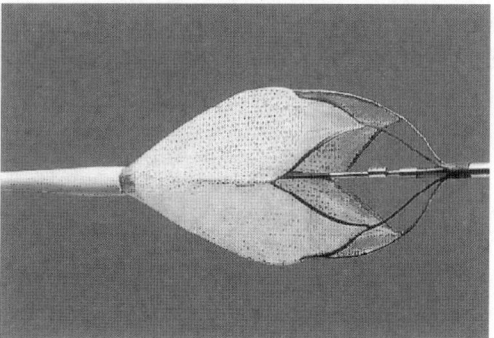

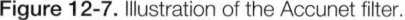

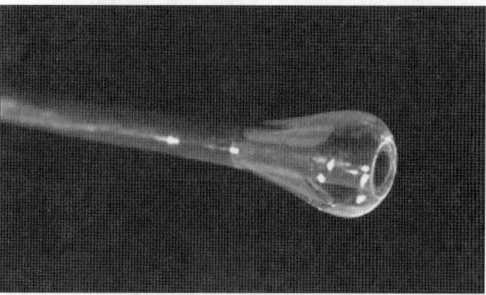

Figure 12-9. Funnel shape balloon at the end of the PAES to direct particles inside the lumen of the catheter.

Figure 12-8. Illustration of the Filter-wire filter.

3. Filters can become full of material and this excess material remains in the lumen of the artery. Particles can be extruded from the filter when the latter is closed.

4. Filters may not appose completely to the circumference of the ICA, leaving a gap between the artery and the filter. This occurs with all filters in different degrees.

5. Filters can damage the intima of the distal ICA.

6. Filters can be caught by the edge or the struts of the stent.

7. Only large particles are captured by filters depending on porous size, which is typically 100 microns. In animal studies, particles of 50 microns produced ischemic lesions.[11] Multiple small- and medium-size particles pass the filter. Consequences of these emboli are still in study. Although knowing the sensitivity to ischemia of the neural issue, it is reasonable to think that those thousand of small- and medium-size particulates would produce temporary or permanent cerebral damage. Recent studies using DWMRI disclosed new lesions in 22.7% of the cases in which a filter was used during CAS.[12]

The above mentioned data do not invalidate the use of distal protection devices since they prove to decrease the incidence of complications related to embolization to the brain during CAS. However, more subtle changes as those detected by DWMRI or detailed cognitive studies are increasingly being quoted in the literature. In a classical study performed in Leicester, more than 10 particles produced significant changes in cognitive studies.[13]

REVERSAL FLOW

Our last stage using CPD during CAS involved the use of reversal of flow to prevent cerebral embolization during CAS. The development of the system and method was based on the observation of reversal of flow during open endarterectomies using temporary shunt (Figure 12–10). When the arteries were clamped and the arteriotomy performed, insertion of a shunt in the distal ICA, leaving the other end of the shunt open, consistently produced reversal of flow in the MCA as demonstrated by TCD (Figure 12–11).

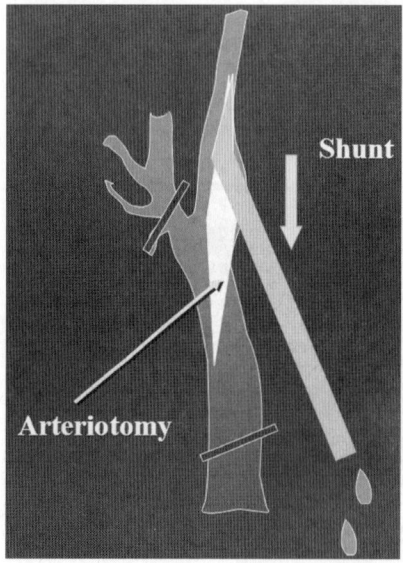

Figure 12-10. Illustration of the observation of reversal of flow in the MCA. During an open endarterectomy while the common and external carotid arteries are clamped, insertion of a shunt into the distal ICA leaving the other side open produced reversal of flow in the ipsilateral ICA and MCA

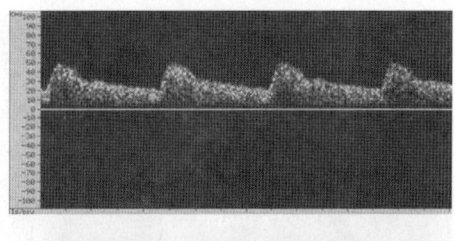

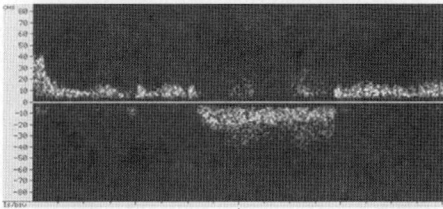

Figure 12-11. Note antegrade flow in the MCA (Top) and reversal of flow (Bottom) after inserting the shunt as described in Figure 10.

The same situation was created percutaneously by introducing an 9 Fr guiding catheter from the groin in the ipsilateral common carotid artery (CCA). The catheter has a balloon at the end that was inflated, and a second balloon placed at the end of an hypotube was inflated in the ECA (Figure 12-12). The side port of the guiding catheter was then connected with the side port of an adjacent venous line. A blood filter was interposed between the two ports to capture particles flowing back from the artery coming into the vein (Figure 12–13). The system was carefully evaluated in two animal experiments, and then clinical application proved that flow reversal is a very valid alternative for cerebral protection since no particles can reach the brain when flow reversal is established.[14]

The advantages of the system soon became evident. Protection started before any interaction with the lesion, and control of the CCA, ECA, and ICA was now possible. Fine coronary guidewires can be used to advance balloons and stents. No damage of

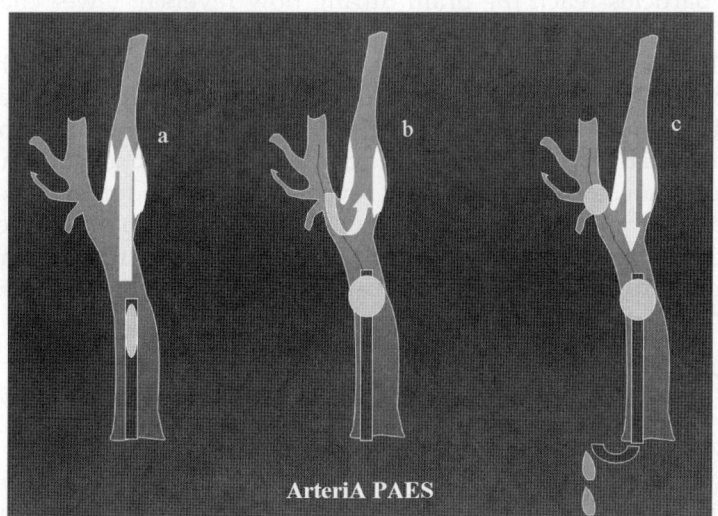

Figure 12-12. Mechanism of flow reversal using the PAES-ArteriA device. **A.** guidecatheter in the CCA, flow is antegrade. **B.** Balloon inflated in the CCA, retrograde flow from the ECA into the ICA. **C.** Second balloon is inflated in the ECA and sideport open promoting flow reversal

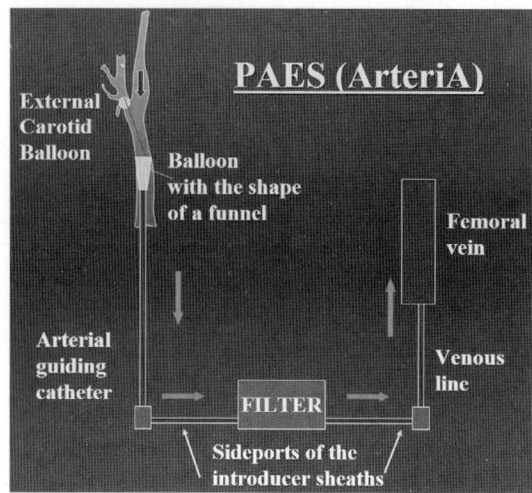

Figure 12-13. PAES in position: PAEC introduced from the femoral artery, both balloons are inflated, the side port of the PAES is connected to the side port of a venous line inserted in the femoral vein. A filter is interposed between the sides.

the distal ICA can occur and particles of all sizes can be effectively removed from the circulation. Amazingly, reversal of flow is very well tolerated, and according to a study performed by Enrique Criado, it is better tolerated than balloon occlusion of the ICA, possibly by promoting collateral flow by the flow reversal (personal communication). Additionally, floating thrombus can be fragmented and aspirated safely reversing the flow, irregular stenosis suggesting the presence of thrombus is not longer a contraindication for CAS. Lesions in tortuous proximal ICA, also considered a contraindication for CAS under distal protection, are easily treated using flow reversal.

Drawbacks of the system are related to the large size of the sheath (9.5 Fr outer diameter) and the potential intolerance of the application of flow reversal. A lower profile system is being developed that will overcome the drawbacks of the large size of the current PAES-ArteriA device (ArteriA, San Francisco, CA).

Since no particles reach the brain during flow reversal, fewer changes such as DWMRI defects and cognitive deficits are expected to occur after its use. Our analysis of the initial 108 consecutive cases using the PAES-ArteriA device, which will be soon published, showed no ipsilateral stroke, one minor contralateral stroke after a combined procedure with CABG, one hyperperfusion syndrome with hemorrhage, and one acute myocardial infarction (AMI). Incidence of AMI/Stroke and death was 2.7%.

We proposed a combination of flow reversal and filters for the rare occasions in which intolerance could be predicted. Flow reversal was established before crossing the lesion with the filter. Once the filter was opened, flow was reestablished, and at the end of the procedure, the filter was closed and retrieved under flow reversal.[15]

CONCLUSION

There is growing evidence that cerebral protection produces benefits. Recently, the safety committee of the EVA-3S trial (symptomatic severe carotid stenosis), which was taking place in Europe, recommended stopping unprotected CAS because the 30-day rate of stroke was 3.9 (0.9 to 16.7) times higher than that of CAS with cerebral protection (four out of 15 versus five out of 58 patients, respectively). Although this result was not based on a randomized comparison of unprotected versus protected CAS, it suggests that the use of cerebral protection devices during CAS reduces periproce-dural strokes[16]. In the registry of carotid stenting, Wholey reported in 12,392 patients a stroke mortality of 2.23% with protection and 5.29% without protection[17]. In summary, all CPD provide relative but effective protection against stroke caused by embolization and will become mandatory during CAS.

REFERENCES

1. Ohki T, et al. Ex vivo human carotid artery bifurcation stenting: correlation of lesion charac-teristics with embolic potential. J Vasc Surg. 1998;27(3):463–471.
2. Coggia M, et al. Embolic risk of the different stages of carotid bifurcation balloon angio-plasty: an experimental study. J Vasc Surg. 2000;31(3):550–557.
3. Rapp, JH, et al. Atheroemboli to the brain: size threshold for causing acute neuronal cell death. J Vasc Surg. 2000;32(1):68–76.
4. Parodi JC, et al. Initial evaluation of carotid angioplasty and stenting with three different cerebral protection devices. J Vasc Surg. 2000;32(6):1127–1136.
5. Whitlow PL, et al. Carotid artery stenting protected with an emboli containment system. Stroke. 2002;33(5):1308–14.
6. Al-Mubarak N, et al. Embolization Via Collateral Circulation During Carotid Stenting With the Distal Balloon Protection System. J EndovascTher. 2001;8(4): 354–357.
7. Milei J, et al. Atherosclerotic plaque rupture and intraplaque hemorrhage do not correlate with symptoms in carotid artery stenosis. J Vasc Surg. 2003;38(6):1241–1247.
8. Bassiouny HS, et al. Critical carotid stenoses: morphologic and chemical similarity between symptomatic and asymptomatic plaques. J Vasc Surg. 1989;9(2):202–212.
9. Ohki T, et al. Efficacy of a filter device in the prevention of embolic events during carotid angioplasty and stenting: An ex vivo analysis. J Vasc Surg. 1999;30(6):1034–1044.
10. Mathias K. in ESVS. Lucerne Switzerland;2001.
11. Heistad D. in Cerebral metabolism and neural function, J. Passoneau, et al., eds. Williams and Wilkins: Baltimore; 1990:202–211.
12. Schluter M, et al. Focal ischemia of the brain after neuroprotected carotid artery stenting. J Am Coll Cardiol. 2003;42(6):1007–1013.
13. Gaunt ME, et al. Role of completion angioscopy in detecting technical error after carotid en-darterectomy. Br J Surg, 1994. 81(1): p. 42–44.
14. Bates MC, et al. Reversal of the direction of internal carotid artery blood flow by occlusion of the common and external carotid arteries in a swine model. Catheter Cardiovasc Interv. 2003;60(2):270–275.
15. Parodi JC, et al. "Seat belt and air bag" technique for cerebral protection during carotid stenting. J Endovasc Ther. 2002;9(1):20–24.
16. Mas JL, Chatellier G, Beyssen B. Carotid angioplasty and stenting with and without cerebral protection: clinical alert from the Endarterectomy Versus Angioplasty in Patients With Symptomatic Severe Carotid Stenosis (EVA-3S) trial. Stroke. 2004;35(1):e18–e20.
17. Wholey MH , Al-Mubarek N. Updated review of the global carotid artery stent registry. Catheter Cardiovasc Interv. 2003;60(2):259–266.

13

Single Center Experience of Carotid Artery Stenting

*G. Matthew Longo, M.D.,
and Mark K. Eskandari, M.D.*

INTRODUCTION

Since Thomas Willis's monumental publication of *Cerebri Anatome*[1] in 1664, physicians and scientists have attempted to elucidate the pathophysiology of cerebral ischemia and infarction. The relatively common problem of cervical carotid artery stenosis, particularly involving the origin of the internal carotid artery, can present as an asymptomatic lesion, bruit, transient ischemic attack (TIA) secondary to embolization or hypoperfusion, or ischemic stroke. Approximately 750,000 strokes occur in the United States annually and 150,000 of these are fatal. Surgical treatment of carotid occlusive disease was given its greatest impetus by Eastcott, Pickering, and Robb's report[2] in November of 1954. The works of Carrea, Molins, and Murphy in Buenos Aires[3], and DeBakey in Houston[4], were later published. Since then the primary treatment modality of severe extracranial carotid artery lesions has been carotid endarterectomy (CEA). This procedure has been substantiated by several multi-center randomized prospective trials demonstrating its efficacy in a subset of symptomatic and asymptomatic patients (NASCET[5], ACAS[6], ECST[7], VA Symptomatic Trial[8]).

The last decade has witnessed an exponential growth in the field of percutaneous transluminal arterial interventions, which has permeated into cervical carotid artery disease. Despite early descriptions of carotid balloon angioplasty and stenting (CAS), only in the last few years has there been widespread interest in this modality.[9-10] Vascular surgeons, neurosurgeons, interventional cardiologists, neuroradiologists, and neurologists recognize the seriousness of the changing technology and have called for and begun prospective randomized studies with rigorous oversight to help guide the debate surrounding CAS.[11] Unfortunately, vascular surgeons, representing the minority performing CAS, remain staunch advocates of CEA and have largely scorned CAS. The tide may change with the recently presented results of two trials showing better outcomes in high-risk patients treated with CAS[12-13] In light of this, we review our experience with CAS performed exclusively by vascular surgeons in an operating room angiosuite, with emphasis on the technical procedure, peri-operative complications, and post-operative results.

MATERIALS AND METHODS

Patients

From April 2001 to May 2001-April 2009, 386 consecutive cervical carotid artery lesions were treated with CAS at Northwestern Memorial Hospital, the VA Lakeside Medical Center, and the Westside VA Medical Center. All patients were treated using a mechanical embolic protection device (EPD) and a self-expanding stent.

Patients either had symptomatic (≥ 50% diameter) or asymptomatic (≥80% diameter) stenoses of the carotid artery. Patients were excluded if they had a major neurologic deficit or illness impeding informed consent, or peripheral vascular disease precluding femoral artery access. All patients were reviewed under protocols approved by the Institutional Review Boards at the listed institutions. The risks and benefits of CAS were explained, and all patients were given informed consent.

Operative Procedure

CAS was performed in an operating room with dedicated endovascular capabilities. Preoperatively, the patients' diagnostic studies included a carotid duplex ultrasonography with a magnetic resonance angiography of the neck and cerebral circulation or a carotid/cerebral angiogram. All patients were loaded with clopidogrel (Plavix) at least 24 hours prior to stenting, and each patient was also given Plavix (75 mg) daily, including the morning of the procedure. In addition, each patient was given aspirin (325 mg) on the morning of the procedure.

Percutaneous access was obtained through a common femoral artery puncture. A J-wire (0.035") and then a short 6 Fr sheath were used to secure access. A marker pigtail catheter (5 Fr, 110 cm long) was placed in the ascending arch under fluoroscopy. A left anterior oblique aortogram at an angle of 30° was obtained. Selection of the common carotid artery was achieved using a Vitek Catheter (Cook, Inc., Bloomington, IN) or a DAV catheter (Cook, Inc.). Systemic heparin (100 units/kg IV) was given to obtain an activated clotting time of 250-300 seconds. A 0.035" Storq wire (300 cm long, Cordis Corporation, a Johnson & Johnson Company, Miami Lakes, FL) was used to cannulate the common carotid artery and then "buried" distally in the external carotid artery. With the Storq wire in place, the short 6 Fr sheath was replaced with a 100 cm length 6 or 7 Fr Shuttle Sheath (Cook, Inc.). The distal tip of the shuttle sheath was placed 2-4 cm proximal to the carotid bifurcation. Angiograms of the intra-cranial and the extra-cranial arteries were performed with at least two different views, AP and lateral.

The lesion was then crossed with the 0.014" wire, as part of one of several EPDs: PercuSurge Guardwire (Medtronic AVE, Santa Rosa, CA) protection system, Accunet (Abbott Vascular, Santa Rosa, CA), Emboshield (Abbott Vascular), Angioguard (Cordis, a Johnson and Johnson Company, Miami, FL). Atropine (1 mg IV) was given before pre-dilatation. The EPD was deployed and angiographic documentation was obtained. The stenosis was then pre-dilated with a low-profile monorail 4 x 20 mm balloon. Stent size was based on the diameter of the trailing end of the stenotic segment. The self-expanding nitinol stent was deployed, and then post-dilated using a 5 x 20 mm balloon. Any released debris was aspirated from the stagnant column of blood below the occlusion balloon, and the PercuSurge balloon was deflated or trapped and removed when using a distal filter EPD. Completion angiograms of the intra-cranial and extra-cranial vessels were done, employing AP and lateral views (Figure 13–1).

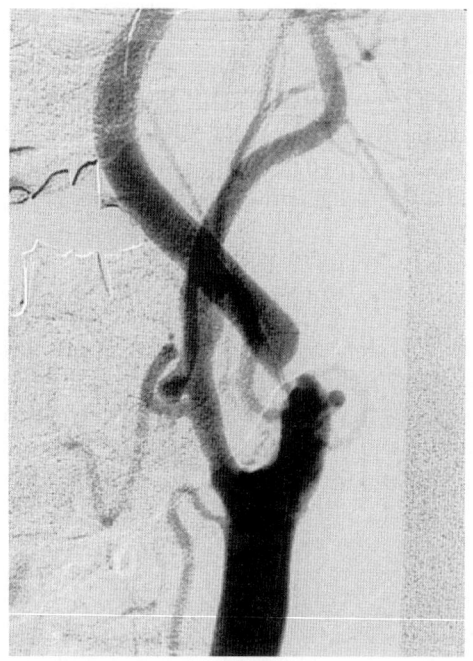
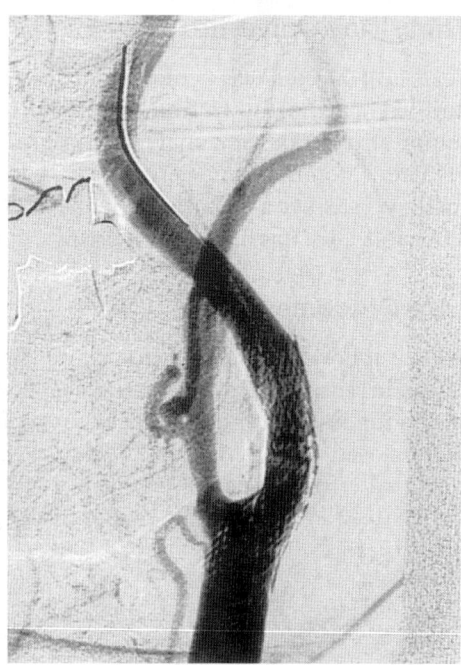

Figure 13-1. Digital subtraction angiography of the right common, internal, and external artery. **A)** Demonstrating a >90% stenosis of the internal carotid artery. **B)** Following angioplasty and stenting, with a good result. The PercuSurge Guardwire occlusion balloon is deflated.

Post-operatively, the patients were sent to the recovery room. If the patient remained hemodynamically stable, he/she was then sent to the regular ward. On postoperative day one, the patients underwent carotid duplex ultrasonography as a baseline study. Surveillance carotid duplex ultrasound was performed at 3, 6, 9, 12, 18, and 24 months, and then annually. Daily Plavix (75 mg) and aspirin (325 mg) were prescribed for at least one month and preferably indefinitely.

Statistical Analysis

All statistical analyses were performed with SPSS software (SPSS, Chicago, IL). Data are expressed as mean±SEM. All probability values were two-tailed and values of $p<0.05$ were considered statistically significant.

RESULTS

Patient Characteristics

A total of 386 procedures were performed and the mean age was 71 years. Among the entire cohort, 82% were men and 18% women, 19% were > 80 years of age, and 31% had a prior history of CEA or external beam neck irradiation (XRT). The mean carotid stenosis was 80% and asymptomatic lesions represent 69% of the group.

Thirty-Day Outcome

Technical success was achieved in all 384 cases (99%). Overall 30-day rates of death, stroke, and myocardial infarction are 0.5%, 1.8% and 0.8%, respectively. The 30-day major/minor stroke rates for analyzed subgroups are statistically significantly different only for recurrent stenosis/XRT versus *de novo* lesion, 0% and 2.7% (p=0.038), but not for asymptomatic versus symptomatic patients, 1.96% and 1.80% (p=0.45) and age <80 versus ≥ 80, 2.0% and 1.4% (p=0.37), respectively.

Late Outcomes

At late follow-up, the restenosis rate (defined as ≥ 80% stenosis) is 3.3%. Restenosis rates for recurrent stenosis/XRT versus *de novo* lesions are 2.7% and 3.4% (p=0.39) Among the restenotic lesions were 2 associate type III stent fractures in *de novo* lesions, both of which were closed cell stents. No additional stent fractures have since been identified. The late death rate for the entire group is 14.0% with no stent-related deaths. One stent-related stroke (0.02%) did occur at 19 months.

DISCUSSION

Technology continues to advance at a rapid pace and provides the surgeon with new therapeutic modalities for the treatment of stroke. Minimally invasive techniques have given the surgeon the tools to treat carotid plaques by using balloon angioplasty and stents. This new treatment strategy is one of the most exciting developments in the surgical treatment of stroke, but it must undergo the same scrutiny as CEA before it becomes widely practiced as a treatment option. Despite several large reports of the outcome of CAS, it should not be put

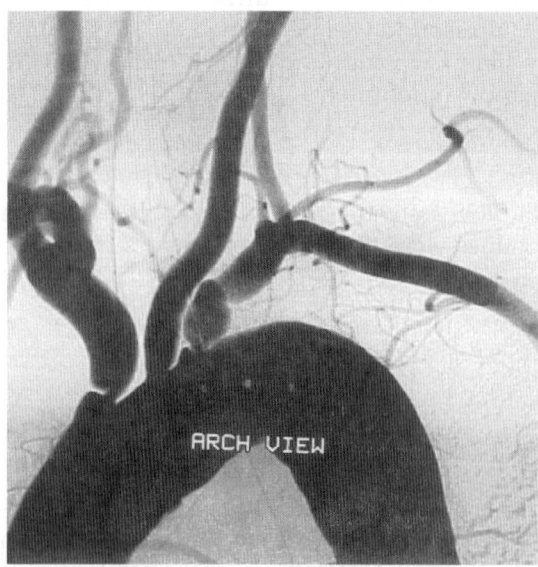 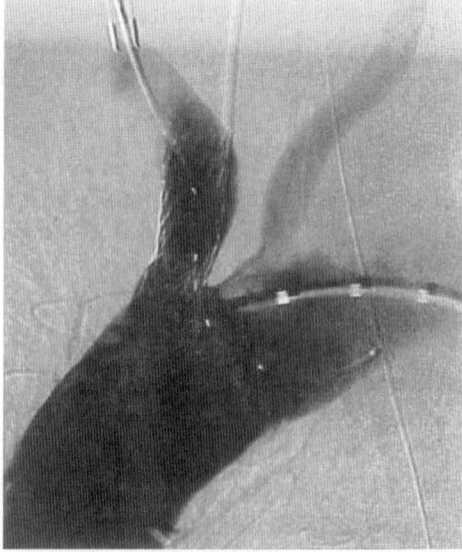

Figure 13-2. Digital subtraction angiography of the aortic. **A.** Demonstrating a stenosis of the innominate artery. **B.** Following angioplasty and stenting, using a retrograde approach.

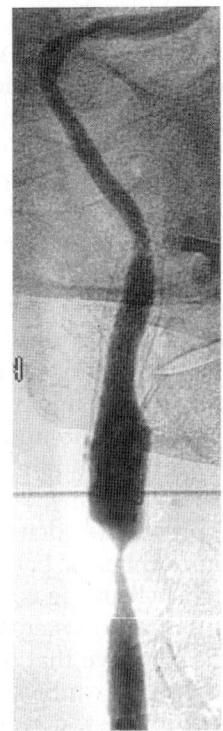 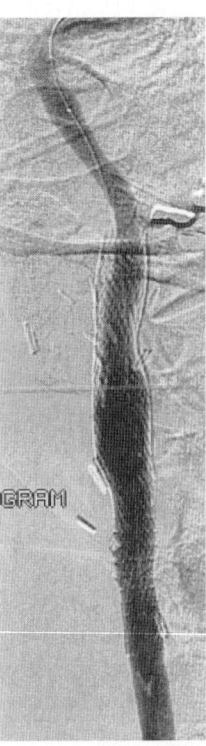

Figure 13-3. Digital subtraction angiography of the right common and internal carotid artery. **A)** Recurrent 80% stenosis in the common carotid artery proximal to the stented segment, but within the prior endarterectomy site. **B)** Following angioplasty and stenting with the PercuSurge Guardwire occlusion balloon deflated.

into widespread practice until the results of randomized trials are completed.[14-16] Although alarming to surgeons, current evidence raises the specter of the end of CEA as the gold standard.[17] To date, the general consensus of CAS based on a multi-speciality review is that it is currently appropriate treatment for high-risk patients at experienced centers, but is not generally appropriate for low-risk patients.[18-19] High-risk patients may include patients with multiple medical comorbidities, restenosis, high and inaccessible carotid lesions, carotid stenosis in a radiated neck, or a previously operated neck. Additionally, concomitant use of mechanical cerebral protection devices is strongly advocated in conjunction with CAS. Multiple groups have demonstrated that cerebral protection devices (distal filter, distal occlusion, or flow-reversal system) do prevent embolization during CAS and should be considered the standard of care when performing these procedures.[20-21]

One of the first and largest randomized trials that evaluated the role of CAS was the Carotid and Vertebral Artery Transluminal Angioplasty Study (CAVATAS).[22] This multi-center trial randomly assigned 504 patients to endovascular treatment (n=251) versus CEA (n=253). Only 26% of the endovascular-treated group were treated with a stent while the other 76% were treated with angioplasty alone. The stroke and death rate between the two groups within 30 days of treatment was not different: 10% in the endovascular group versus 9.9% in the CEA group. At 3 years follow-up the rate of death or stroke was 14.3% in the endovascular group and 14.2% in the surgery group. The investigators concluded that there was no difference in the major risks of either treatment group. A major criticism of this study is the peri-procedural complication rate of 9.9% in the CEA group, which is much higher than published reports for CEA. In addition, only a small portion of the endovascular group was treated with angioplasty and stenting. Several other early studies lacking brain protection demonstrated unacceptably high periprocedural neurologic complication rates. These are exemplified by the Leicester trial, which was prematurely terminated after enrolling 17 patients when 5 of the 7 patients treated with unprotected CAS developed a periprocedural neurologic event.[23] This unfortunate study was followed by the WALLSTENT trial, which was stopped prematurely when the 30-day stroke and death rate of 12.1% for unprotected CAS was compared to a 4.5% rate in the CEA arm.[24]

The results have vastly improved with the incorporation of low-profile balloons, stents, and mechanical cerebral protections systems. In fact, a recent publication by Wholey et al.[25] evaluated the global experience of carotid artery stent placement in a survey study of 36 major centers across the world performing this procedure. Overall, there were 4,749 patients with 5,210 diseased carotid arteries who underwent CAS. The combined minor and major strokes and procedure-related death rate was 4.63% for the study based on vessels treated and 5.07% based on patient volume. The total stroke and death rate, which included deaths not related to the procedure such as cardiac deaths, was 5.74% based on procedures and 6.30% based on number of patients. This survey suggests that CAS may be safely performed, but there is a learning curve in performing the procedure. The centers that performed less than 50 carotid stents had the highest complication rate. Most surgeons and interventionalists believe that the learning curve is about 20-25 cases in the hands of someone possessing advanced percutaneous endovascular skills. While the results of this survey are of interest, surveys cannot replace controlled clinical trials in assessing the value of major procedures.

The two recent high-risk trials – SAPPHIRE and ARCHeR – lend additional support to the efficacy of CAS using cerebral protection devices with reported embolic retrieval in 57%-60% of cases.[12-13] The early results of SAPPHIRE showed a 30-day combined death, stroke, and/or myocardial infarction (MI) rate (including non-Q wave MI) of 5.8% in the CAS group versus 12.6% for CEA (p=0.047).[13] Although this was statistically different, the difference was primarily due to the inclusion of non-Q wave MI's. The 12-month results showed a continued benefit in the CAS group with a major adverse event rate of 11.9% in the CAS group compared to 19.9% in CEA patients.[26] Importantly, a statistically significant difference was again only seen when analyzing myocardial infarction rates (2.5%-CAS versus 7.9%-CEA, p=0.04). The Acculink for Revascularization of Carotids in High Risk Patients (ARCHeR) demonstrated a 30-day major adverse event rate of 7.8%.[12] In similar high-risk CEA patient cohorts, stroke, death, and myocardial infarction (MI) rates are equivalent or higher.[27] The International Society of Endovascular Specialists (ISES) has established the Carotid Revascularization with Endarterectomy and Stenting Systems (CARESS) Trial. This is a multicenter trial investigating the feasibility of new devices that may prevent stroke associated with angioplasty and stenting the cervical carotid artery. The lead-in, feasibility trial for CARESS enrolled 287 CEA patients and 152 CAS patients between April 2001 and December 2002. The results demonstrated no significant difference in the 30-day all-cause mortality or the 30-day combined all-cause mortality, stroke, and myocardial infarction rates between CEA (3%) and CAS (2%). The pivotal study of this trial will enroll approximately 2,500 patients in up to 30 centers.[28] Ultimately, the Carotid Revascularization Endarterectomy versus Stent Trial (CREST) investigators[29] will provide the necessary information about the true efficacy of CAS in symptomatic patients. Funded by the National of Health (NIH) and the National Institute of Neurological

Disorders and Stroke (NINDS), this study will prospectively randomize 2,500 symptomatic patients to either CAS or CEA, 1-year results are expected to be reported in the fourth quarter of 2009. Additionally, the ACT I (Asymptomatic Carotid Stent Trial), which randomizes asymptomatic standard risk patients to CEA or CAS, should conclude enrollment by the end of 2009 with 30-day results expected in early 2010.

When comparing the results of this review with NASCET and ACAS, the rate of stroke and death are comparable. The 30-day major stroke death rate in the NASCET trial was 2.1% compared to 2.3% in the ACAS over the same time period.[5-6] Our own experience has shown that CAS has nearly equivalent results with CAS or CEA among asymptomatic patients with regards to periprocedural stroke rates (1.7% versus 1.0%, respectively).[30] Carotid in-stent restenosis is another critical concern, which does not seem to mirror the experience of coronary interventions. In a previous report by our group, we that the occurrence of restenosis to be low and was not adversely effected by a prior history of CEA or XRT.[31] Our restenosis rate of 3.3% corroborates the mid-term experience of others.[25] Overall, the results of this study demonstrate that carotid artery angioplasty and stenting using cerebral protection can be performed safely with results comparable to CEA. Furthermore, this study underscores the need for vascular surgeons treating carotid artery occlusive disease to possess advanced catheter-based skills and to be trained specifically in carotid angioplasty and stenting techniques. As the true efficacy and durability of carotid stenting becomes elucidated through ongoing national trials, individuals from several different specialties will continue to perform these procedures both within the trial setting and independently. The lay press has even begun to predict the end of carotid endarterectomy while noting that tremendous battles will begin to determine who treats carotid disease.[32] Each group will attempt to claim exclusive rights over CAS, and the group able to perform these procedures with complication rates less than what is seen in CEA will have the most legitimate argument.

REFERENCES

1. Willis T. Cerebri Anatome: The Anatomy of the Brain and Nerves. Feindel W, ed. Montreal, Quebec: McGill University Press, 1965.
2. Eastcott HHG, Pickering GW, Rob CG. Reconstruction of internal carotid artery in a patient with intermittent attacks of hemiplegia. *Lancet* 1954;2:994–996.
3. Carrea R, Molins M, Murphy G. Surgical treatment of spontaneous thrombosis of the internal carotid artery in the neck. Carotidcarotidal anastomosis. Report of a case. *ACTA Neurol Latin Am.* 1955;1:71–78.
4. DeBakey ME. Successful carotid endarterectomy for cerebrovascular insufficiency: Nineteen-year follow-up. *JAMA* 1975;233:1083–1085.
5. North American Symptomatic Carotid Endarterectomy Trial Collaborators. Beneficial effect of carotid endarterectomy in symptomatic patients with high-grade carotid stenosis. *N Engl J Med* 1991;325:445–453.
6. Executive Committee for the Asymptomatic Carotid Atherosclerosis Study. Endarterectomy for asymptomatic carotid artery stenosis. *JAMA* 1995;273:1421–1428.
7. European Carotid Surgery Trialists' Collaborative Group. Randomised trial of endarterectomy for recently symptomatic carotid stenosis: Final results of the MRC European Carotid Surgery Trial (ECST). *Lancet* 1998;351:1379–1387.
8. Mayberg MR, Wilson SE, Yatsu F, et al. for the Veterans Affairs Cooperative Studies Program 309 Trialist Group. Carotid endarterectomy and prevention of cerebral ischemia in symptomatic carotid stenosis. *JAMA.* 1991;266:3289–3294.

9. Mathias K, Bockenheimer S, von Reutern G, et al. Catheter dilatation of arteries supplying the brain. Radiologie 1983;23:208–214.

10. Diethrich EB, Gordon MH, Lopez-Galarza LA, et al. Intraluminal Palmaz stent implantation for treatment of recurrent carotid artery occlusive disease: A plan for the future. J Interv Cardiol 1995;8:213–218.

11. Bettman MA, Katzen BT, Whisnant J, et al. Carotid stenting and angioplasty: A statement for healthcare professionals from the Councils on Cardiovascular Radiology, Stroke, Cardio-Thoracic and Vascular Surgery, Epidemiology and Prevention, and Clinical Cardiology, American Heart Association. *Stroke* 1998;29:336–338.

12. Wholey MH. The ARCHeR trial: Results for carotid stenting in high risk surgical patients: Preliminary 30-day results. Presented at the American College of Cardiology Scientific Meeting; March 30, 2003; Chicago, IL.

13. Yadav JS. The 30-day SAPPHIRE results. Presented at the American Heart Association 2002 Annual Meeting; November 17-20, 2002; Chicago, IL.

14. Roubin GS, New G, Iyer SS, et al. Immediate and late clinical outcomes of carotid artery stenting in patients with symptomatic and asymptomatic carotid artery stenosis: A 5-year prospective analysis. *Circ* 2001;103:532–537.

15. Gable DR, Bergamini T, Garrett WV, et al. Immediate follow-up of carotid artery stent placement. *Am J Surg* 2003;185:183–187.

16. Eskandari MK, Longo GM, Vijungco JD, et al. Does carotid stenting measure up to endarterectomy? A vascular surgeon's perspective. *Arch Surg*, in press.

17. White CJ. Another nail in the coffin of carotid endarterectomy. Editorial comment. *J Amer Coll Card* 2001;38:1596–1597.

18. Veith FJ, Amor M, Ohki T, et al. Current status of carotid bifurcation angioplasty and stenting based on a consensus of opinion leaders. *J Vasc Surg* 2001;33:S111–S116.

19. Barr JD, Connors JJ 3rd, Sacks D, et al. Quality improvement guidelines for the performance of cervical carotid angioplasty and stent placement. *J Vasc Interv Radiol* 2003;14:1079–1093.

20. Ohki T, Veith FJ, Grenell S, et al. Initial experience with cerebral protection devices to prevent embolization during carotid artery stenting. *J Vasc Surg* 2002;36:1175–1185.

21. Reimers B, Corvaja N, Moshiri S, et al. Cerebral protection with filter devices during carotid artery stenting. *Circ* 2001;104:12–15

22. CAVATAS Investigators. Endovascular versus surgical treatment in patients with carotid stenosis in the Carotid and Vertebral Artery Transluminal Angioplasty Study (CAVATAS): a randomised trial. *Lancet* 2001;357:1729–1737.

23. Naylor AR, Bolia A, Abbott RJ, et al. Randomized study of carotid angioplasty and stenting versus carotid endarterectomy: A stopped trial. *J Vasc Surg* 1998;28:326–334.

24. Alberts MJ. Results of a multicenter prospective randomized trial of carotid artery stenting vs. carotid endarterectomy [abstract]. *Stroke* 2001;32:325d.

25. Wholey MH, Wholey M, Mathias K, et al. Global experience in cervical carotid artery stent placement. *Cathet Cardiovasc Intervent* 2000;50:160–167.

26. Yadav JS, The 12-month SAPPHIRE results. Presented at the Transcatheter Cardiovascular Therapeutics 2003 Annual Meeting; September 15-19, 2003; Washington, D.C.

27. Ouriel K, Hertzer NR, Beven EG, et al. Preprocedural risk stratification: Identifying an appropriate population for carotid stenting. *J Vasc Surg* 2001;33:728–732.

28. CARESS Steering Committee. Carotid revascularization using endarterectomy or stenting systems: Phase I clinical trial. *J Endovasc Ther* 2003;10:1021–1030.

29. Hobson RW, Brott T, Ferguson R, et al. CREST: Carotid Revascularization Endarterectomy Versus Stent Trial *Cardiovasc Surg* 1997;5:457–458.

30. Tang GL, Matsumura JS, Morasch MD, Pearce WH, Nguyen A, Amaranto D, Eskandari MK, Carotid angioplasty and stenting vs carotid endarterectomy for treatment of asymptomatic disease: single-center experience. *Arch Surg*, 143(7):653–8, 2008

31. Eskandari MK, Brown KE, Kibbe MR, Morasch MD, Matsumura JS, Pearce WH. Restenosis after carotid stent placement in patients with previous neck irradiation or endarterectomy. *J Vasc Interv Radiol* 18(11):1368–74, 2007.

32. Sternberg S. Science clearing the way for a shift in fighting stroke. *USA Today* April 27, 2004.

Carotid Stent Trials

14

Should NASCET and ACAS be Repeated?

Wesley S. Moore, MD

SHOULD NASCET AND ACAS BE REPEATED?

The North American Symptomatic Carotid Endarterectomy Trial (NASCET) and the Asymptomatic Carotid Atherosclerosis Study (ACAS) were large, well-organized trials, which have had a major impact on the management of extracranial carotid atherosclerosis. Both trials had clearly defined patient populations in which the results of carotid endarterectomy were compared with then-available best medical management. It is my contention that both trials were well designed, appropriately performed, and that their results continue to be applicable today. I do not believe that a repeat of either trial is either ethical or scientifically justified.[1]

A repeat of any clinical trial must not be treated lightly when one considers patient commitment and possible sacrifice, the use of professional time, and cost burden to the United States by expenditure of NIH research dollars. Before addressing the specific question, we need to examine the potential reasons to repeat a clinical trial as they apply to each of the two trials in question, as well as the reasons not to repeat a clinical trial.

REASONS TO REPEAT A CLINICAL TRIAL

Design Flaw

If it can be shown that one of the trials suffered from an error in design, which led to an erroneous conclusion, that would be a basis for considering redo of the trial.

Improved Medical Management

As time has passed since the completion of the two trials, new approaches to medical management and stroke prevention have occurred. These include the addition of new and better antiplatelet drug regimens, and recognition of the importance of the use of statins as well as the importance of beta blockers or ace inhibitors in the reduction of atherosclerotic risk factors.

Improved Surgical Management and Results

Clearly, the quality of surgical management of carotid bifurcation disease has continued to improve over the years. This will have a positive benefit in reduction of surgical risk and has the potential of even increasing the benefit of surgery when compared with medical management alone. Improvement in surgical results probably reflects improved training of surgeons performing carotid endarterectomy as well as better pre- and postoperative care.

Change in the Natural History of Disease

It would seem unlikely that the risk of carotid bifurcation disease, in and of itself, has changed, independent of factors that would affect risk factor management. The latest data from the American Heart Association indicate that there continue to be 700,000 new or recurrent strokes in the United States each year. Of these, 150,000 are fatal, which continue to make stroke the third leading cause of death in the United States each year. The survivors of acute stroke continue to be added to approximately 4 million stroke survivors, which makes stroke the leading cause of adult disability in the United States.

Questions Regarding Statistical Analysis

If it can be shown that the statistical analysis of either study was faulty and that this led to an erroneous conclusion, then clearly this would be justification for a new study.

New Data

If there were newer studies that show contrary or conflicting results, then it would be reasonable to enter into a discussion concerning the need to repeat a previous Level-1 study.

Alternative Interventional Management

An alternative interventional technique, in and of itself, would not justify a repeat of a surgical versus medical management trial. However, it will serve as a basis for a trial comparing the alternative interventional technique with a standard surgical approach.

REASONS NOT TO REPEAT A TRIAL

Potential Detriment to the Control Group

Unless it could be shown that one of the trials is highly flawed, then the initiation of a new trial places the control group, those patients randomized to medical therapy, at increased risk. It is highly unlikely that a new trial could be started when the available evidence is examined since the basis of a new trial would have to be the establishment of clinical equipoise. Since current Level-I data have established proof of the lack of equipoise, then this would never pass an ethics committee evaluation of the National Institutes of Health.

Furthermore, it will never pass individual hospital ethics committee analysis in the absence of compelling evidence to show that something had changed in the interval such that the control group would not knowingly be placed at increased risk as documented by prior Level-I evidence studies.

Cost

It has been estimated that the NASCET trial cost the U.S. taxpayer nearly $38 million dollars and the ACAS trial cost in excess of $24 million dollars. Keep in mind that these costs do not reflect current rates of inflation. The cost to carry out a large trial increases on an annual basis. Therefore, the cost to repeat a trial in today's dollars would incur an even greater expense. This expenditure could not be justified in the absence of compelling evidence to suggest that a new trial would be likely to yield a different result.

Let us now examine each of the two trials regarding each of the above points.

THE NASCET TRIAL

Possibility of a Design Flaw

A careful review of the multiple reports from NASCET indicates that the hypothesis that was tested was well defined and that the study was carefully designed to test the hypothesis. The designers of the trial were particularly clever in that they stratified patients into two groups based on the percent stenosis of the studied carotid artery. A high-grade carotid stenosis group with lesions in the 70%–99% category underwent a separate randomization from a second group of patients with lesser degrees of stenosis falling in the 30%–69% category. Therefore, the benefit of carotid endarterectomy, when compared with best medical management, could be separately identified and analyzed. The benefit of carotid endarterectomy in the high-grade stenosis group became rapidly apparent and permitted the Data and Safe Monitoring Committee of the NIH to impose a stopping rule of that portion of the trial after only 18 months. An analysis of the data demonstrated that carotid endarterectomy produced an absolute risk reduction of death and stroke of 17% and a relative risk reduction of 67%.[2] These results were consistent with multiple retrospective studies using Level-III analysis. However, the NASCET study, for the first time, presented Level-I evidence in favor of carotid endarterectomy. Patients with the lesser degree of stenosis in the 30%–69% category did not demonstrate an obvious difference with the same degree of rapidity. In this group of patients, the study actually went on to full completion, and only on a subsequent analysis, demonstrated a beneficial effect in favor of carotid endarterectomy beginning with a 50% stenosis threshold. Patients with stenoses in the 50%–69% category, treated surgically, had a 15.7% five-year ipsilateral stroke and death rate when compared to those treated medically, who had a 22.2% ipsilateral stroke and death rate. These differences were statistically significant in favor of carotid endarterectomy, but were not nearly as dramatic as those in the high-grade stenosis group.[3] However, had the initial decision to stratify randomization into two groups not been followed, there would have been a dilution effect between patients with high-grade stenosis and lesser degrees of stenosis, which would have led to a greater delay in identifying the high-risk patient with stenosis in the 70%–99% category who benefited the most from carotid endarterectomy. Clearly, there was no design flaw in the NASCET trial.

Improved Medical Management

The most compelling reason to consider a new study is the possibility that medical management has improved sufficiently to erase the beneficial difference between carotid endarterectomy and medical management. There are now more potent antiplatelet drugs than aspirin. Ticlopidine was demonstrated in the TASS study to have a slightly better outcome in preventing TIA and stroke when compared with aspirin. However, this comes at the risk of bone marrow suppression. Therefore, Ticlid was primarily used with aspirin failure rather than the primary drug of choice.[4] The newer generation drug—Clopidogrel or Plavix—was also shown to be superior to aspirin in the CAPRIE study.[5] Both Ticlid and Plavix have been shown to be somewhat superior to aspirin, but with only a small absolute risk reduction benefit when evaluating adverse outcome events compared with aspirin. The use of statins and beta blockers have been shown to have a beneficial effect in reducing the risk of death and stroke in the populations being studied. It should be kept in mind that the use of all these newer drugs also benefit those patients being treated surgically and would not be restricted to the medical arm alone. Thus, it could be argued that while the absolute risk of untoward events might be lowered in the overall study, it is unlikely that the absolute risk reduction and benefit of the surgical arm would change relative to the group randomized to medical management alone.

Improved Surgical Management and Results

The results of carotid endarterectomy have clearly improved since the publication of the trial. There are many reasons for this including improved training of surgeons, not only in the technical aspects of the operation, but also in diagnosis and patient selection. Improved pre- and postoperative care—including the use of statins, beta blockers, and the perioperative use of antiplatlet drugs—have all contributed to improved surgical results. Advances in anesthesia have had a major impact on the reduction of morbidity and mortality.

Do these improved results justify a repeat trial? Clearly not. Since surgery was shown to be superior to medical management alone, improved surgical results could only make the comparison more compelling.

Change in the Natural History of Disease

It is unlikely that the natural history of the plaque itself has changed, independent of newer drugs or risk factor modification. An analysis of mortality due to cardiovascular causes has demonstrated that there has been a consistent decline in death rate from various cardiovascular causes, including stroke. However, this decline in mortality has not been accompanied with a decline in the incidence of events. This is particularly true for stroke. In fact, recent data suggest that there may actually be an increase in event rate.[6] Irrespective of whether or not there is an event rate change, there has not been sufficient change in the natural history to justify a new trial.

Errors in Statistical Analysis

The NASCET trial had an outstanding team of statisticians involved in both trial design and data analysis. Their work was carefully prepared and critically reviewed both before and after publication. It is highly unlikely that there is an error in analysis that would lead to an erroneous conclusion.

NEW DATA

There are no new data suggesting that carotid endarterectomy is inferior to medical management. In fact, the opposite is true. Both the ECST (European)[7] and VA Symptomatic trials[8] fully support NASCET results.

Alternative Interventional Management

Alternative interventional approaches to carotid bifurcation disease in the form of carotid angioplasty and stenting have been anecdotally applied. Preliminary data suggest that there is clinical equipoise between carotid endarterectomy and angioplasty. However, this is not a reason to repeat the NASCET trial. It is a good reason to carry out a trial comparing carotid endarterectomy with angioplasty, and, in fact, such a trial is underway as the CREST trial.[9]

Potential Detriment to the Control Group

With three trials providing Level-I proof of the efficacy of carotid endarterectomy in reducing the risk of death and stroke when compared with medical management alone, what patient would be willing to volunteer to participate in a new randomized trial with the risk that he or she would be randomized to the less efficacious form of treatment? Likewise, I would find it difficult to believe that the ethics committee of a funding agency or a participating hospital would be willing to participate in such a study unless there was overwhelming evidence to suggest that a new study was indicated. There is no such evidence.

Cost

At the time the NASCET was performed, over a decade ago, the cost to the American taxpayer thru the NIH granting mechanism was $38 million dollars. At the present time, factoring in inflation as well as the increased cost of medical care, the cost of a new NASCET trial would likely be double that figure.

THE ACAS TRIAL

Possibility of a Design Flaw

The hypothesis that was tested in ACAS was that patients who had hemodynamically significant stenoses of the internal carotid artery, as documented by the presence of a 60% diameter reducing stenosis or greater and as measured by contrast angiography using the North American method of measurement, would have fewer fatal and non-fatal strokes following carotid endarterectomy together with best medical management, than those treated with best medical management alone, including aspirin as an antiplatelet regimen. The decision to set the threshold at 60% was based on two factors: (1) the then current practice of surgeons who advocated operating on asymptomatic patients was the presence of a 50% stenosis or greater bulb stenosis; and (2) a 60% diameter reducing bulb stenosis is the minimum required to produce a pressure gradient and hence, by definition, a hemodynamically significant stenosis. Currently, most surgeons are basing their decision to operate on a duplex scan. The duplex scan criterion for the asymptomatic patient is an

80%–99% percent category using the Strandness definition. In spite of this, the results of the ACAS trial demonstrated an absolute risk reduction in favor of operation of 5.9% and a relative risk reduction of 53%.[10] If we were to design a new trial today, we would probably raise the percent stenosis threshold. However, since the previous trial was clearly positive with lesser stenoses, it is most likely that a new trial with higher grade stenoses would show an even more beneficial difference. Thus, if there was a design flaw in terms of percent stenosis, correction of that would be likely to make the trial show an even greater benefit of operation. Therefore, there is nothing to be gained in repeating the trial based on a new design.

Improved Medical Management

The discussion here is similar to the material discussed under the NASCET trial heading. Therefore, any benefit in improved medical management would likely benefit both groups, thus leaving the relative benefit in favor of operation the same. The recently completed trial sponsored by the Medical Research Council of Great Britain documented exactly that finding. When they did a subset analysis in which asymptomatic patients who were on statins and beta blockers were randomized to surgery versus medical management, the results continued to show the same relative benefit in favor of carotid endarterectomy.[11] Therefore, the rationale of repeating the study because there is now better medical management is not justified.

Improved Surgical Management and Results

The same argument applies here as it does to the symptomatic trial. Improvements in surgical management and results would only widen the difference in results in favor of surgical management. One of the criticisms of the ACAS trial was that the surgical results were "too good." The 30-day stroke morbidity and mortality of patients randomized to surgical management was 2.3%. However, when the results were examined for patients actually undergoing carotid endarterectomy, the 30-day stroke morbidity and mortality was only 1.5%. The balance represented the complications associated with contrast angiography. The critics of the ACAS trial stated that careful selection of surgeons participating in the trial lead to unrealistically good results that are unlikely to be repeated when applied to the community of surgeons as a group. This has not turned out to be the case. Asymptomatic patients have been shown to be the safest group to operate on, and routinely have the lowest complication rates as reported from both individual series or community based studies. Thus, there is no justification for repeating the trial based on the possibility that new surgical results might be worse than the original ACAS report.

Change in the Natural History of Disease

There is no evidence that there has been a change in the natural history of the asymptomatic carotid stenosis. An analysis of the control group of the more recent ACST trial shows the same incidence of stroke morbidity and mortality as the control group of ACAS.[11] Therefore, this factor cannot be used as a justification to repeat the trial.

Errors in Statistical Analysis

Critics of the ACAS trial have tried to attack the results based on whatthey considered to be a flawed statistical analysis. However, each attack has been satisfactorily answered, and independent statisticians have upheld the validity of design and analysis. Therefore, there is no justification in calling for a new trial based on questions regarding statistical analysis.

New Data

There are indeed new data, and the new data are in concurrence with and further validate the findings and conclusions of the ACAS trial. The Medical Research Council (MRC) of Great Britain sponsored a prospective randomized trial with a similar design to ACAS. Between April 1993 and July of 2003, 3,120 patients from 126 centers in 30 countries were entered. Patients were randomized to immediate carotid endarterectomy (1,560) or delayed carotid endarterectomy (1,560) should symptoms develop. The results of this very large trial were remarkably similar to ACAS. The risk of death and stroke were statistically significantly reduced from 12% in the medically managed group to 6% in the surgically managed group, including perioperative events. The MRC study was also able to show that both men and women benefited equally from operation. This newer and more contemporary study published in 2004 should, once and for all, put to rest any concerns about the validity of the ACAS trial.[11]

CONCLUSION

Both the NASCET and ACAS trials were well designed, carefully controlled, and meticulously scrutinized. Their results and conclusions are as valid today as they were when the results were first published. Any proposal to repeat either trial lacks justification, would never gain funding, and in the opinion of most dispassionate observers, would be unethical in that there is virtually no likelihood that a repeat trial would yield different or compelling scientific information.

REFERENCES

1. Moore WS. Resolved: NASCET and ACAS need not be repeated - The affirmative position. *Arch Neurol*. 2003;60:775–778.
2. North American Symptomatic Carotid Endarterectomy Trial Collaborators. Beneficial effect of carotid endarterectomy in symptomatic patients with high-grade carotid stenosis. *N Engl J Med*. 1991;325:445–453.
3. Barnett HJM, Taylor DW, Eliasziw M, et al. The benefit of carotid endarterectomy in patients with symptomatic moderate or severe stenosis. *New Engl J Med*. 1998;339:1415–1425.
4. Hass WK, Easton JD, Adams HP Jr, et al. A randomized trial comparing ticlopidine hydrochloride with aspirin for the prevention of stroke in high risk patients. *N Engl J Med*. 1989;321:501–507.
5. Ringled PA, Bhatt DL, Hirsch AT, et al. Benefit of clopidogrel over aspirin is amplified in patients with history of ischemic events. *Stroke*. 2004;35:528–532.
6. Wolf PA, O'Neal A, D'Agostino RV, et al. Declining mortality, not declining incidence of stroke: The Framingham Study. *Stroke*. 1989;20–29.
7. Randomized trial of endarterectomy for recently symptomatic carotid stenosis: Final results of the MRC European Carotid Surgery Trial. *Lancet*. 1998;351:1379–1387.
8. Mayberg MR, Wilson SE, Yatsu F, and the VA Symptomatic Carotid Stenosis Group. Carotid endarterectomy and prevention of cerebral ischemia in symptomatic carotid stenosis. *JAMA*. 1991;266:3289–3294.

9. Hobson RW. CREST (Carotid Revascularization Endarterectomy versus Stent Trial): Background, design, and current status. *Semin Vasc Surg*. 2000;13:139–143.

10. Executive Committee for the Asymptomatic Carotid Atherosclerosis (ACAS) Study. Endarterectomy for asymptomatic carotid artery stenosis. *JAMA*. 1995;273:1421–1428.

11. MRC Asymptomatic carotid surgery trial (ACST) Collaborative group. Prevention of disabling and fatal strokes by successful carotid endarterectomy in patients without recent neurologic symptoms: Randomized control trial. *Lancet*. 2004;363:1491–1502.

15

Current Status of CREST (Carotid Revascularization Endarterectomy vs. Stent Trial)

Robert W. Hobson II, M.D.

Clinical trial methodology was used during the last two decades to establish the efficacy of carotid endarterectomy (CEA) when combined with best medical care over optimal medical management alone in the treatment of patients with symptomatic[1-3] and asymptomatic[4-5] extracranial carotid occlusive disease. Some investigators have recommended carotid artery stenting (CAS) as an alternative to CEA[6] suggesting that the procedure is less invasive and particularly useful in patients at high risk for carotid endarterectomy.[7] Results from two randomized clinical trials have suggested comparability or noninferiority of CAS in comparison with CEA in good risk as well as high-risk patients.[7-8] The emergence of clinical equipoise has emphasized the need for an efficacy comparison of carotid endarterectomy and stenting.[9]

Currently, three large randomized clinical trials are being conducted to evaluate the efficacy of CAS in comparison to CEA in conventional risk patients.[8, 10-11] In North America, the CREST (Carotid Revascularization Endarterectomy versus Stent Trial, NINDS, NIH, (R01 NS38384-01, NINDS, NIH) protocol is being conducted in approximately 70 centers in the United States and Canada.[10] In the United Kingdom and Europe, the CAVATAS (Carotid and Vertebral Artery Transluminal Angioplasty Study) II investigators are randomizing good risk patients between CAS and CEA and have currently randomized over 300 patients.[8] In Germany, the SPACE (Stent-Protected percutaneous Angioplasty of the Carotid versus Endarterectomy) investigators are randomizing symptomatic better risk patients between the two procedures and have now randomized over 500 patients.[11] The purpose of this chapter will be to provide an update on the status of CREST and its early results with its lead-in credentialing registry.

CURRENT TECHNICAL CONSIDERATIONS IN PERFORMANCE OF CAS

Current practice suggests consideration for CAS for several indications: high-risk patients with medical comorbidities, carotid restenosis following prior CEA, radiation-induced carotid stenosis, and anatomically high internal carotid stenoses.[12] Medical comorbidities include factors such as age over 80 years, coronary artery disease with AMI within the prior four weeks or CABG within the prior six weeks, congestive heart failure (Class II/IV), congestive heart failure with ejection fraction of <30%, dialysis dependent renal failure, and COPD with FEV1.0 of <1.0L. Local factors increasing the risk of CEA include carotid restenosis after CEA, anatomically high lesions (above C_2), contralateral occlusion or laryngeal nerve palsy, and radiation induced stenosis (particularly with prior neck dissection, permanent tracheal stoma, or cervical scarring). These indications were considered and approved by a multidisciplinary consensus panel[12] and represent a reasonable approach in view of the American Heart Association's position[13] against use of CAS for symptomatic carotid stenosis unless a part of an approved randomized clinical trial.

During our early clinical experience, we restricted use of CAS primarily to carotid restenosis after CEA.[14] Symptomatic or asymptomatic carotid restenoses after CEA are relatively uncommon and are generally attributed to myointimal hyperplasia during the early postoperative period (within 36 months) or recurrent atherosclerosis thereafter. Surgical management of carotid restenosis is controversial for two major reasons.[15-17] First, indications for operative management in the asymptomatic patient with high-grade (80%) restenosis remain controversial due to the low risk of stroke or progression to total occlusion.[15, 17] Second, reoperation is associated with an increased risk of perioperative neurological events and cranial nerve palsies.[16, 17] Because of these issues, some authors recommend CAS as an alternative to operative management.[18-20]

We prospectively collected data and intervened using endovascular techniques on patients with symptomatic and asymptomatic (>80%) carotid restenosis due to myointimal hyperplasia for the purpose of defining technical feasibility and periprocedural outcomes.[14] Examples of pre- and postprocedural arteriograms (Figure 15–1) are presented and demonstrate placement of a 10 mm x 20 mm WallStent® (Boston Scientific Vascular, Natick, MA). A 3 mm low profile balloon was used to initially dilate the lesions followed by placement of the WallStent® with poststent balloon dilatation to obtain the final result. Intravascular ultrasound was utilized to ensure adequate apposition of the stent to the arterial wall. In these cases and all but one other case, stents were placed across the carotid bifurcation. Serial postprocedural duplex ultrasonography has demonstrated patency of all external and internal carotid arteries.

Our clinical series[21, 22] has been expanded to 105 high-risk patients and recently 177 patients (194 CAS procedures), using nitinol self-expanding stents and cerebral protection (Table 15–1). Indications for CAS included restenosis after prior CEA (57%), primary stenosis (Figure 15–2) in patients with medical comorbidities (27%) and those randomized to CAS with conventional risk profiles (4.5%), radiation-induced stenosis (7%), in-stent restenoses (3%), and anatomically high bifurcation (1.5%). In cases of restenosis after prior CEA, the original method of closure of the endarterectomy site does not influence results.[23] Primary closure and synthetic or autologous patching had comparable CAS results. No arterial dissections or disruptions were observed. Overall thirty-day stroke and death was 2.85%.[21] In-stent restenosis (Figure 15–3) was observed by serial duplex ultrasonography at 6.4% projected over a five-year follow-up

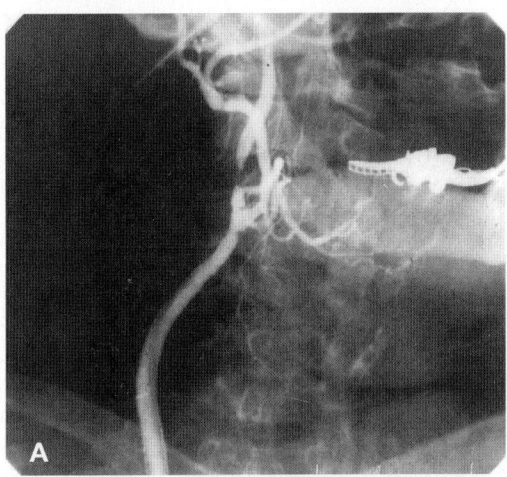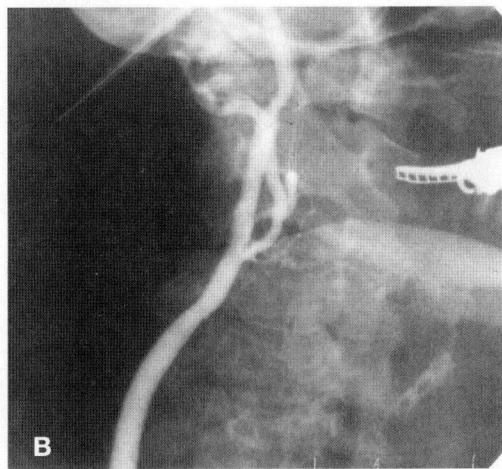

Figure 15-1. A. Preprocedural stenosis in a symptomatic restenosis patient (with permission: Hobson RW II et al. *J Vasc Surg.* 1999;29:228-238). **B.** Post-carotid angioplasty-stenting result using an 8 x 20 mm WallStent® (demonstrated by means of selective arteriography (with permission: Hobson RW II et al. *J Vasc Surg.* 1999;29:228-238).

TABLE 15-1. UPDATED PROTOCOL FOR CAROTID STENT (CAS) PROCEDURES (INNOVATIONS UNDERLINED)*

- Preprocedural Aspirin (325 mg p.o. qd or b.i.d.) and Clopidogrel (75 mg p.o. qd.).

- Transfemoral approach.

- Heparinization to <u>ACT 225-250</u> (with introduction of anti-embolic device)

- 5F Vitek catheter for cannulation of aortic arch branches.

- 0.035in. coated Terumo long exchange guidewire to external carotid artery.

- <u>6F guide sheath</u> (100 cm length) to common carotid artery proximal to lesion; occasional use of the 0.035 in. Amplatz stiff guidewire is recommended to advance the Vitek catheter or 6F guide sheath, into the common carotid artery.

- 0.014in guidewire to cross common-internal carotid stenosis, and place an <u>antiembolic device</u> (ACCUNET, Guidant, Santa Clara, CA); 3 or 4 mm low profile balloon for pre-deployment dilatation as required.

- Deployment of a <u>nitinol self-expanding stent</u> (ACCULINK, Guidant, Santa Clara, CA).

- Poststent dilatation using 5.0–5.5 mm balloons.

- Intermittent hand-injection angiography during procedure; utilize bony landmarks for balloon and stent placements.

- Routine use of <u>femoral closure device</u> (Angioseal, St. Jude Medical, Minnetonka, MN); aspirin and Clopidogrel are continued for a minimum of one month after CAS.

*Modified/Updated from Hobson RW et al. *J Vasc Surg* 1999; 29:228-238.23

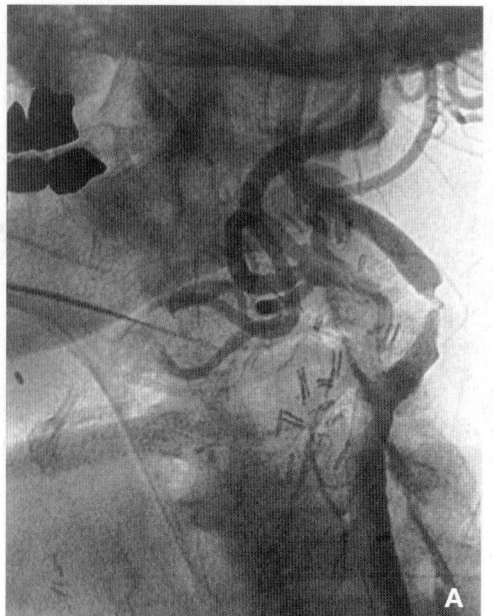 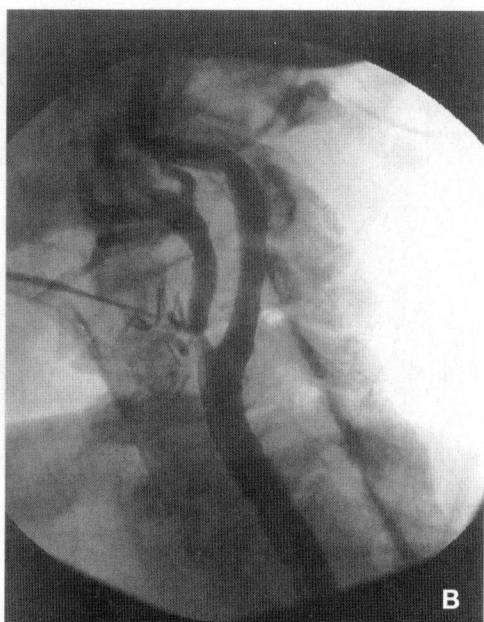

Figure 15-2. A. Selective lateral carotid angiogram shows high-grade stenosis in proximal internal carotid artery. **B.** Selective angiogram shows results after placement of a self-expandable nitinol stent **B.** An antiembolic device (ACCUNET) was used during the procedure.

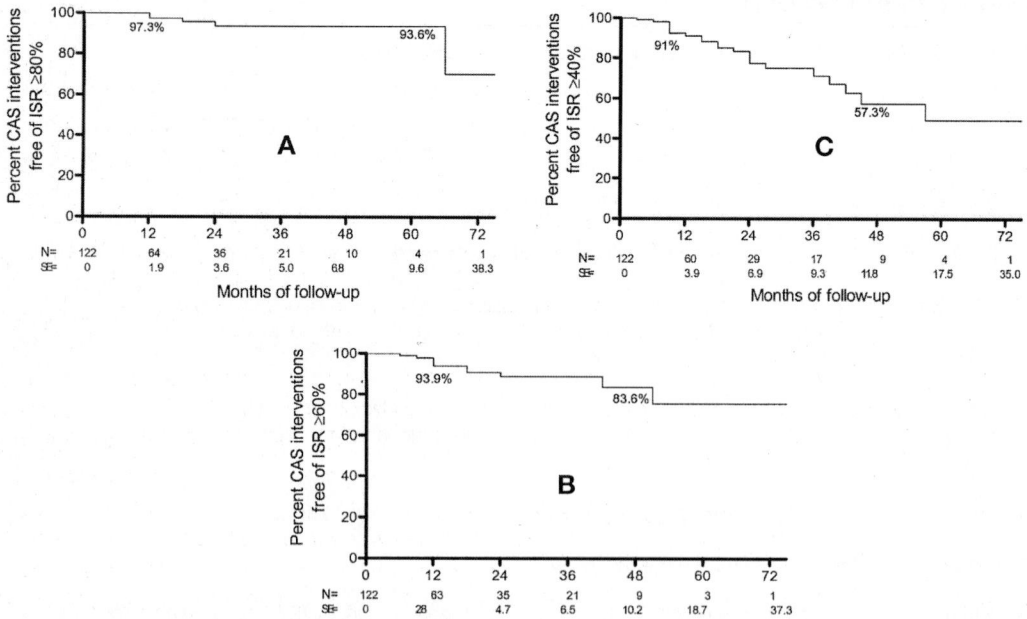

Figure 15-3. Cumulative life table analysis. **A.** Projected recurrence rates for 1 and 5 years were 2.7% and 6.4%, respectively, for clinically significant disease (in-stent recurrent stenosis ≥80%). Cumulative rates of in-stent recurrent stenosis 60% or greater **B.** at 1 and 4 years were 6.2% and 16.4%, respectively, and of in-stent recurrent stenosis 40% or greater (**C**) were 9.0% and 42.7%, respectively (with permission from Lal BK, Hobson RW II et al. *J Vasc Surg*. 2003;38:1162-1169).

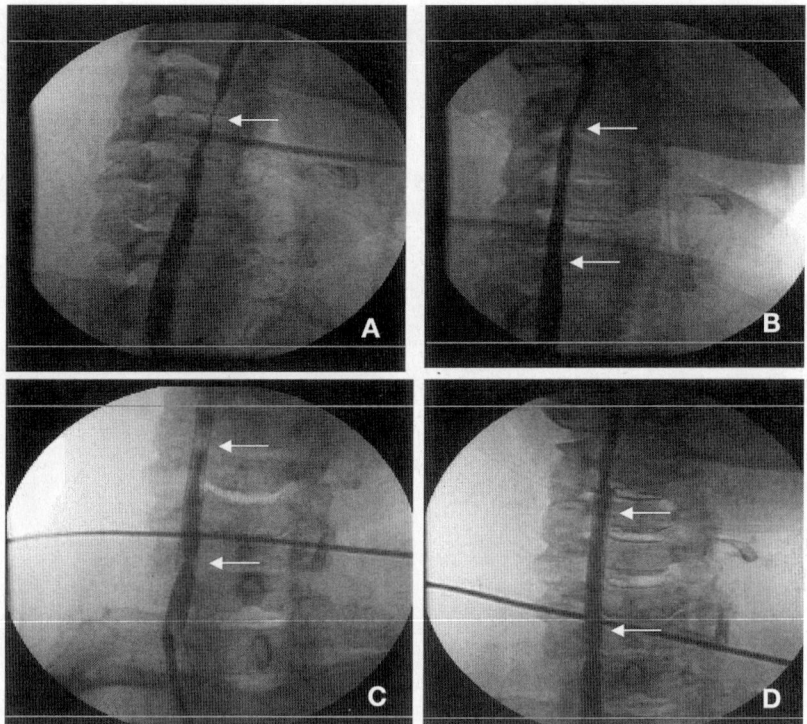

Figure 15-4. A. B. Selective angiogram of a lengthy symptomatic restenotic lesion after CEA treated by Wallstent®. **C. D.** In-stent restenosis 12 months later treated by balloon dilatation alone without subsequent recurrence.

(≥80%).[24] Management of in-stent restenosis (Figure 15–4) by repeat balloon angioplasty with or without placement of a second stent appears to be effective.

Advanced endovascular techniques have been used in 50/194 procedures (26%) of patients.[22] Cannulation of the common carotid artery has been facilitated by use of catheters other than the routinely employed Vitek catheter (Table 15–1) in12/50 cases (24%). These have included catheters such as the JB 1 or 2, Simmons, or Berenstein (Figure 15–5). Abnormal arch anatomy (bovine origin of the left common carotid from the innominate artery or more proximal origin of the innominate and left common carotid arteries from the ascending aorta) can result in difficulty with cannulation. A knowledge of various catheters will facilitate these maneuvers in most patients. We have also used 0.014 "buddy" wires in 24/50 cases (48%) of high-grade stenosis with internal carotid lumenal diameters of <1.0 mm (Figure 15–6). Predilatation is performed with low profile 2–3 mm balloons followed by placement of the antiembolic device. However, reduction in the profile of cerebral protection devices will facilitate performance of CAS without need for predilatation. An appreciation of contraindications to CAS including severe tortuosity or circumferential calcification (Figure 15–7), accounting for 4/50 cases (8%) is important. These cases are best treated by CEA. An analysis of CAS procedures using standard techniques (Group 1, n = 144, 74%) as compared with the group requiring advanced methods (Group 2, n = 50, 26%) demonstrated comparable 30-day stroke and death rates (Group 1 = 3.1%, Group 2 = 2.0%, p = 0.56).[22] Knowledge of these techniques will increase the number of cases for management by CAS without increasing the periprocedural risks.

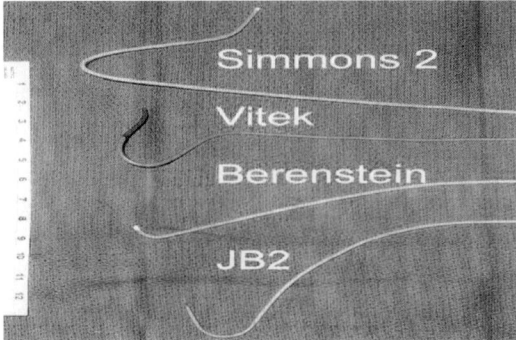

Figure 15-5. Catheters for cannulation of aortic arch branches.

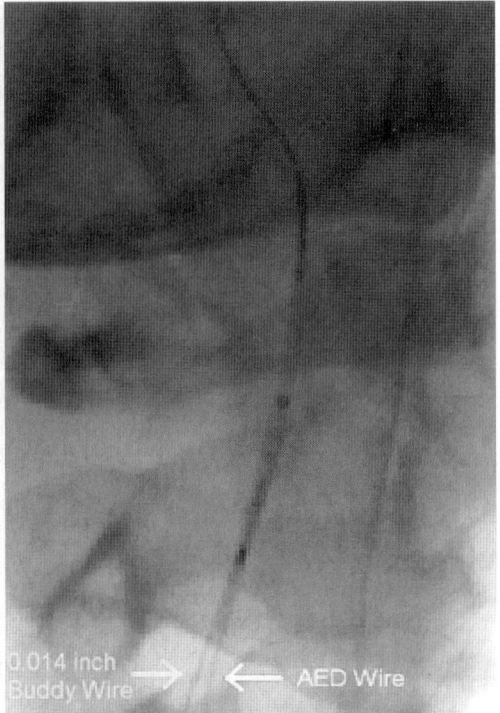

Figure 15-6. Cervical roentgenogram demonstrating placement of an 0.014 in "buddy" wire to allow pre-dilatation of a stenotic lesion and facilitate passage of an antiembolic device (AED).

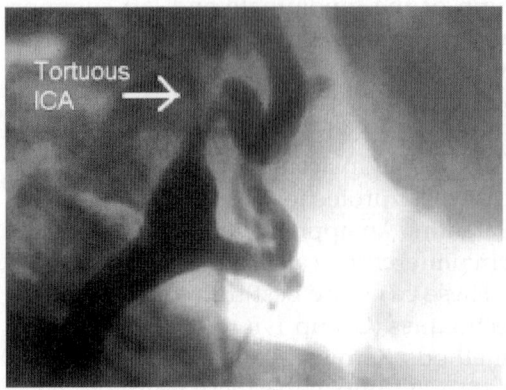

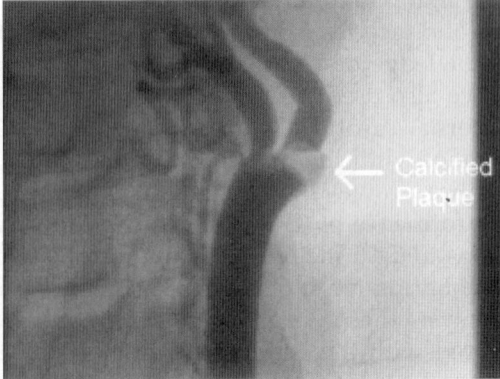

Figure 15-7. A: Selective carotid angiogram demonstrating severe tortuosity above a high-grade stenosis. B: Selective carotid angiogram identified a circumferentially calcified plaque.

Based on our experience with these subsets of patients as well as a review of published reports, data suggest that an efficacy trial such as CREST comparing the efficacy of CEA and CAS should proceed in this country.

CREST ORGANIZATION PLAN

The CREST investigators received approval for funding from the NINDS, NIH for a trial to compare efficacy of CEA and CAS in conventional symptomatic patients with stenoses to >50%.[10] However, recognizing that CAS is a relatively new procedure; each participating center was required to complete a credentialing phase so as to reassure clinicians that the safety of these procedures had been reviewed and established before proceeding with the randomized phase of the trial.

A lead-in or credentialing phase that requires performance of up to 20 interventional procedures at each of 60–70 participating centers is nearing completion to the satisfaction of the study's Interventional Management Committee, and randomization of patients between the two treatments was initiated in 2002. The primary outcome events for this clinical trial will include (1) any stroke, myocardial infarction, or death during the 30-day perioperative or periprocedural period, or (2) ipsilateral stroke after 30 days. Endpoints will be reviewed by an Adjudication Committee blinded to the assigned treatment. Stroke will be determined by a positive TIA/stroke questionnaire confirmed by an evaluation of a neurologist. Myocardial infarction will be determined by EKG and enzyme abnormalities. Secondary goals include (1) describing differential efficacy of the two treatments in men and women, (2) contrasting perioperative-procedural (30-day) morbidity and post-procedural (after 30 days) mortality for CEA and CAS, (3) estimating and contrasting the restenosis rates for the two procedures, (4) identifying subgroups of participants at differential risk for the two procedures, and (5) evaluating differences in health related quality of life issues and cost-effectiveness.

Differential efficacy assessment of CEA and CAS based on gender is a secondary goal for CREST. In patients with high-grade asymptomatic stenosis reported by ACAS, CEA offered a 66% reduction in events over a five-year period for men, but only a 17% reduction for women.[5] In NASCET, while no differential gender effects were reported among symptomatic patients with stenosis greater than 70%,[1] male patients demonstrated greater benefit after CEA than women for stenoses of 50–69%.[25] While the causes for these examples of differential efficacy between genders are not well understood, the effect may be attributed to a higher complication rate for CEA in women, possibly caused by their reported smaller arterial sizes and a greater surgical morbidity.[5] Unfortunately, neither ACAS or NASCET suspected the possibility of a differential gender effect. However, given the results of these two randomized clinical trials, a requirement for *a priori* plans to evaluate the possibility of a differential gender effect has become an important component of CREST. Centers are being selected with a goal of recruiting a patient sample with as high as 40% women in the randomized phase.

Patients will be evaluated at baseline, 24-hours postprocedure, 30 days, six months and thereafter at six-month intervals. Baseline procedures will include a brief medical history and physical examination, a risk factor evaluation, performance of neurological status questionnaires, a neurological examination, electrocardiogram (ECG), and a baseline carotid duplex scan. The 30-day follow-up will include evaluation of the neurological status through questionnaires, ECG, and a follow-up carotid duplex scan. All six month follow-up visits will include a brief physical, completion of the neurological questionnaire, risk factor evaluation, and carotid duplex scan. All patients with a positive neurological status questionnaire will be evaluated by a neurologist. The sample size for the study is approximately 2,500 symptomatic patients, which provides a 90% power to detect difference of greater than 1.2% per year in primary endpoints. Lesser differences would be considered sufficiently small to declare the treatments equivalent. Thus far, over 900 patients have been entered into the CREST lead-in or credentialing registry, while over 200 patients have been randomized.

RESULTS FROM THE CREST LEAD-IN REGISTRY

As noted in the organizational plan, interventionalists were credentialed by the performance of up to 20 CAS procedures in symptomatic (stenosis >50%) or asymptomatic patients (stenosis > 70%). Two-thirds of the patients in this registry[26] were asymptomatic stenosis patients and the remainder were entered with symptoms of amaurosis fugax, transient ischemic attack, or nondisabling stroke within the prior 180 days. Updated thirty-day stroke and death as well as stroke, MI, and death data are available on these groups of patients. As of March 2004, 845 patients from 57 centers have been entered into the CREST lead-in phase (208 randomizations). The 30-day combined stroke and death rate was 3.4% (95% CI: 1.7, 5.0). Myocardial infarctions were observed in 4 patients (<1%). For symptomatic patients, the 30-day stroke and death rate was 5.6% (CI 95%: 2.0, 9.2) and for asymptomatic patients the rate was 2.4% (95% CI 0.6, 4.1). These data included octogenarians, a group not previously included in NASCET or ACAS. However, 30-day stroke-death rates for the group have been reported as increased[27] and care must be exercised in recommending CAS for this high-risk subset. CREST reported an initial 30-day stroke and death rate among octogenarians of 11.8%,[27] significantly higher than observed for patients 70–79 (5.3%), 60–69 (1.3%), or less than 60 years old (1.7%).

CONCLUSIONS

Opinions have varied about the participation of interventionalists and vascular surgeons in randomized clinical trials comparing CEA and CAS. However, the emergence of clinical equipoise[9] between CEA and CAS as supported by a rigorous credentialing phase of CREST should reassure our colleagues about their participation as well as the ethical conduct of this trial. Clinical data from CREST confirm the opinion of increasing comparability between CEA and CAS, thereby reinforcing the need for an efficacy trial in good-risk patients.

REFERENCES

1. North American Symptomatic Carotid Endarterectomy Trial Collaborators. Beneficial effect of carotid endarterectomy in symptomatic patients with high-grade carotid stenosis. *N Engl J Med*. 1991;325:445–453.

2. European Carotid Surgery Trialists' Collaborative Group. MCR European Carotid Surgery Trial: Interim results for symptomatic patients with severe (70-99%) or with mild (0-29%) carotid stenosis. *Lancet*. 1991;337:1235–1243.

3. Mayberg MR, Wilson SE, Yatsu F and the VA Symptomatic Carotid Stenosis Group. Carotid endarterectomy and prevention of cerebral ischemia in symptomatic carotid stenosis. *JAMA*. 1991; 266:3289–3294.

4. Hobson RW II, Weiss DG, Fields WS, et al, and the Veterans Affairs Cooperative Study Group. Efficacy of carotid endarterectomy for asymptomatic carotid stenosis. *N Engl J Med*. 1993;328:221–227.

5. Executive Committee for the Asymptomatic Carotid Atherosclerosis Study: Endarterectomy for asymptomatic carotid stenosis. *JAMA*. 1995;273:1421–1428.

6. Roubin GS, New G, Iyer SS, et al. Immediate and late clinical outcomes of carotid artery stenting in patients with symptomatic and asymptomatic carotid artery stenosis: a 5-year prospective analysis. *Circulation*. 2001;103:532–537.

7. Yadav JS. Stenting and angioplasty with protection in patients at high risk from endarterectomy: The SAPPHIRE study. *Circulation*. 2002;106:2986a.

8. Brown MM, Rogers J, Bland JM and the CAVATAS Investigators: Endovascular versus surgical treatment in patients with carotid stenosis in the carotid and vertebral artery transluminal angioplasty study (CAVATAS): A randomized trial. *Lancet*. 2001;357:1729–1737.

9. Freedman B. Equipoise and the ethics of clinical research. *N Engl J Med*. 1987;317:141–145.

10. Hobson RW II. Update on the Carotid Revascularization Endarterectomy versus Stent Trial (CREST) protocol. *J Am Coll Surg*. 2002;194(1 Suppl):S9–14.

11. Kunze AK, Ringleb PA, Hacke W, et al. The SPACE Study (Stent-Protected percutaneous Angioplasty of the Carotid vs. Endarterectomy). Poster presentation, 28th International Stroke Conference, February, 2003, Phoenix, AZ.

12. Veith FJ, Amor M, Ohki T, et al. Current status of carotid bifurcation angioplasty and stenting based on a consensus of opinion leaders. *J Vasc Surg*. 2001;33:S111–116.

13. Bettmann MA, Katzen BT, Whisnant J, et al. Carotid stenting and angioplasty; A statement from the Councils on Cardiovascular Radiology, Stroke, Cardio-thoracic and Vascular Surgery, Epidemiology and Prevention, and Clinical Cardiology, American Heart Association. *Stroke*.1998;29:336–346.

14. Hobson RW II, Goldstein JE, Jamil Z, et al. Carotid restenosis: Operative and endovascular management. *J Vasc Surg*. 1999;29:228–238.

15. Lattimer CR, Burnand KG. Recurrent carotid stenosis after carotid endarterectomy. *Br J Surg*. 1997;84:1206–1219.

16. Stoney RJ, String ST. Recurrent carotid stenosis. *Surgery*. 1976;80(6):705–710.

17. Bartlett FF, Rapp JH, Goldstone J, et al. Recurrent carotid stenosis: Operative strategy and late results. *J Vasc Surg*. 1987;5:452–456.

18. Bergeron P, Chambran P, Benichou H, Alessandri C. Recurrent carotid disease: Will stents be an alternative to surgery? *J Endovasc Surg*. 1996; 3:76–79.

19. Yadav JS, Roubin GS, King P, et al. Angioplasty and stenting for restenosis after carotid endarterectomy. Initial experience. *Stroke*. 1996; 27:2075–2079.

20. Chakhtoura EY, Hobson RW II, Goldstein J, et al. In-stent restenosis after carotid angioplasty stenting: Incidence and management. *J Vasc Surg*. 2001;33:220–226.

21. Hobson RW II, Lal BK, Chakhtoura E, et al. Carotid artery stenting: Analysis of 105 high-risk patients. *J Vasc Surg*. 2003;37:1234–1239.

22. Choi HM, Hobson RW II, Goldstein J, et al. Technical challenges encountered in a program of carotid stenting. *J Vasc Surg*. 2004;40:746–751.

23. Hobson RW II, Lal BK, Chakhtoura EY, et al. Carotid artery closure for endarterectomy does not influence results of angioplasty-stenting for restenosis. *J Vasc Surg*. 2002;35:435–438.

24. Lal Bk, Hobson RW II, Goldstein J, et al. In-stent restenosis after carotid artery stenting: Life table analysis and clinical relevance. *J Vasc Surg*. 2003;38:1162–1169.

25. Barnett HJM, Taylor DW, Eliasziw M, et al for the North American Symptomatic Carotid Endarterectomy Trial Collaborators. Benefit of carotid endarterectomy in patients with symptomatic moderate or severe stenosis. *N Engl J Med*. 1998;339:1415–1425.

26. Hobson RW II, Brott TG, Roubin GS, et al. Carotid stenting in the CREST lead-in phase: Periprocedural stroke myocardial infarction, and death rates are lower than reported for preceding stent trials. *Circulation*. 2003;108(17):IV604.
27. Howard G, Hobson RW II, Brott TG, et al for the CREST Investigators. Does the stroke risk of stenting increase at older ages? Thirty-day stroke - death rates in the CREST Lead-in phase. *Circulation*. 2003;108 (17):IV688.

16

Update on ACT I

Jon S. Matsumura, M.D.
Kenneth Rosenfield, M.D.
Gary M. Ansel, M.D., F.A.C.C.
Seemant Chaturvedi, M.D.
William A. Gray, M.D.
Thomas S. Riles, M.D.
Lawrence R. Wechsler, M.D.

ACAS and ACST are large pivotal randomized trials that established indications for carotid endarterectomy (CEA) in selected patients with asymptomatic stenosis of >/=60%.[1-2] Treatment guidelines of the Society for Vascular Surgery published in 2008 have found "low quality evidence" for recommending against carotid artery stenting (CAS) for asymptomatic patients who are not high anatomic risk for CEA.[3] This is because randomized trials that directly compare CEA to CAS have included remarkably few asymptomatic patients.[4-6] This chapter will review the paucity of existing data, and describe clinical trials in progress to more completely explore the role of CAS in asymptomatic standard risk patients. In contrast, four randomized trials focused on symptomatic standard risk subjects have failed to show noninferiority between CEA and CAS.

Carotid and Vertebral Artery Transluminal Angioplasty Study (CAVATAS) randomized 504 subjects; only 60 (12%) were asymptomatic to CEA or carotid angioplasty with and without stenting (74% had angioplasty alone).[4] None had embolic protection (EPD). Prior experience records of investigators were reviewed and some centers received assistance from veteran centers. Thirty-day stroke (defined as symptoms for more than seven days) and death rates were 9.9% in the open surgery group and 10% in the endovascular arm. Restenosis was more common in the angioplasty arm, but there was no difference in stroke rate at three years after randomization. While this trial was a randomized trial that showed similar results, CAS technology has matured significantly with routine use of stenting and EPD. In fact, a second follow-up trial with routine stenting (CAVATAS-2) is underway although embolic protection is not routinely recommended.

A single center randomized trial was performed in Kentucky in 85 asymptomatic patients.[5] There were no complications in the CEA or endovascular arm. Although these results also showed similar outcomes between treatments, it is striking how much better the outcomes are when compared to the CAVATAS trial.

The Stenting and Angioplasty with Protection in Patients at High Risk for Endarterectomy (SAPPHIRE) trial randomized 334 subjects; 71% were asymptomatic to receive CEA or CAS with routine EPD.[6] This trial is different because it included patients who had criteria that were deemed to make them high risk for CEA. Also, SAPPHIRE had one of the highest preexisting CAS volumes, along with a quality threshold. Interventionalists were required to have < 6% periprocedural stroke/death; median prior experience of physicians was 64 cases with a range of 20–700 CAS procedures. In comparison, the median annual volume of each surgeon was 30 cases. In the entire cohort, 30-day composite stroke/death/myocardial infarction rates were 12.6% with CEA and 5.8% with CAS. The 30-day stroke/death rates were 5.4% with CEA and 4.8% with CAS. In this trial of very experienced operators with known complication rates of <6%, noninferiority of CAS and CEA was demonstrated in patients at high risk for CEA.

The lead-in phase for the Carotid Revascularization Endarterectomy vs. Stenting Trial (CREST) required interventionalists to submit results from 10–30 CAS cases.[7,8] The initial design was focused on symptomatic patients only, and there was a quality threshold of 30-day stroke/death rate <6% for symptomatic patients and satisfactory performance in the lead-in phase. The lead-in portion of the trial included patients at high and low risk for CEA and a mix of asymptomatic and symptomatic patients. Thirty-day stroke/death rate was about 4.6% in an earlier publication of lead-in data. Initially, a study of standard risk patients with symptomatic stenosis, CREST was subsequently modified to include enrollment of both symptomatic and asymptomatic patients to improve the pace of enrollment. In 2008, CREST completed enrollment with over 1,300 symptomatic patients and about 1,200 asymptomatic patients, but the preliminary results of the randomized phase will not be available until late 2009.

HIGH RISK FOR CAS CONCEPT

Published randomized trials with asymptomatic patients have shown similar results with CEA and CAS, although they have heterogeneous outcome rates. Process of care improvements over several decades have led to optimizing CEA outcomes using patient and physician selection criteria, advances in perioperative medical management, systemic heparin anticoagulation, routine patching or eversion technique, shunting routines, and anesthetic preference. CAS is comparatively new, and optimal CAS techniques are emerging.

Postmarket registries, like the CAPTURE trial, provide the largest databases of contemporary CAS procedures with routine use of embolic protection.[9] CAPTURE has independent neurologic assessment that is recommended in society-endorsed guidelines and often leads to better detection of procedural stroke compared to population-based studies. Because of its size, there is adequate statistical power for multivariate analysis to identify variables that predict stroke. A multivariate model was created using stepwise regression using initial univariate analysis at P<0.25. Only patients with complete data for all selected variables were included and missing data were not imputed. The final multivariate model included parameters with P<0.05. These independent predictors are age > 80 years, symptomatic status, balloon predilation without EPD, and multiple stents. Experienced clinicians, reflecting their observations from practice, have published criteria of high-risk factors for CAS, including octogenarians, recent symptoms, severe tortuousity and calcification (the latter anatomic situations are conditions associated with multiple stents or precluding EPD).[10]

ACT I

The Asymptomatic Carotid Stenosis: Stenting versus Endarterectomy Trial (ACT I) was conceived on this background of recognizing factors that are high risk for CEA or CAS. Specifically, ACT I is a prospective, randomized, multicenter trial comparing CEA and CAS for the treatment of asymptomatic patients with significant unilateral carotid stenosis who are at standard risk for both CEA and CAS. Exclusion criteria include prior CEA, high-risk anatomy, octogenarians, and symptomatic carotid disease. Site selection involves detailed screening of training, experience, and outcomes of both surgeons and interventionalists. The weighted randomization ratio is 1 CEA:3 CAS in up to 1,658 subjects. Prior trials have generated a wealth of information on CEA, and the weighted randomization will provide a larger sample size of CAS patients to assess uncommon CAS issues. Contemporary CEA and CAS techniques, such as routine EPD and adjunctive medical therapy, are expressly prescribed. Figure 16–1 illustrates a patient with high-grade stenosis treated with CAS and EP. The primary outcome is a composite of any stroke, myocardial infarction, and death during a 30-day postprocedural period and ipsilateral stroke between 31 and 365 days postprocedure. All patients have independent neurologic examination at 24 hours, 30 days, six months, and annually for five years (Table 16–1). Further, there are committees for independent data safety monitoring, surgical management, interventional management, and clinical events adjudication; and corelabs for electrocardiograms, duplex ultrasounds, and angiograms. ACT I is sponsored by Abbott Vascular.

TABLE 16-1. ACT I FOLLOW-UP EVALUATION SCHEDULE

Evaluation	30 Days (±7 days)	6 Months (±14 days)	12 Months and Annually for Four Additional Years Years (±30 days)
Independent Neurological Examination	√	√	√
NIH Stroke Scale / Barthel Index / Modified Rankin Scale	√	√	√
Fasting Lipid Panel		√	√
Electrocardiogram	√		
Bilateral carotid duplex ultrasound	√		√

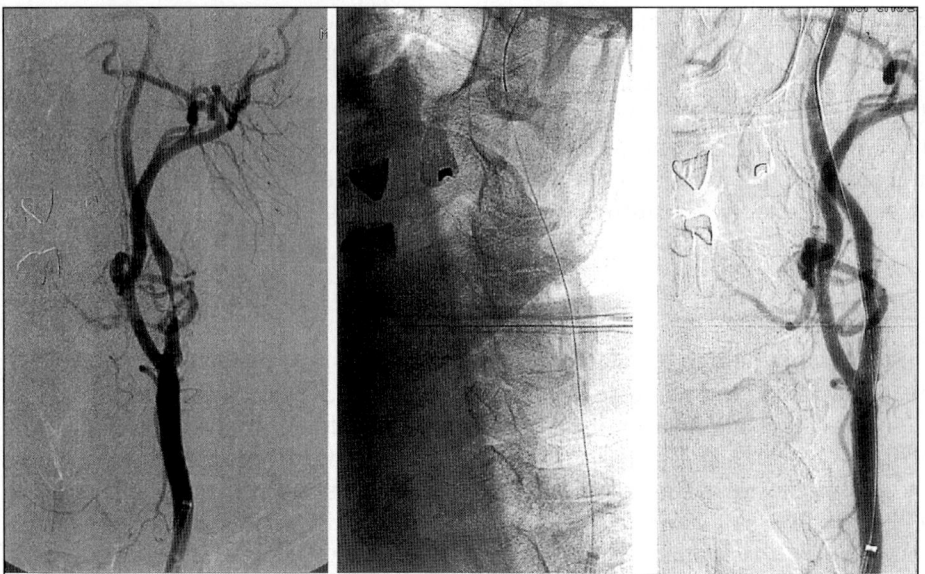

Figure 16-1. Left panel is selective left carotid arteriogram of subject with a high grade carotid stenosis. Center panel shows deployment of barewire for embolic protection filter in the distal internal carotid artery. Right panel is arteriogram after placement of tapered, closed cell carotid stent.

SUMMARY

Process of care is evolving with CAS, and the concept of high-risk CAS has emerged. Early trials with relatively inexperienced interventionalists, absent embolic protection, angioplasty alone or with nondedicated stents, and unselected application in all patients have shown suboptimal outcomes with CAS, and many were stopped. Randomized trials provide the best evidence to compare treatment strategies, and ACT I will evaluate contemporary techniques of CAS compared to CEA in the asymptomatic patient who is standard risk for both procedures. These trials must be large and have long follow-up to be adequately powered to detect the margins of benefit with intervention on asymptomatic patients with severe carotid stenosis. Current treatment recommendations are based on the committed work of previous investigators in ACAS and ACST, and large trials like ACT I should be supported and completed in order to gain evidence for the best future treatment of patients with carotid stenosis.

REFERENCES

1. Executive Committee for the Asymptomatic Carotid Atherosclerosis Study. Endarterectomy for Asymptomatic Carotid Artery Stenosis. *JAMA*. 1995;273:1421–28.
2. MRC Asymptomatic Carotid Surgery Trial (ACST) Collaborative Group. *The Lancet*. 363: May 2004. 1491–1502.
3. Hobson RW, Mackey WC, Ascher E, et al. Management of atherosclerotic carotid artery disease: Clinical practice guidelines of the Society for Vascular Surgery. *J Vasc Surg*. 2008;48: 480–6.

4. CAVATAS Investigators. Endovascular versus surgical treatment in patients with carotid stenosis in the carotid and vertebral artery transluminal angioplasty study: a randomized trial. *Lancet*. 2001;35:1729–37.

5. Brooks WH, McClure RR, Jones MR, et al. Carotid angioplasty and stenting versus carotid endarterectomy: randomized trial in a community hospital. *J Am Coll Cardiol*. 2001;38: 1589–95.

6. Yadav JS, Wholey MH, Kuntz RE, et al. Protected carotid-artery stenting versus endarterectomy in high-risk patients. *N Engl J Med*. 2004;351:1493–501.

7. Hobson RW II, Howard VJ, Roubin GS et al. Carotid artery stenting is associated with increased complications in octogenarians: 30-day stroke and death rates in the CREST lead-in phase. *J Vasc Surg*. 2004;40:1106–11.

8. Hobson RW II, Howard Virginia, Roubin GS et al. Credentialing of surgeons as interventionalists for carotid artery stenting: Experience from the lead-in phase of CREST. *J Vasc Surg*. 2004;40:952–7.

9. Roubin GS, Iyer S, Halkin A, Vitek J, Brennan C. Realizing the potential of carotid artery stenting: Proposed paradigms for patient selection and procedural technique. *Circulation*. 2006;113:2021–30.

10. Gray W. The CAPTURE Registry: Predictors of Outcomes in Carotid Artery Stenting with Embolic Protection for High Surgical Risk Patients in the Early Post-Approval Setting. *Cathetet Cardiovasc Intervent*. 70:1025–1033 (2007).

17

Lessons Learned from Italian Registry for Carotid Stenting (RISC) in 1,000 Cases

GM Biasi M.D., F.A.C.S., F.R.C.S., G Deleo M.D.,
L Inglese M.D., A Cremonesi M.D., A Froio M.D.,
V Camesasca M.D., C Piazzoni M.D., and A Liloia M.D.,
for the RISC Investigators

The effectiveness of carotid endarterectomy (CEA) in the prevention of stroke in symptomatic and asymptomatic patients with carotid stenosis has been demonstrated by several randomized studies.[1-2] Carotid artery stenting (CAS) is an alternative technique that gives favorable results when associated with the use of brain protection devices (BPD).[3]

Recent randomized studies tend to demonstrate the noninferiority of carotid artery stenting (CAS) compared to carotid endarterectomy for the treatment of carotid stenosis.[4] Nevertheless, a review of the randomized evidence does not support changes in clinical practice, apart from recommending carotid endarterectomy as the treatment of choice for suitable carotid artery stenosis.[5]

Several ongoing randomized trials are now comparing CEA with CAS in order to establish the gold standard in the prevention of stroke,[6-7] and the results are expected to be published in four or five years' time. After such a long period, it is probable that the stent and the BPD used in those trials will have become obsolete. The establishment of a registry has been considered in order to obtain results in a shorter lapse of time, without limitations due to the fact that in a randomized study, the type of the stent and the BPD cannot change throughout the trial.

The Italian Registry for Carotid Stenting (RISC: Registro Italiano per lo Stenting Carotideo) has been proposed by specialists of different disciplines interested and directly involved in Italy in the prevention of stroke due to carotid plaques through stenting of carotid lesions. The aim of the Study was to constitute a multidisciplinary working group collecting data on carotid stenting procedures performed by different specialists with different techniques, outside randomized clinical trials, in the "real word" settings.

METHODS

The Registry

A national multicenter, multidisciplinary, nonrandomized, prospective study was created in May 2001, with the collaboration of Vascular Surgeons (VS), Interventional Radiologists (IR), Cardiologists (IC), and Neuroradiologists (INR). The Registry has been endorsed by four Italian Societies: Società Italiana di Chirurgia Vascolare ed Endovascolare (SICVE, for Vascular Surgery), Società Italiana di Cardiologia Invasiva (GISE, for Interventional Cardiology), Società Italiana di Radiologia Medica (SIRM, for Radiology) and Associazione Italiana di Neuro-radiologia (AINR, for Neuroradiology). Each Society provided its contribution in the planning stage.

The four disciplines are represented in the Executive Committee (EC) and in the Scientific Committee (SC) of the Registry.

One representative from each company sponsoring the initiative (Boston Scientific Italia S.p.A., Cordis Italia S.p.A., Endotech, Guidant Italia S.r.l., Medtronic Italia S.p.A.) is included in the EC. All companies manufacturing carotid stents have been involved in order to provide the most recent updates on devices, and to ensure impartiality and transparency in the registry. It is important to stress that companies will not be involved in any way in data collection, elaboration, and analysis.

The SC, completely independent of EC, will check that the enrolling criteria are fulfilled and will enforce each defaulting Center to strictly observe the protocol. Moreover, the SC will convene on a regular basis, providing a thorough control of data, and with on-site visits and inspections.

Center Selection

Inclusion criteria for centers were the following:

- At least 10 carotid stenting procedures in the last 12 months.
- A multidisciplinary team including a vascular surgeon and a neurologist.

Patient Enrollment and Online Database:

Patients were recruited before the procedure by fax. The procedure was the following:

- Introduction by the participating center of demographic information of the patient using the online database (https://www.risc.unimib.org/default.htm).
- Fax form printing from the Web site.
- Fax-sending to the Data Coordinating Center.
- Code assignment.
- Patient enrollment.

All steps were completed before the procedure.

Clinical and periprocedural data were collected within 72 hours after the procedure through the Web site.

Patient Evaluation

The following evaluations were performed before the procedure:

- Blood sampling.
- Cardiologic and neurological examination.

- Carotid duplex scanning with description of characteristics of carotid plaques (echogenicity, homogeneity, surface).
- Brain CT or MRI scan.
- Supra-aortic vessel angiography with intracranial views.

Endovascular Procedures:

Indications to treatment were based on the guidelines of the respective societies.

Each center was free to use different techniques and devices (guidewires, catheters, balloons, stents, brain protection devices).

Endpoints and Follow-up

The primary endpoint of the study will be:

- Any stroke (both minor/major and ipsicontralateral) and any death within 30 days.
- Rate of restenosis after six, 12 and 24 months.
- Rate of ipsilateral stroke after six, 12 and 24 months.

A TIA will be defined as a focal neurologic deficit lasting less than 24 hours. A stroke will be considered disabling (major) with a Rankin Score of 3 or more at 90 days.

A fatal stroke will be defined as death attributed to an ischemic stroke or intracerebral hemorrhagic stroke.

The follow-up will be scheduled as follows:

- A physical examination and a carotid duplex scan will be performed by a medical doctor (no technicians) at one, six, 12, and 24 months.
- The occurrence of any stroke and transient ischemic attack (TIA) during the procedure, at discharge, and during follow-up, will be carefully evaluated by means of CT or MRI, and by an independent neurologist who will be blind to clinical data and outcome of stenting procedure.
- Restenosis will be defined as a reduction of internal carotid lumen > 50% on duplex imaging.

Data Collection and Analysis

Fondazione Villa Maria (FVM), a nonprofit organization with clinical and managerial experience in managing databases, was identified and hired to collect and analyze the RISC data in order to guarantee transparency and independency.

RESULTS

One thousand four hundred fifty-four (1,454) CAS procedures were performed, 244 patients were excluded after recruitment due to protocol violation, and 1,210 patients entered the registry. Twenty-eight percent of procedures were performed by vascular surgeons, 36% by cardiologists, and 36% by radiologists.

Asymptomatic patients were 863/1,210 (71.3%), primitive lesions 1042/1210 (86.1%), positive pre-procedural cerebral CT scan 418/1,210 (34.5%).

Technical success was achieved in 1,195/1,210 patients (98.7%). A brain protection device was used in 1,107/1,210 patients (91.5%). The 30-day death rate was 0.7%, the stroke rate was 1.2% for a combined rate of 1.9%. Six hundred twenty-three, 367, and 131 patients were analyzed at six months, 12 months, and two years of follow-up. The ipsilateral stroke and neurological death rate was 0.3%, 0.7%, and 0.7% after six months, 12 months, and two years, respectively. The restenosis rate was 6.0%, 3.0%, 2.4%, and 0.8% after one month, six months, 12 months, and two years, respectively.

DISCUSSION

Data from international, multicenter, and prospective studies has proved the effectiveness of CAS, especially when performed under brain protection, in preventing brain embolization from carotid plaques with results that seem to match those obtained with CEA.[3,8]

The role of carotid plaque echolucency as a predictor of stroke during CAS has recently been demonstrated.[9] The Gray Scale Median (GSM), a computer-assisted objective index of carotid echolucency, has been used to identify plaques at different risk of stroke. Patients with a GSM value lower than 25 had a higher risk of stroke compared to those with a GSM value higher than 25.

There is, at present, no randomized evidence that CAS provides better results as compared with CEA in the prevention of brain embolization from carotid plaques.[5,10-11] Indication to CEA or CAS is not supported by solid data and is still very controversial. A correct selection or nonselection of patients, like the concept of "the real population," might put a final word to this challenging situation, but for the time being, registries are likely to produce more rapidly reliable information.

The RISC registry was the first multidisciplinary trial, endorsed by societies of four different specialties (Vascular Surgery, Cardiology, Radiology, and Neuroradiology). Centers were not obliged to use a specific stent from the sponsoring company. In this trial, *all* carotid stent manufacturing companies have been involved in order to guarantee transparency and the highest level of technology. The online database provided an accurate tool to collect data.

CONCLUSION

CAS is a safe procedure with good results in the "real world" setting outside clinical trials as evidenced by this multicenter, multidisciplinary registry. Brain protection devices are useful in reducing the rate of neurological complications, even if neurological death and stroke still persist, which stresses the importance of carotid plaque evaluation to reduce the embolic load to the brain.

RISC INVESTIGATORS

Istituto Policlinico San Donato, U.O. di Chirurgia Vascolare 1a—San Donato Milanese—
    D. Tealdi M.D.

Istituto Policlinico San Donato, Servizio di Emodinamica e Radiologia Interventistica—San Donato Milanese—L. Inglese M.D.

Azienda Ospedaliera G. Salvini, U.O. di Chirurgia Vascolare—Garbagnate Milanese—R. Mattassi M.D.

Ospedale Maggiore C.A. Pizzardi, Servizio di Radiologia 2a—Bologna, A. Ziosi M.D.

Centro Nazionale per il Salvataggio d'Arto—Milano—E. Calabrese M.D.

EMO Centro Cuore Columbus—Milano—A. Colombo M.D.

Policlinico Le Scotte, U.O. di Chirurgia Vascolare—Siena—C. Setacci, M.D.

Azienda Ospedaliera C‡ Granda Niguarda, U.O. di Chirurgia Vascolare—Milano—M. Puttini M.D.

Casa Sollievo della Sofferenza, Servizio di Radiologia Interventistica—San Giovanni Rotondo—W. Lauriola M.D.

Cliniche Gavazzeni, U.O. di Neuroradiologia—Bergamo—P. Sganzerla M.D.

Ospedale Maggiore San Giovanni Battista Molinette, Servizio di Angioradiologia Interventistica—Torino—C. Rabbia M.D.

Ospedale Mauriziano Umberto I, Servizio di Radiologia—Torino—P. Carbonatto M.D.

Azienda Ospedaliera San Gerardo Ospedale Bassini, U.O. di Chirurgia Vascolare—Cinisello Balsamo—G. Deleo M.D.

Ospedale Civile Sant'Agostino, U.O. di Chirurgia Vascolare—Modena—G. Coppi MD;

Policlinico Tor Vergata, Servizio di Radiologia—Roma—G. Simonetti MD;

Policlinico Umberto I, U.O. di Chirurgia Vascolare—Roma—F. Benedetti Valentini M.D.

Policlinico Sant'Orsola, U.O. di Chirurgia Vascolare—Bologna—M. D'Addato M.D.

Villa Maria Cecilia Hospital, Servizio di Emodinamica—Cotignola—A. Cremonesi M.D.

Azienda Ospedaliera Santissima Annunziata, Servizio di Radiologia—Taranto—M. Resta M.D.

Policlinico Le Scotte, U.O. di Neuroradiologia—Siena—C. Venturi M.D.

Azienda Ospedaliera Sant'Anna, Servizio di Emodinamica—Como—R. Galli M.D.

Ospedale di Careggi, U.O. Cardiologia 2a—Firenze—M. Santoro M.D.

Azienda Ospedaliera Manzoni, U.O. di Chirurgia Vascolare—Lecco - G. Lorenzi M.D.

REFERENCES

1. Ferguson GG, Eliasziw M, Barr HW et al. The North American Symptomatic Carotid Endarterectomy Trial : surgical results in 1415 patients. *Stroke*. 1999;30(9):1751–1758.
2. Halliday A, Mansfield A, Marro J, et al. MRC Asymptomatic Carotid Surgery Trial (ACST) Collaborative Group. Prevention of disabling and fatal strokes by successful carotid endarterectomy in patients without recent neurological symptoms: randomised controlled trial. *Lancet*. 2004;363(9420):1491–1502.
3. Cremonesi A, Manetti R, Setacci F et al. Protected carotid stenting: clinical advantages and complications of embolic protection devices in 442 consecutive patients. *Stroke*. 2003;34(8): 1936–1941. Epub 2003 Jul 3.
4. Yadav JS, Wholey MH, Kuntz RE et al. Stenting and Angioplasty with Protection in Patients at High Risk for Endarterectomy Investigators. Protected carotid-artery stenting versus endarterectomy in high-risk patients. *N Engl J Med*. 2004;351(15):1493–1501.
5. Coward LJ, Featherstone RL, Brown MM. Safety and efficacy of endovascular treatment of carotid artery stenosis compared with carotid endarterectomy: a Cochrane systematic review of the randomized evidence. *Stroke*. 2005;36(4):905–911. Epub 2005 Mar 3.
6. Hobson RW 2nd, Howard VJ, Roubin GS et al. CREST Investigators. *J Vasc Surg*. 2004;40(6): 1106–1111.

7 CARESS Steering Committee. Carotid revascularization using endarterectomy or stenting systems (CARESS): phase I clinical trial. *J Endovasc Ther.* 2003;10(6):1021–1030.

8. Roubin GS, New G, Iyer SS et al. Immediate and late clinical outcomes of carotid artery stenting in patients with symptomatic and asymptomatic carotid artery stenosis: a 5-year prospective analysis. *Circulation.* 2001;103(4):532–537.

9. Biasi GM, Froio A, Diethrich EB et al. Carotid plaque echolucency increases the risk of stroke in carotid stenting: the Imaging in Carotid Angioplasty and Risk of Stroke (ICAROS) study. *Circulation.* 2004;110(6):756–762.

10. Cambria RP. Stenting for carotid-artery stenosis. *N Engl J Med.* 2004;351(15):1565-7.

11. Eliasziw M, Barnett HJ. Carotid-artery stenting versus endarterectomy. *N Engl J Med.* 2005;352(6):624–7; author reply 624–7.

SECTION V

Perioperative Care after Carotid Stent Intervention

18

Preventable Complications of Carotid Stenting

Katherine E. Brown, D.O.
and Mark K. Eskandari, M.D.

Advances in endovascular therapies have allowed for carotid artery angioplasty and stenting (CAS) to now be recognized as an acceptable alternative for treating extracranial carotid artery stenosis. Notable trials comparing CAS to carotid endarterectomy (CEA) in both high-risk populations and the community at large have been published with compelling results.[1-5] SAPPHIRE randomized high-risk patients to either CAS with embolic protection versus CEA, and showed that CAS was not inferior to CEA when the combined endpoints of myocardial infarction (MI), stroke, and death were examined.[1] ARCHeR also concluded that, when compared to high-risk CEA historical controls, CAS with cerebral protection was not inferior to CEA using similar primary endpoints. CaRESS,[3] a nonrandomized, equivalence cohort study, showed that the patients who underwent CAS with various forms of mechanical embolic protection had similar rates of 30-day outcomes as did patients in earlier CEA studies.[6,7]

Fortunately, vascular surgeons have embraced this technologic leap of faith and are rapidly achieving a greater presence among the various subspecialty physicians performing CAS with good outcomes.[8,9] As the application of CAS continues to gain momentum, a larger body of data is available for review, which will be helpful in detecting the causes of failures. This chapter will provide an overview of some of the more common problems and challenges associated with CAS, as well as potential solutions.

IATROGENIC ARTERIAL INJURY (LOCAL AND REMOTE)

Access Site Vessels

As with any interventional procedure, access to the arterial system has its own unique set of complications. Typically, femoral arterial access is used for CAS. Many such

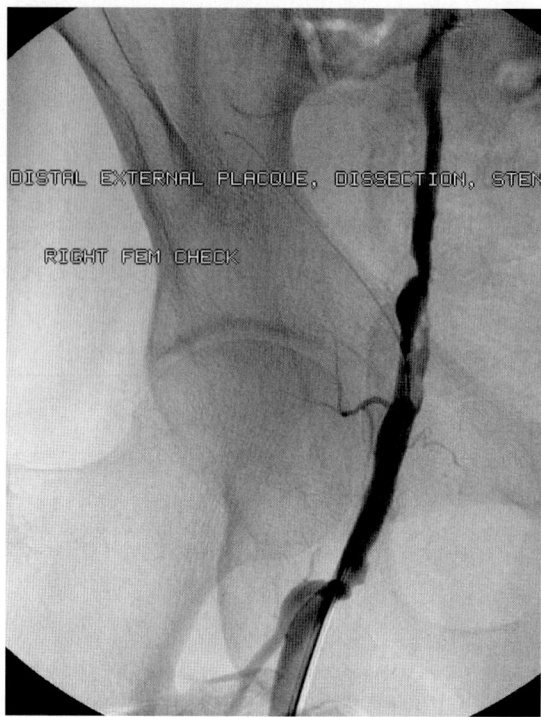

DISTAL EXTERNAL PLACQUE, DISSECTION, STEN

RIGHT FEM CHECK

Figure 18-1. Angiogram of an iatrogenic external iliac artery dissection.

patients will have coexisting peripheral vascular occlusive disease, which may predispose them to increased risks of dissection (Figure 18-1), infection, hematoma, pseudoaneurysm, arteriovenous fistula, thrombosis, and retroperitoneal hematoma following any percutaneous intervention. A recent study showed that operative repair is required for complications arising from endoluminal procedures at a rate of 0.7% for diagnostic angiography alone, to as high as 3.4% after interventional therapies.[10] The use of large diameter sheaths and concomitant systemic anticoagulation are known to result in higher periprocedural complications.[10-12]

Pseudoaneurysm and Arteriovenous Fistula

Femoral pseudoaneurysms (FPAs) are one of the more frequent of the vascular complications requiring treatment after percutaneous interventions. A recent report documents the rate of FPAs to be 1.7% for all angiographic procedures. Of these, the incidence of FPAs that required surgical repair was 1.1% after diagnostic procedures and 4.7% following interventional procedures.[13] Identified risk factors were noted to be presence of hypertension, high body mass index (BMI), sheath sizes exceeding 7Fr, improper location of arterial puncture site (either in the external iliac artery or below the common femoral bifurcation), inadequate compression of the vessel at completion of the procedure, and excessive anticoagulation. The majority of small (<3 cm), nonenlarging, asymptomatic FPAs can be managed expectantly, with many thrombosing spontaneously over one to two weeks.[14,15] For FPAs that do not thrombose spontaneously, alternative therapy is indicated. Proposed options have evolved over the last decade from surgical repair to ultrasound guided compression, and now ultrasound guided thrombin injection achieving prompt durable results.[16,17] On the other hand, iatrogenic arteriovenous fistulae, which occur with less frequency, typically require operative repair.

Hematoma (Local and Retroperitoneal)

Similarly, groin hematomas and retroperitoneal hematomas are a direct result of improper puncture technique or inadequate compression of the vessel on removal of the sheath. Groin hematomas, the most common complication, can occur in up to 10% of angiographic procedures, but those requiring transfusion or surgical intervention account for less than 0.5% of cases.[18] The incidence of retroperitoneal hematoma is reported at 0.15% but requires consideration as a life-threatening complication. Unless a high index of suspicion is maintained, many retroperitoneal hematomas go unrecognized until hemodynamic instability from hemorrhagic shock occurs. This can be a devastating complication and is best assessed by clinical evaluation coupled with imaging, preferably an intravenous contrast enhanced computed tomography (CT) scan (Figure 18-2). Use of a percutaneous closure device may lessen the occurrence of these problems.

Brachial Access

When dealing with patients in whom femoral arterial access is not possible, brachial artery access is another option. This location carries a similar set of complications as femoral access including hematoma, arterial dissection, nerve injury, or inadequate vessel diameter for delivery sheaths. Complications related to arterial access are best avoided by proper patient selection and careful access to the vessel, as well as careful hemostasis at completion of the procedure. Adjunctive use of ultrasound guidance allows measurement of the target vessel size and ensures accurate placement of the sheath. Unlike femoral artery access, the most worrisome complication of brachial

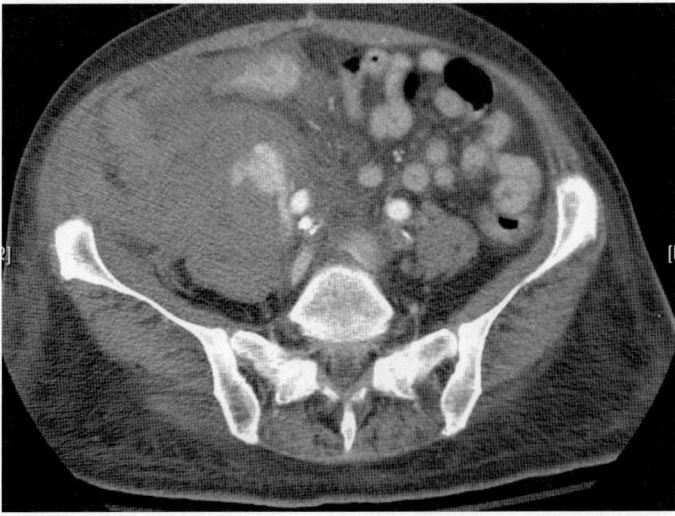

Figure 18-2. CT scan of an iatrogenic retroperitoneal bleed from the limb of an aortobifemoral bypass graft showing active extravasation and a larger retroperitoneal hematoma.

access is the development of a small brachial sheath hematoma, which can be visually unapparent yet can compress the median nerve and result in permanent neurolgic impairment. Any clinical stigmata of nerve impingement mandates prompt exploration and evacuation of the hematoma.

Arch and Brachiocephalic Vessels

It must be remembered that *all* phases of CAS are associated with the risk of distal embolization and neurologic compromise. This even includes the diagnostic arch aortogram. Careful placement of the catheter in the aortic arch and removal of air from the line is essential. When attempting to cannulate the arch vessels for either imaging or intervention, direct injury (dissection or embolization) can be averted with good techniques. Among elderly patients, excessive tortuosity, angulation, and/or calcification can make tracking of catheters and wires particularly difficult and, thus, create a higher risk of embolization or local arterial injury (Figure 18-3).[19] Not surprisingly, one study demonstrated that 90% of embolic events recorded during coronary angiography occurred either during contrast injection or during manipulation of catheters and wires around the aortic arch, yet resulted in no neurologic sequelae. It cannot be emphasized enough that attempts at CAS in elderly patients (>80 years of age) with heavily calcified and tortuous aortic arch anatomy should be performed by highly experienced interventionalists or avoided altogether.

Internal Carotid Artery

The extracranial internal carotid artery (ICA) is also prone to local traumatic injury, particularly with the widespread use of mechanical embolic protection devices (EPDs).

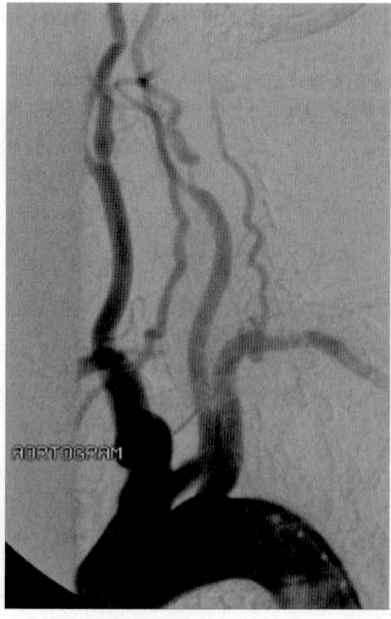

Figure 18-3. Arch aortogram showing a true "bovine" arch with the left common carotid artery arising from the innominate artery.

Spasm in the form of either true vasospasm or pseudospasm can occur from wire placement alone, but more characteristically manifests after placement of distal filtration devices.[20-21] True vasospasm can be so severe that it can result in flow arrest in the distal ICA and possible ICA thrombosis. Fortunately, as reported by Reimers et al., the majority of cases quickly abate with intra-arterial administration of nitrates.[21] Similarly, Cremonesi et al. observed spasm of the ICA, which resolved with nitrates, related to the protection device in 7.9% of their stent procedures.[22] These same investigators found that, when flow impairment continued despite intra-arterial nitrate, occlusion of the filter from debris or clot was evident and flow was normalized when the filter was retrieved. On the other hand, pseudospasm occurs because of the placement of a rigid system (i.e., wire or EPD) within an angulated distal ICA, which causes the vessel to accordion on itself. The worrisome aspect of this is the potential of forming clot within the small cul-de-sacs or causing a localized dissection. This form of spasm is not relieved with vasodilators and will improve only with removal of the offending element. Dissection of the distal ICA can also occur with stiff wires or filters in sharply angulated vessels, and with distal balloon occlusion systems from overinflation of the occlusion balloon.

HIGH-RISK TARGET LESIONS (ANATOMIC AND PATHOLOGIC)

Vessel Tortuosity

In the ideal circumstances, the target lesion for CAS will be straight, focal, and heterogeneous in its pathologic makeup. From a practical point of view, this is a rare occurrence. In fact, vessel tortuosity is far more common and, in some cases, can be so severe that it precludes any attempt at CAS. Once the common carotid artery (CCA) is cannulated with either a guiding catheter or sheath, the next step is crossing and treating the offending lesion. Surprisingly, moderate degrees of angulation of the common carotid and ICA can be exaggerated after placement of rigid sheaths and wires. The end result is inability to cross the lesion with either an EPD or a bare wire. An additional concern is kinking of the leading edge of the stent if it is placed at a natural bend in the ICA. Coils, kinks, and severe tortuosity of the ICA should be avoided when considering CAS.

Plaque Characteristics

It is not unusual for carotid bifurcation disease to be a mix of soft and calcified plaque, but too much of either one is a predictor of poorer outcomes after CAS. It has been demonstrated that echolucent or severely stenotic plaques in the ICA carry a higher risk of embolic events during CAS.[23] This is further supported by Mathur et al., who found in their series of 231 stent procedures, that there was a relationship between increased incidence of procedural stroke in lesions that were categorized as long/multiple (>10 mm in length and/or >1 lesion separated by normal vessel wall) as well as lesions that were ≥90% stenotic.[24] Presumably, these types of lesions have increased embolic potential due to plaque burden and severe stenosis, making traversing them with protection devices more risky. The ICAROS study sought to find a relationship between the gray-scale median (GSM) as an indicator of echogenicity of plaques and risk of CVA during CAS.[25] These investigators found that lesions with a GSM = 25,

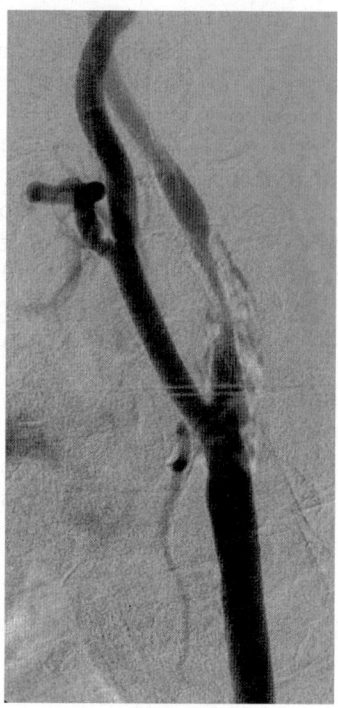

Figure 18-4. Digital subtraction carotid angiogram showing a bifurcation stenosis with extensive circumferential plaque calcification.

correlating with a predominantly echolucent plaque, and lesions with a higher degree of stenosis carried a higher risk of stroke during CAS. Moreover, utilization of EPDs increased the risk of adverse events, suggesting that crossing these lesions with devices is hazardous. This has important implications for the selection of patients for CAS. The implication is that lesions that are echolucent and severely stenotic carry a higher risk of procedural stroke from embolic events. It is in these patients that CAS may have a higher risk of CVA versus CEA, and they should not be considered candidates for an endovascular approach.[26] Similarly, heavily calcified lesions are to be avoided (Figure 18-4). The two primary concerns are inability to fully expand the stent and embolization from a friable plaque.

EPDS AND STENTS

Mechanical Cerebral Protection

The recognized potential for cerebral emboli from thrombus or intra-arterial atheromatous debris during CAS fostered development of three main types of embolic protection devices: 1) distal balloon occlusion, 2) filters, and 3) proximal balloon occlusion.[27,28] There are limitations to each device and each carries its own set of technical considerations.

Distal filtration devices consist of a nitinol skeleton covered with a porous polyurethane filter that is designed to trap released embolic debris while maintaining antegrade cerebral flow. In general, these devices have a large crossing profile, making it more difficult to cross extremely tight lesions without prior angioplasty. Therefore, tight lesions may require predilation with a small balloon (2 or 3 mm) to assist in delivery of the filter element. Obviously, "predilation" is prone to the risk of embolic complications. In cases of sharply angulated target lesions, use of a "buddy wire" to facilitate placement of filter devices may be beneficial. It is essential that an appropriately sized filter device be placed in a relatively straight portion of the distal ICA to ensure good wall apposition, precluding passage of debris around the system. Ideally, filters should be oversized 0.3 mm–1 mm larger than the ICA diameter in the intended landing zone. The filter device should remain in place without excessive movement. There is evidence to suggest that even slight movement of the filter device can cause intimal damage and increase the amount of embolic particles released.[29] In order to keep the filter location constant, CCA sheath location must also remain constant. Prolapse of the guiding sheath into the arch or excessive movement of the sheath can result in possible filter basket detachment, stent entanglement, or guide wire damage (Figure 18-5).

Distal balloon occlusion devices have the advantage of lower crossing profiles and usually do not require predilation to cross the target lesion. Flow arrest must be documented after the occlusion balloon is inflated in order to ensure adequate wall apposition with the distal ICA. After angioplasty and placement of the stent, the static column of blood is aspirated before resumption of flow to the cerebral circulation. The protective effect of the system relies on cessation of flow to the cerebral circulation during the intervention, thereby eliminating the risk of cerebral emboli. Not all

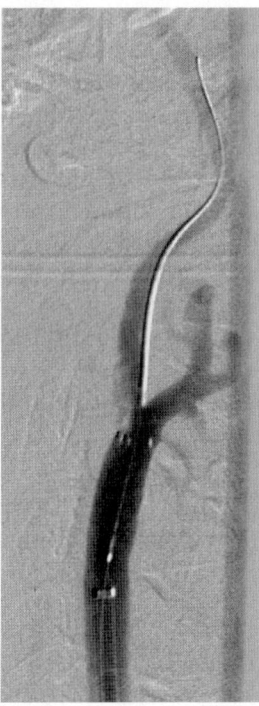

Figure 18-5. Carotid angiogram showing a deployed filter basket inadvertently pulled down to the carotid bifurcation.

patients can tolerate flow arrest. In fact, a recent study evaluating patients undergoing CAS with a balloon occlusion device (PercuSurge Guardwire, PercuSurge, Minneapolis, MN) reported an incidence of neurologic "intolerance" in 10/43 patients during CAS.[30] Fortunately, all neurologic events were transient and resolved with resumption of intracerebral flow. An incomplete circle of Willis was identified in the majority of patients experiencing procedural neurological compromise. Maintenance of adequate blood pressure and intravascular volume status during CAS, as well as prevention of bradycardia, ameliorates cerebral hypoperfusion that may also contribute to neurological compromise.

Proximal balloon occlusion and flow reversal is a novel approach to CAS analogous to the methods employed during traditional CEA, the theoretic benefit being establishing cerebral protection with flow reversal prior to actually crossing the target lesion. Furthermore, intolerance occurs less frequently with flow reversal than with flow cessation,[31] and this form of protection allows for the capture of all particulate debris, regardless of size. The first generation designs were cumbersome, rigid, and required large delivery sheaths (10Fr). Newer systems are easier to use and lower in profile. Unfortunately, not enough data are available to precisely assess their true benefit.

Filter Retrieval Failure

Conversion to open CEA may be required if the distal protection device cannot be safely recovered after stenting is completed. Removal of the filtration device is difficult when large amounts of thrombus or atheromatous debris fill the filter basket to a point that it cannot be collapsed enough to be captured with the retrieval catheter. Prevention of this problem is multifactorial including good technique (i.e., avoidance of overdilating the artery), adequate antiplatelet therapy, and full systemic anticoagulation during the procedure (target ACT 250-300). When retrieving the filter device, care must be taken to avoid prematurely retracting the filter before it is properly sheathed; otherwise, the filter element can become entangled within the stent struts.[32,33] A dreaded complication is detachment of the filter element after entanglement. The recommendations for such a problem are to trap the filter by placing an additional stent to "plaster" it against the arterial wall and prevent migration. In tortuous vessels, the retrieval sheath may be difficult to maneuver across the stented ICA, and advancement of another type or size of sheath for recovery has been described. It may also be helpful to move the patient's head or have the patient swallow to assist in advancement of the catheter past the stent. If these solutions are not successful, emergent conversion to open surgical repair is advocated. Good case planning and selection should avert the need for such dire options.

SYSTEMIC COMPLICATIONS

Stroke

The primary objective of CAS is stroke prevention. In order to achieve this, a procedural risk of stroke is a recognized complication. The etiology of CAS-associated strokes is most frequently embolic in nature, arising from either atheroemboli, fresh clot, or air. All three are preventable with good interventional techniques. The treatment of stroke from the first two remains controversial, but most would pursue systemic therapy (i.e., anticoagulation, permissive hypertension) over catheter-directed lysis. Stroke from air emboli is a unique and unusual situation that is best treated with hyperbaric oxygen therapy (Figure 18-6).

Hemodynamic Instability

Periprocedural hemodynamic instability after CAS can manifest as hypertension, hypotension, or bradycardia, with an incidence ranging from 13% to 68%.[34-37] Many of these are a direct result of stretch on the carotid sinus and stimulation of the baroreflex. The resultant effect is a decrease in sympathetic tone and a temporary increase in parasympathetic stimulation resulting in hypotension and bradycardia. Attempts to elucidate the risk factors for these hemodynamic changes during CAS have revealed results with some common themes. One study that evaluated 140 CAS procedures found that balloon expandable stents and larger diameter balloon expansion resulted in a higher incidence of postoperative hypotension.[34] Similarly, Mendelsohn et al. found a relationship between the need for dopamine infusion during the postdilation period in patients who had placement of stents that were ≥10 mm in width or ≥40 mm in length as opposed to patients with smaller stents who required no additional treatment for hypotension.[36] There is evidence that patients >80 years old, female patients, and patients who have had a previous myocardial infarction have an increased risk of experiencing hypotension during the procedure, and they were more likely to remain hypotensive in the postoperative period.[37-38] Another finding among several studies was that patients who required treatment for intraprocedural hypotension were more likely to have postoperative hypotension that required ICU monitoring and additional medications.[36-38] Avoiding oversized stents and maintaining adequate intravascular volume are measures that may avoid hypotension requiring prolonged vasopressor medications in the postoperative period. Being prepared for these events by having vasopressor agents on hand is essential in avoiding profound hypotension and possible resultant cerebral ischemia.

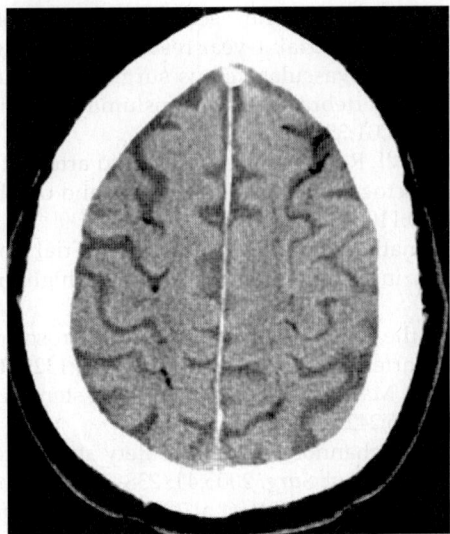

Figure 18-6. Head CT scan showing bilateral intracerebral air after an arch aortogram.

Bradycardia

Bradycardia also occurs quite frequently and often in conjunction with hypotension. Many advocate use of prophylactic atropine dosing prior to angioplasty and stent placement. Although there are no randomized studies evaluating the efficacy of pre-medication with atropine, there is a suggestion that it decreases the incidence of intraprocedural bradycardia and hence prevents additional cardiac stress. This is especially true in patients undergoing CAS who have primary carotid stenosis.[39] At the least, the addition of 0.5 mg–1.0 mg of prophylactic atropine intravenously prior to balloon dilation and stent placement has not had any deleterious effects or caused any adverse cardiac events that have been reported.

CONCLUSION

CAS remains a viable alternative to CEA in certain subgroups of patients with cervical carotid stenosis. While randomized trials continue to clarify its role in other populations, evaluation of periprocedural failures may help reduce associated complications. Clearly, experience, judgement, case planning, and case selection influence the overall outcomes of CAS. It is hoped that this chapter sheds some light on recognized preventable complications and will assist future interventionalists wishing to pursue this mode of therapy.

REFERENCES

1. Yadav JS, Wholey MH, Kuntz RE, et al. Protected carotid-artery stenting versus endarterectomy in high-risk patients. *N Eng J Med.* 2004;351:1493–1501.
2. Roubin GS, New G, Iyer SS, et al. Immediate and late clinical outcomes of carotid artery stenting in patients with symptomatic and asymptomatic carotid artery stenosis. *Circulation.* 2001;103:532–537.
3. CaRESS Steering Committee. Carotid Revascularization using Endarterectomy or Stenting Systems (CaRESS) phase I clinical trial: 1-year results. *J Vasc Surg.* 2005;42:213–219.
4. CAVATAS Investigators. Endovascular versus surgical treatment in patients with carotid stenosis in the Carotid and Vertebral Artery Transluminal Angioplasty Study (CAVATAS): a randomised trial. *Lancet.* 2001;357:1729–1737.
5. Hobson RW 2nd, Howard VJ, Roubin GS, et al. Carotid artery stenting is associated with increased complications in octogenarians: 30-day stroke and death rates in the CREST lead-in phase. *J Vasc Surg.* 2004;40:1106–1111.
6. North American Symptomatic Carotid Endarterectomy Trial Collaborators. Beneficial effect of carotid endarterectomy in symptomatic patients with high-grade carotid stenosis. *N Eng J Med.* 1991;325:445–453.
7. Executive Committee for the Asymptomatic Carotid Atherosclerosis Study. Endarterectomy for asymptomatic carotid artery stenosis. *JAMA.* 1995;273:1421–1428.
8. Eskandari MK, Longo GM, Matsumura JS, et al. Carotid stenting done exclusively by vascular surgeons. *Ann Surg.* 2005;242:431–438.
9. Schneider PA, Silva MB Jr, Bohannon WT, et al. Safety and efficacy of carotid arteriography in vascular surgery practice. *J Vasc Surg.* 2005;41: 238–245.
10. Messina LM, Brothers TE, Wakefield TW, et al. Clinical characteristics and surgical management of vascular complications in patients undergoing cardiac catheterization: Interventional versus diagnostic procedures. *J Vasc Surg.* 1991;13:593–600.

11. Ricci MA, Trevisani GT, Pilcher DB. Vascular complications of cardiac catheterization. *Am J Surg*. 1994;167:375–378.
12. Fransson SG, Nylander E. Vascular injury following cardiac catheterization, coronary angiography, and coronary angioplasty. *European Heart Journal*. 1994;15:232–235.
13. Ates M, Sahin S, Konuralp C, et al. Evaluation of risk factors associated with femoral pseudoaneurysms after cardiac catheterization. *J Vasc Surg*. 2006;43:520–524.
14. Kresowik TF, Khoury MD, Miller BV, et al. A prospective study of the incidence and natural history of femoral vascular complications after percutaneous transluminal coronary angioplasty. *J Vasc Surg*. 1991;13:328–333.
15. Kent KC, McArdle CR, Kennedy B, et al. A prospective study of the clinical outcome of femoral pseudoaneurysms and arteriovenous fistulas induced by arterial puncture. *J Vasc Surg*. 1993;17:125–131.
16. Kumins NH, Landau DS, Montalvo J, et al. Expanded indications for the treatment of post catheterization femoral pseudoaneurysms with ultrasound-guided compression. *Am J Surg*. 1998;176:131–136.
17. Liau CS, Ho FM, Chen MF, et al. Treatment of iatrogenic femoral artery pseudoaneurysm with percutaneous thrombin injection. *J Vasc Surg*. 1997;26:18–23.
18. Singh H, Cardella JF, Cole PE, et al. Quality improvement guidelines for diagnostic arteriography. *J Vasc Radiol*. 2002;13:1–6.
19. Bladin CF, Bingham L, Grigg L, et al. Transcranial Doppler detection of microemboli during percutaneous transluminal coronary angioplasty. *Stroke*. 1998;29:2367–2370.
20. Cardaioli P, Giordan M, Panfili M, et al. Complication with an embolic protection device during carotid angioplasty. *Catheterization and Cardiovascular Interventions*. 2004;62: 234–236.
21. Reimers B, Corvaja N, Moshiri S, et al. Cerebral protection with filter devices during carotid artery stenting. *Circulation*. 2001;104:12–15.
22. Cremonesi A, Manetti R, Setacci F, et al. Protected carotid stenting: clinical advantages and complications of embolic protection devices in 442 consecutive patients. *Stroke*. 2003;34: 1936–1941.
23. Ohki T, Marin ML, Lyon RT, et al. Ex vivo human carotid artery bifurcation stenting: correlation of lesion characteristics with embolic potential. *J Vasc Surg*. 1998;27:463–471.
24. Mathur A, Roubin GS, Iyer SS, et al. Predictors of stroke complicating carotid artery stenting. *Circulation*. 1998;97:1239–1245.
25. Biasi G, Froio A, Diethrich E, et al. Carotid plaque echolucency increases the risk of stroke in carotid stenting the Imaging in Carotid Angioplasty and Risk of Stroke (ICAROS) study. *Circulation*. 2004;110:756–762.
26. Roubin GS, Iyer S, Halkin A, et al. Realizing the potential of carotid artery stenting: proposed paradigms for patient selection and procedural technique. *Circulation*. 2006;113: 2021–2030.
27. Al-Mubarak N, Roubin GS, Vitek JJ, et al. Effect of the distal-balloon protection system on microembolization during carotid stenting. *Circulation*. 2001;104:1999–2002.
28. Eskandari MK. Cerebral embolic protection. *Sem Vasc Surg*. 2005;18:95–100.
29. Muller-Hulsbeck S, Stolzmann P, Liess C, et al. Vessel wall damage caused by cerebral protection devices: ex vivo evaluation in porcine carotid arteries. *Radiology*. 2005;235:454–460.
30. Chaer RA, Trocciola S, DeRubertis B, et al. Cerebral ischemia associated with PercuSurge balloon occlusion balloon during carotid stenting: incidence and possible mechanisms. *J Vasc Surg*. 2006;43:946–952.
31. Parodi JC, Ferreira LM, Sicard G, et al. Cerebral protection during carotid stenting using flow reversal. *J Vasc Surg*. 2005;41:416–422.
32. Ganim RP, Muench A, Giesler GM, et al. Difficult retrieval of the EPI Filterwire with a 5 French coronary catheter following carotid stenting. *Catheter Cardiovasc Interv*. 2006;67: 309–311.
33. Shilling K, Uretsky BF, Hunter GC. Entrapment of a cerebral embolic protection device. *Vasc Endovasc Surg*. 2006;40:229–233.

34. Dangas G, Laird JR Jr, Satler LF, et al. Postprocedural hypotension after carotid artery stent placement: predictors and short- and long-term clinical outcomes. *Radiology.* 2000;215: 677–683.
35. Park B, Shapiro D, Dahn M, Arici M. Carotid artery angioplasty with stenting and postprocedure hypotension. *Am J Surg.* 2005;190:691–695.
36. Mendelsohn FO, Weissman NS, Lederman RJ, et al. Acute hemodynamic changes during carotid artery stenting. *Am J Cardiol.* 1998:82:1077–1081.
37. Qureshi AI, Luft AR, Sharma M. Frequency and determinants of postprocedural homodynamic instability after carotid angioplasty and stenting. *Stroke.* 1999;30:2086–2093.
38. Trocciola SM, Chaer RA, Lin SC, et al. Analysis of parameters associated with hypotension requiring vasopressor support after carotid angioplasty and stenting. *J Vasc Surg.* 2006;43:714–720.
39. Cayne NS, Faries PL, Trocciola SM, et al. Carotid angioplasty and stent-induced bradycardia and hypotension: impact of prophylactic atropine administration and prior carotid endarterectomy. *J Vasc Surg.* 2005;41:956–961.

19

Nonneurologic Complications Associated with Carotid Stenting

Mark A. Patterson, M.D.
and William D. Jordan, Jr., M.D.

Carotid endarterectomy remains the standard treatment for stenoses involving the extracranial carotid arteries. Subsequent to initial reports detailing success with carotid angioplasty and stenting, intense clinical and research efforts have focused on defining the most appropriate role for percutaneous intervention in this anatomic region. Initial effort was primarily aimed toward confirming the feasibility of nonsurgical therapy for carotid stenosis. Feasibility efforts by and large have given way to comparison studies whose immediate goals were to prove equivalence or noninferiority in comparison to carotid endarterectomy.[1] As the most appropriate role for percutaneous carotid artery intervention continues to evolve, the basis of comparison to open surgery has centered primarily on neurologic complications-such as major and minor stroke, transient ischemia, as well as their impact on patient and procedural outcomes. An often neglected endpoint among series detailing experience with carotid angioplasty and stenting involves nonneurologic complications that develop in the acute and delayed setting in relation to percutaneous carotid procedures. This chapter details the prevalence, diagnosis, and management of nonneurologic complications that have arisen in relation to carotid artery stenting.

ACUTE PROCEDURAL/TECHNICAL COMPLICATIONS

Access-related Complications

The most commonly used route for accessing the arterial tree and subsequently the supra-aortic vessels is via retrograde common femoral puncture. Direct antegrade puncture of the cervical carotid artery described in early reports detailing carotid intervention is presently most often used as an alternative when femoral access is difficult or unsuccessful. Additionally, isolated reports exist describing brachial artery access for carotid angioplasty secondary to inability to gain femoral access.[2] While the brachial approach is feasible, these smaller arteries are subject to higher rates of thrombosis, perforation, and bleeding. The decision to pursue carotid intervention via questionable or risky access should provoke the clinician to reevaluate the relative risk of percutaneous carotid therapy perhaps in favor of more direct access as is capable with carotid endarterectomy. One death early in the UAB experience resulted from carotid thrombosis after failed direct common carotid puncture and secondary femoral puncture through severe aortoiliac occlusive disease resulted in retroperitoneal hematoma and hypotension.

Technical difficulty in traversing the aorta and successfully cannulating the supra-aortic branch vessels has decreased following development of shape-specific selective catheters and lower profile devices. Improved trackability and various catheter options for cannulation have produced relative comfort with the femoral approach. Most clinicians embarking on percutaneous carotid interventions have accumulated extensive experience obtaining arterial access. Regardless of this fact, every percutaneous procedure cannot proceed until safe arterial cannulation is achieved. Experience with percutaneous procedures in alternate vascular regions has demonstrated greater incidence of groin-related complications following therapeutic procedures in comparison to strictly diagnostic procedures.[3] This higher complication rate is likely related to the larger access sheath requirement during therapeutic procedures. Groin-related complications include hematoma, hemorrhage, pseudoaneurysm development, arteriovenous fistula, lower extremity ischemia, and retroperitoneal hematoma (Figure 19-1). Access injuries are usually categorized as minor or major depending on transfusion requirement, need for surgical intervention, and prolongation of hospital stay. Review of current series describing carotid angioplasty and stenting reveals an incidence of groin-related complications ranging from 0% to 7.8%.[4,5] Predisposing factors for groin artery complications include multiple needle punctures during access acquisition,

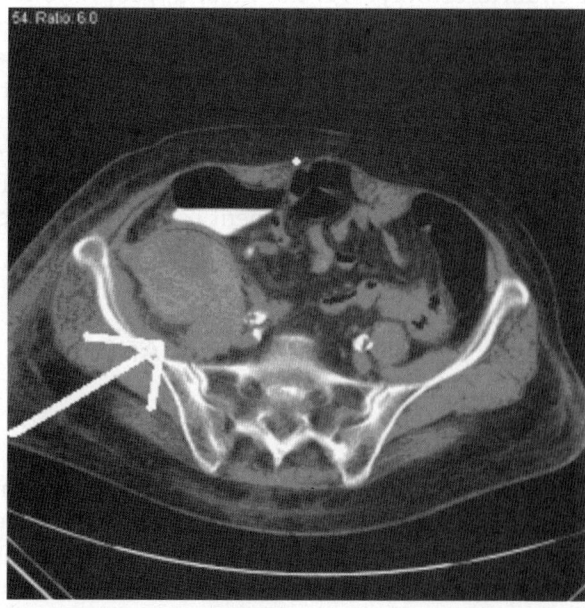

Figure 19-1. Retroperitoneal hematoma following CAS.

patient obesity, and groin artery calcification, as well as procedural anticoagulation and antiplatelet requirements. Use of arterial closure devices has reduced, but not eliminated, groin-related complications. Additionally, despite improved access site hemostasis with closure devices, more common use of these devices has been linked to increased instances of primary arterial infection.[6]

Supra-aortic Arterial Access Failure

The most commonly reported etiology for procedural failure during carotid stenting procedures is inability to successfully place a guide catheter or sheath in the common carotid artery.[7-8] Improvements in catheter design have yielded more flexible and specifically shaped catheters leading to easier branch artery access. Use of long sheaths or shape-specific guide catheters may enhance consistent, atraumatic entry of devices into the target vessels. Quick and atraumatic entry into the supra-aortic vessels can limit the embolic risk from aortic arch plaque as well as reduce the risk of branch vessel dissection (Figure 19-2). Additionally, shaped guides and sheaths may be critical to cannulation success in the steep, angulated arch where the target artery originates below the inferior curve of the arch. Early reports detailed target artery access failures as high as 15%, while more current studies report access failure in the 0% to 3% range.[8] An additional feature of decreased target artery access failure no doubt relates to increased comfort and familiarity with navigating difficult arch anatomy as experience with the procedure has increased.

Aside from increased familiarity with navigating the aortic arch and cannulation of the arch vessels, attention to arch anatomy based on angulation of the arch with respect to target vessel takeoff has further impacted cannulation success. Separation of diagnostic angiography and therapeutic procedures can allow time for patient-specific preintervention planning, further enhancing the ability to achieve appropriate guide catheter or sheath placement.

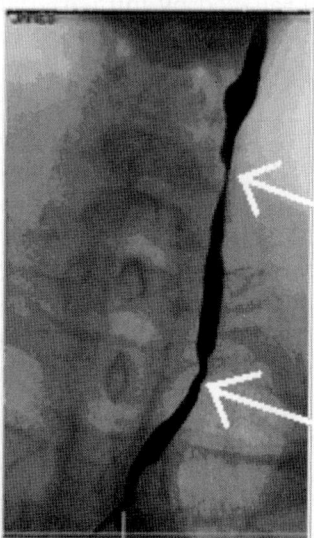

Figure 19-2A. Proximal CCA dissection created during CCA access.

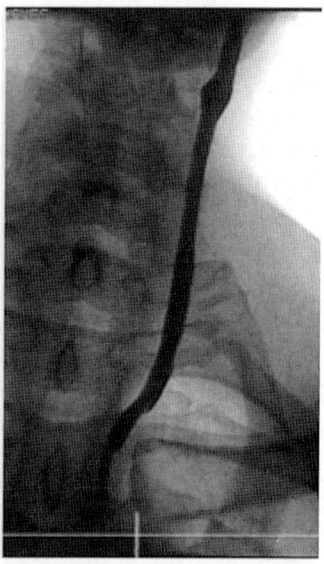

Figure 19-2B. CCA dissection treated with stenting.

Carotid Lesion or Stent Site Complications

Once the arch branch vessel has been successfully cannulated and an appropriate guiding catheter has been advanced to a satisfactory position within the target common carotid artery, attention is focused on addressing the stenosis. Reported complications arising at this portion of the procedure include perforation, dissection, and embolization, as well as inability to successfully engage and cross the lesion. External carotid perforation has been documented in instances in which the artery is used as an "anchor" for catheter exchange and advancement. Perforation of the internal carotid artery may occur during attempts to cross tight stenoses or as the result of plaque/adventitial fractures immediately following stent placement across densely calcified lesions. While fortunately rare in occurrence, methods of management have included both catheter-based techniques and surgical conversion.[8,9]

Similar to perforation, dissection of the common and internal carotid vessels represents a potentially lethal complication. After the fifth case of carotid angioplasty at UAB in 1994 resulted in dissection, occlusion, and major stroke, stenting of carotid stenoses has become routine. Subsequently, procedure-related dissection or acute occlusion has been significantly reduced (<1%).[8] Risk factors for dissection include difficult arch anatomy as well as proximal common carotid calcification or stenosis. While internal carotid dissection may occur during lesion predilation, primary stenting has nearly eliminated this problem. Guide wire injury and plaque fracture at the edges of the stent following deployment represent additional factors contributing to procedure-related arterial dissection.[9-11]

Arterial Spasm, Acute Vessel Thrombosis

Arterial spasm, when observed, typically involves the distal nondiseased portion of the internal carotid artery following balloon or stent manipulation. Spasm may occur distal to the implanted stent immediately following deployment or in conjunction with cerebral protection device deployment and retrieval (Figure 19-3). Literature reports indicate that arterial spasm is usually transient and may be relieved by intra-arterial vasodilator administration. Currently reported incidence of arterial spasm is 2% to 3.6%.[9-11] Fortunately, acute vessel or in-stent thrombosis is a rare event. Most series report isolated instances of acute thrombosis, many of which may be resolved with neurorescue efforts via direct thrombin inhibitor or thrombolytic agent administration. Mechanical thrombectomy devices have also been successfully used.[12]

Arterial Kinks, External Carotid Occlusion

In addition to arterial spasm, kinking of the internal carotid artery has also been documented during carotid stenting. While most commonly observed during treatment of tortuous vessels, overaggressive stent length may contribute by extension of the stent more distally into the internal carotid artery than desired. Additional stent placement may resolve the kink while open conversion has also been necessary.[13]

The specific character and anatomy of the arterial stenosis deserves consideration in order to limit postprocedure arterial kinks. Stenting of carotid stenoses harboring kinks at the diseased site prior to treatment often leads to transmission of the kink to the distal end of the stent following deployment (Figure 19-4) Such preprocedure anatomic findings may represent indication for surgical carotid reconstruction as opposed to catheter-based therapy. Plaque-related kinks may also limit or preclude distal

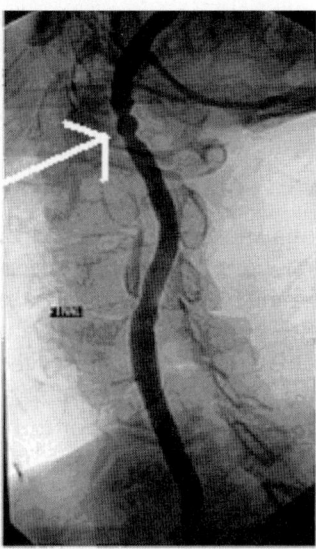

Figure 19-3. Spasm of distal ICA, following retrieval of cerebral protection device.

embolic protection device use leading to increased risk for procedural related neurologic complications.

External carotid artery occlusion is most commonly observed when bifurcation lesions originate in the distal common carotid artery, and appropriate stent placement requires the stent to cross or "jail" the external carotid origin. While most frequently

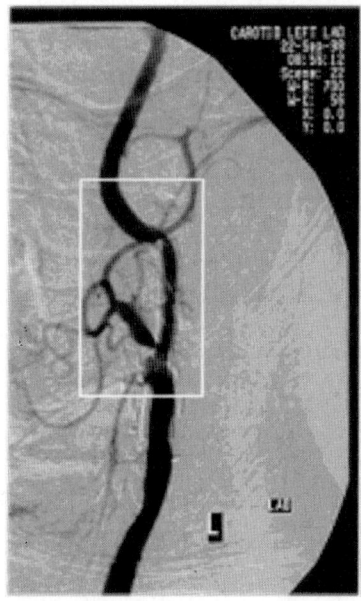

Figure 19-4A. Transmission of arterial kink to distal end of stent.

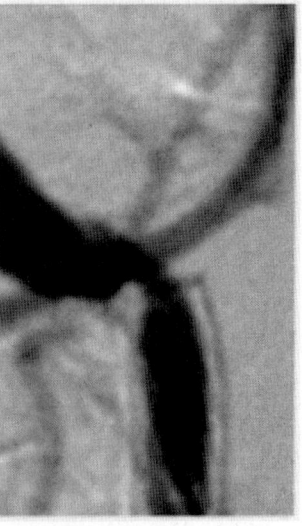

Figure 19-4B. Magnified view of kink (inset).

identified on follow-up duplex evaluations, no significant clinical consequence has been reported. External carotid occlusions may also occur as a result of unappreciated dissection in the ECA during procedures in which wire advancement into the vessel is required to anchor the guide wire for catheter exchange or advancement.

Acute Systemic Procedural Events

The very nature of percutaneous therapy for carotid bifurcation disease implies manipulation of the carotid sinus, which houses baroreceptors important for blood pressure control and activation of parasympathetic reflexes influencing heart rate. Early series detailing experience with carotid angioplasty and stenting documented hypotension and bradycardia as frequent events observed in as many as 71% of procedures.[10] In the initial UAB reports, as many as 32% of patients developed some systemic effect that required additional treatment or in-hospital monitoring (Table 19-1). Most commonly, these patients developed bradycardia that was sometimes associated with hypotension requiring vasoactive medications. The etiology for these events involves distention of the carotid sinus during dilatation of the bifurcation lesion both prior to and following stent placement. Literature review suggests a trend toward less severe episodes of both hypotension and bradycardia with the more consistent use of self-expanding stents and the practice of downsizing pre- and postdilatory angioplasty balloons.[5,8] Once activated, the hypotensive or bradycardic reflexes are usually transient and readily treated with administration of intravenous or intra-arterial reversal agents. Transient or continuous vasopressor administration may be necessary to reverse hypotension, while temporary or permanent pacemaker placement may be required to treat persistent bradycardia, heart block, or asystole. More current experience has led to pretreatment with atropine or glycopyrrolate prior to balloon angioplasty and stent placement as a means of minimizing procedural-related bradycardia.[4] A recent series by Trocciola et al. evaluating the need for vasopressor support following carotid stenting identified prior myocardial infarction and PercuSurge occlusion balloon use as risk factors associated with the need for short-term vasopressor support (<24 hours), while females greater than 80 years of age were more likely to require va-

TABLE 19-1. NONNEUROLOGIC COMPLICATIONS REQUIRING CARDIOPULMONARY MONITORING AMONG PATIENTS RECEIVING CAROTID ANGIOPLASTY AND STENTING AT UAB, (1994-1997).

	Carotid Artery Stenting (293 procedures)
Hypotension	68
Bradycardia	19 (1 permanent pacemaker)
Hypertension	1*
Hematoma	1*
GI bleeding	3
Anemia	1
Retroperitoneal hematoma	1
Myocardial infarction	1
Pulmonary edema	1
Total	96 (32.8%)

*Patients with more than 1 complication

sopressor support for more than 24 hours. Furthermore, vasopressor use, when necessary, did not lead to increased instances of myocardial infarction or episodes of congestive heart failure.[14]

Complications Related to Cerebral Protection Devices

Prior to development and use of cerebral protection devices, criticism regarding the neurologic complication profile of carotid angioplasty and stenting, particularly among surgeons, centered on the uncertain clinical implications of embolized atheromatous debris. Not only have the devices improved procedural safety, they have initiated more widespread acceptance of percutaneous carotid interventions. Despite improved neurologic complication rates, there are technical issues related to protection device use that may influence the success of stenting procedures. Nonneurologic complications associated with the devices typically involve local problems associated with positioning, deployment, and retrieval. Inability to cross the lesion remains the most common cause for cerebral protection device application failure. Predilation with small diameter (2–3 mm) balloons is frequently employed, but represents an embolic risk. As previously mentioned, positioning and deployment of the device can induce arterial spasm. Despite precise attention to cerebral protection device position, movement of the device within the artery likely occurs and may produce spasm or arterial dissection. Larger series detailing the use of cerebral protection devices describe the incidence of failure to cross lesions in the range of 0% to 4%. Dissections, while relatively uncommon, have also been reported to occur among 1% to 3% of stenting procedures.[9,11]

Inability to appropriately recapture the device has led to stent displacement as well as atheroembolization. A recent report by Chane et al. details an instance in which a protection device became entrapped within the struts of a deployed stent during retrieval.[15] An endovascular grasping device was ultimately required to remove the device. During the additional manipulation, local arterial dissection occurred requiring additional stent placement for resolution. Most instances of problematic device retrieval have been associated with tight stenoses, tortuous arteries, or long lesions originating in the common carotid artery. Fortunately, such events appear to be limited; however, early series report difficulty with device retrieval complicating as many as 8.7 % of carotid interventions.[11]

Despite the demonstrated reduction in procedural neurologic complication rates, consistent cerebral protection device use increases procedural complexity, and emphasizes the necessity of appropriate operator skill and training.

POSTPROCEDURAL/DELAYED EVENTS

Medical or Systemic Complications

In order for carotid angioplasty and stenting to confirm its viability as an alternative to carotid endarterectomy, not only the procedural or technical issues, but also postprocedural systemic or medical complication profiles must be acceptable. In general, percutaneous carotid intervention is viewed as a minimally invasive procedure, performed under local anesthesia with a limited overall medical complication rate. Current series detailing the medical complications arising in patients receiving percutaneous carotid intervention involve cardiac, pulmonary, renal/urinary, and vascular organ systems. Both prospective and retrospective series have documented postprocedural myocardial infarction, pulmonary infection, renal insufficiency, and urinary retention/infection. Groschel et al. demonstrated an overall medical complication rate of 19%. Increased age and symptomatic disease were identified as independent predictors of medical complication development. Review of the early UAB experience likewise demonstrated that 32.8% of patients required additional intervention or monitoring due to a complication postprocedure (Table 19-1). The most commonly encountered events involved blood pressure abnormalities (hypo- and hypertension) and cardiac arrhythmias. The significance of these events becomes most germane as they typically necessitate additional in-hospital cardiopulmonary monitoring often leading to increased length of stay.[1,16-17]

Intracranial Hemorrhage

Experience with carotid angioplasty and stenting has demonstrated that percutaneous carotid intervention is not immune to development of isolated intracranial hemorrhage. As with endarterectomy, the development of intracranial hemorrhage remains low with most series reporting isolated instances. Degree of intracranial bleeding ranges from small punctate hemorrhages to massive bleeding accompanied by mass effect and death. Factors associated with this finding include symptomatic patients, very tight stenoses, contralateral occlusion, and increased age.[18] As prevention strategies continue to develop, the degree to which the currently used antiplatelet regimens contribute to the incidence of intracranial hemorrhage remains to be determined.

Stent Deformation

Postprocedure stent deformation has been identified at various stages of postprocedure surveillance. In the initial experience at UAB, stent deformation represented the most common etiology for early in-stent restenosis. All of the reported deformations in the noted series involved balloon expandable stents (Figure 19-5). Subsequent to this experience, more consistent use of self-expanding stents has nearly eliminated postprocedure stent deformation. Current series report deformation incidence in the range of 1% to 2%. Interventions to address stent deformation have involved repeat angioplasty and stenting, as well as surgical removal.[10]

Recurrent Stenosis

Perhaps the final proving ground for carotid angioplasty and stenting exists in its long term durability in relieving extracranial carotid stenosis, thus providing acceptable long-term stroke risk reduction (Figure 19-6). Appropriate identification of recurrent stenosis implies that a suitable method for poststenting surveillance exists. Duplex ultrasound has proven to be a very useful modality for postendarterectomy surveillance and has been instrumental in establishing appropriate surveillance protocols for monitoring postendarterectomy patients.[19] The application of current duplex velocity criteria for postendarterectomy restenosis to poststenting surveillance has been the subject of considerable debate. The basic tenets of debate center on the difference between the two procedures as it relates to plaque removal. Limited compliance of the stented artery in conjunction with retained plaque burden can lead to elevated velocity measurements in the setting of limited overall reduction of intraluminal surface area.

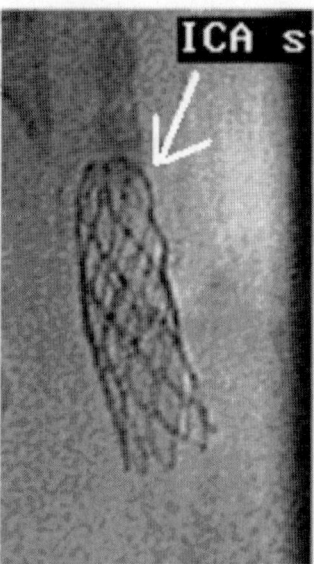

Figure 19-5. Deformed balloon expandable stent creating recurrent stenosis.

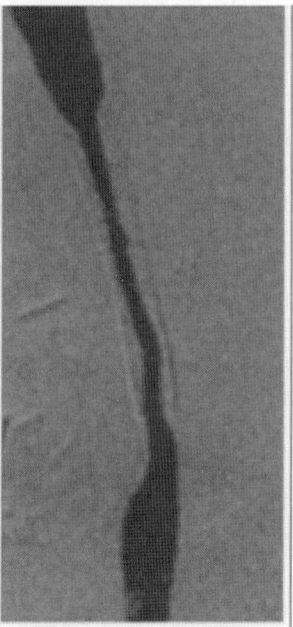

Figure 19-6. In-stent restenosis.

Current series among the surgical and medical literature suggest that overall recurrent stenosis rates are acceptable and rarely associated with neurologic events. Hobson et al. identified restenosis creating greater than 40% intraluminal diameter reduction among 22 of 122 patients. Only six patients (6.4%) developed stenosis producing > 80% intraluminal diameter reduction.[20] UAB experience demonstrates an almost 20% incidence of duplex flow abnormalities (peak velocity > 110 cm/sec) with 8% harboring peak velocity > 170 cm/sec in limited surveillance up to five years.[21] However, the flow velocities have not consistently correlated with angiographic stenoses. Definitive poststenting duplex criteria remain in development at UAB, while additional preliminary criteria have been proposed in other centers.[22]

The Unknown

As with any new intervention, the potential for unique or previously unobserved complications to arise among patients receiving carotid stents will only be fully realized as experience accumulates. One of the most widely accepted indications for carotid stenting involves treatment of carotid stenoses arising subsequent to external beam irradiation. Avoidance of cervical neck incisions in these patients eliminates wound-related morbidity as well as the potential for cranial nerve injury. A recent report by Kaviani et al. details the management of a carotid-cutaneous fistula arising secondary to pseudoaneurysm formation related to an infected carotid stent 20 months after implantation. While the authors propose primary stent infection leading to false aneurysm development with subsequent erosion through the skin as the etiology of the fistula, this case illustrates the possibility for unique stent-related complications to evolve. As is the case with carotid endarterectomy, appropriate long-term poststenting surveillance is mandatory to identify, diagnose, and manage further "unknown" long-term stent-related complications as they arise.[23]

Future Study

Following its initial description, carotid angioplasty and stenting has received considerable scrutiny. The present status of percutaneous carotid intervention continues to develop. Future investigation will center on strategies to limit recurrent stenosis as well as the development of appropriate surveillance duplex ultrasound velocity criteria. While carotid intervention appears to have confirmed noninferiority in comparison to carotid endarterectomy among high-risk patients, continued demonstration of reduced neurologic and nonneurologic complication rates will be necessary to supplant surgical endarterectomy as the standard for managing carotid bifurcation stenosis. Currently ongoing randomized trials will provide substantive data to appropriately direct further clinical decisions regarding the management of patients with extracranial carotid artery occlusive disease.

REFERENCES

1. Yadav JS, Wholey MH, Kuntz RE, et al. Protected carotid-artery stenting versus endarterectomy in high risk patients. *N Engl J Med* 2004, 351(15): 1493–501.
2. Ohki T, Timaran CH, Yadav JS: Technique of Carotid Angioplasty and Stenting. In Moore WS: *Vascular and Endovascular Surgery- A Comprehensive Review*. Philadelphia, Saunders Elsevier, 2006, pp 355–382.
3. Nasser TK, Mohler ER III, Wilensky RL, et al. Peripheral vascular complications following coronary interventional procedures. *Clin Cardiol* 1995 18: 609–15.
4. Al-Mubarak N, Roubin GS, Vitek JJ,et al. Procedural Safety and Short Term Outcome of Ambulatory Carotid Stenting. *Stroke* 2001 32: 2305–09.

5. Tan KT, Cleveland TJ, Berczi V, et al. Timing and frequency of complications after carotid artery stenting: What is the optimal period of observation? *J Vasc Surg* 2003; 38: 236–43.

6. Hollis Jr HW, Rehring TF. Femoral endarteritis associated with percutaneous suture closure: New technology, challenging complications. *J Vasc Surg* 2003; 38–38–7.

7. Wholey MH, Wholey MH, Jarmolowski CR,et al. Endovascular Stents for Carotid Artery Occlusive Disease. *J Endovasc Surg* 1997;326–338.

8. Roubin GS, Gishel N, Iyer SS, et al. Immediate and late clinical outcomes of Carotid Artery Stenting in Patients with Symptomatic and Asymptomatic Carotid Artery Stenosis: A 5-year Prospective Analysis. *Circulation* 2001; 103:532–37.

9. Cremonesi A, Manetti R, Setacci F,et al. Protected Carotid Stenting: Clinical Advantages and Complications of Embolic Protection Devices in 442 Consecutive Patients. *Stroke* 2003; 34: 1936–41.

10. Yadav JS, Roubin GS, Iyer SS, et al. Elective Stenting of Extracranial Carotid Arteries. *Circulation* 1997;95:376–81.

11. Reimers B, Corvaja N, Moshiri S, et al. Cerebral Protection With Filter Devices During Carotid Artery Stenting. *Circulation* 2001;104:12–15.

12. Bush RL, Bhama JK, Lin PH, et al. Transient ischemic attack due to early carotid stent thrombosis: Successful rescue with rheolytic thrombectomy and systemic abciximab. *J Endovasc Ther* 10: 870–874.

13. Choi HM, Hobson II RW, Goldstein J, et al. Technical challenges in a program of carotid artery stenting. *J Vasc Surg* 2004;40:746–51.

14. Trocciola SM, Chaer RA, Lin SC, et al. Analysis of parameters associated with hypotension requiring vasopressor support after carotid angioplasty and stenting. *J Vasc Surg* 2006;43:714–20.

15. Chane M, Ballard A, Vanpatten A, et al. Management of Detached Accunet Embolic Protection Filter During Percutaneous Carotid Artery Intervention. *Vascular Disease Management* 2006 March/April: 218–22.

16. Groeschel K, Ernemann U, Riecker A, et al. Incidence and risk factors for medical complications after carotid artery stenting. *J Vasc Surg* 2005; 42:1101–7.

17. Jordan WD Jr., Voellinger DC, Fisher W, et al. A comparison of carotid angioplasty with stenting versus carotid endarterectomy with regional anesthesia. *J Vasc Surg* 1998; 28: 397–403.

18. McKevitt FM Macdonald S, Venables GS, et al. Complications following Carotid Angioplasty and Carotid Stenting in Patients with Symptomatic Carotid Artery Disease. *Cerebrovascular Diseases* 2004; 17: 28–34.

19. Carballo RE, Towne JB, Seabrook, et al. An outcome analysis of carotid endarterectomy: the incidence and natural history of recurrent stenosis. *J Vasc Surg* 1996 23(5):749–53.

20. Brajesh KL, Hobson RW III, Goldstein J, et al. In stent recurrent stenosis after carotid artery stenting: Life table analysis and clinical relevance. *J Vasc Surg.* 2003; 38: 1162–9.

21. Jordan WD Jr, Alcocer F. Long-term Ultrasound Results of Carotid Stenting. Veith, FJ: *29th Global: Vascular and Endovascular Issues, Techniques and Horizons.*™ Montefiore Medical Center, Albert Einstein College of Medicine, New York, 2002, pp XXII 9.1–9.2.

22. Stanziale SF, Wholey MH, Boules TN, et al. Determining In-Stent Stenosis of Carotid Arteries by Duplex Ultrasound Criteria. *J Endovasc Therapy* 2005; 12: 346–353.

23. Kaviani A, Ouriel K, Kashyap VS. Infected carotid pseudoaneurysm and carotid-cutaneous fistula as a late complication of carotid artery stenting. *J Vasc Surg* 2006; 43: 379–82.

20

Surveillance Duplex Scanning after Carotid Stent Angioplasty

Dennis F. Bandyk, M.D.
Paul A. Armstrong, D.O.

Duplex ultrasound testing, an accurate method to detect and estimate the severity of atherosclerotic internal carotid artery (ICA) stenosis, is recommended to monitor the anatomy of carotid intervention since restenosis is associated with increased stroke risk.[1-5] Testing immediately after carotid artery endarterectomy (CEA) or stent angioplasty (CAS) provides assessment of technical success by excluding residual stenosis.[6,7] The goal of subsequent duplex surveillance is to identify recurrent stenosis, document repair site occlusion, and monitor the contralateral ICA for disease progression. Since the clinical application of CAS has continued to expand, it is prudent to scrutinize the durability and stroke prevention efficacy of this endovascular therapy. The incidence of in-stent stenosis following CAS remains a concern with rates of 1–30% reported, a wide range attributed to variations in diagnostic testing methods, interpretation criteria, and duration of follow-up.[3-5, 8-10] At present, it is recommended that each vascular center performing CAS examine outcomes, including duplex surveillance for stent stenosis or occlusion, and its correlation with neurologic events and stroke-related death.

The accuracy of duplex ultrasound in grading CAS site stenosis has been questioned, especially in interpretation of the 50% diameter-reduction (DR) threshold.[5,10] Correlation of duplex findings with procedural CAS angiography have reported an elevated peak systolic velocity (PSV) in the 150–200 cm/s range when a residual angiogram stenosis of <20–30% DR is left; an observation recorded on the initial duplex examination from 20–30% of ICA stents with <50% DR on angiography.[6,10-11] The type of stent implanted may also influence in-stent PSV values.[6,12] The clinical significance of elevated stent velocity following CAS is unknown as is the significance of moderate 50–75% in-stent stenosis. After surgical endarterectomy (CEA), restenosis of this severity has not been associated with an increased risk for stroke compared to normal

(<50% DR) repairs.[7] High-grade (>75–80% DR) stenosis after CEA or CAS is generally felt to be clinically significant lesion, and has been associated with progression to occlusion and stroke. Most reports on CAS surveillance have not focused on the detection and treatment of high-grade stent stenosis, or recommended a clinically useful algorithm for patient follow-up. Our vascular group has applied a previously validated duplex testing protocol after CEA for CAS surveillance.[7-8] Using serial testing, the prevalence of carotid stent-angioplasty stenosis was studied, including assessment for stent stenosis progression or regression; and the yield of surveillance for detection of high-grade in-stent stenosis or contralateral ICA stenosis progression and their relationship to clinical symptoms.

CAROTID DUPLEX TESTING AND SURVEILLANCE PROTOCOL

Duplex ultrasound testing after CAS should include complete mapping of the extracranial common (CCA), internal, and external carotid (ECA) arteries, and flow assessment in the vertebral and subclavian arteries. Bilateral testing with measurement upper extremity brachial artery systole pressure is standard. Carotid artery imaging is performed in both transverse and saggital planes to assess stent apposition to the CCA and ICA walls, identify stent deformation and/or in-stent intima thickening, and examine for stenosis outside of stented artery segment. In most patients, a linear array transducer (5–10 MHz) is optimal to image artery/stent anatomy and record pulsed Doppler signals. Color or power Doppler imaging are useful in the recognition of focal versus diffuse in-stent stenosis, and to interrogate the site of maximum stenosis for pulsed Doppler velocity spectra changes. Disease classification is based on spectral waveform parameters (PSV, EDV) including the ratio of PSVs recorded from within the stent, and compared to a proximal CCA recording site (Figure 20–1). Velocity spectra are recorded (60° or less Doppler angle) at multiple sites in the CCA, ICA (proximal, mid, distal), and ECA to confirm normal carotid flow or estimate stenosis severity.

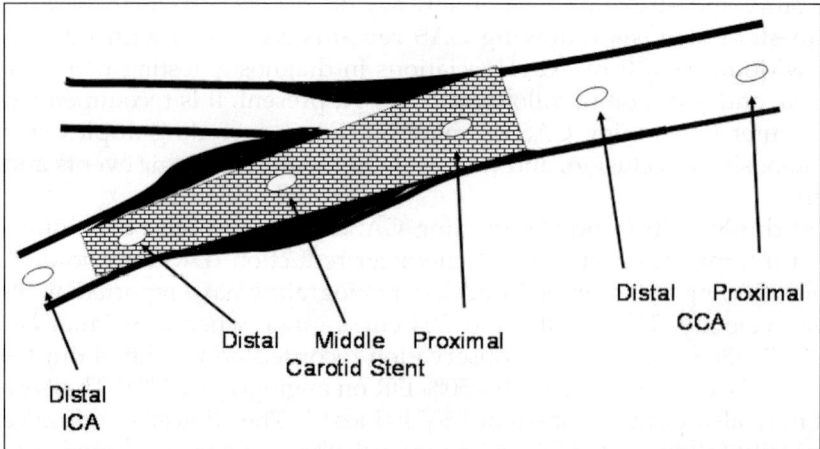

Figure 20-1. Schematic of a carotid stent angioplasty site depicting sites of pulsed Doppler spectral recordings from the common carotid artery (CCA), within the carotid stent (proximal, mid, distal), and from the distal internal carotid artery (ICA).

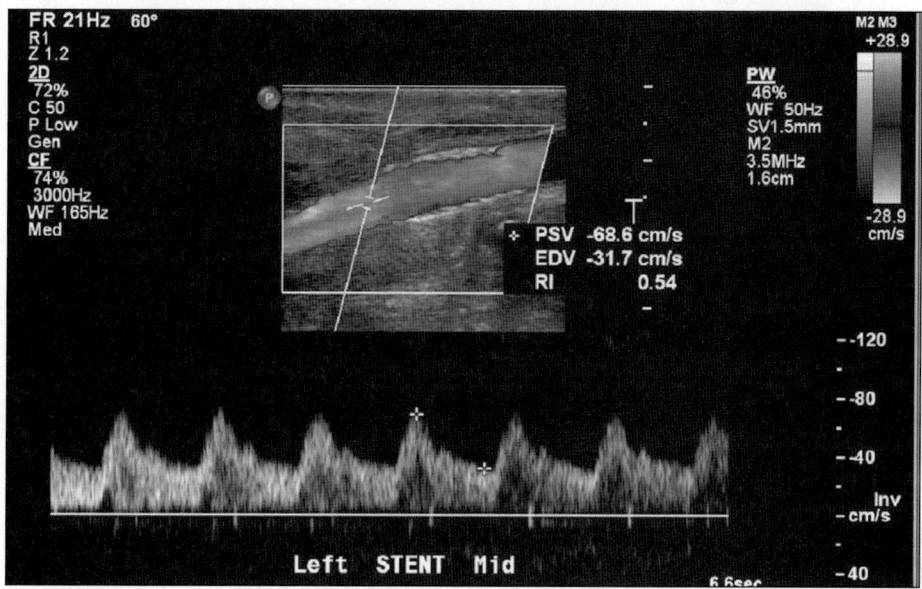

Figure 20-2. Color Doppler image and mid-stent pulsed Doppler velocity recorded after carotid stent angioplasty.

Our vascular group orders a bedside duplex examination to be performed in the postanesthesia care unit (PACU) approximately two to three hours after the CAS procedure. The goal of testing is to exclude a major technical problem prior to femoral artery sheath removal. Attention is focused primarily on the stented carotid segment to document its patency, exclude in-stent thrombus, and verify unobstructed flow based on center-stream velocity spectra recordings from within and downstream of the stent. Using real-time color Doppler, the stented ICA should appear widely patent; that is, not focal stenosis and low-resistance spectral waveform without turbulent flow (Figure 20–2). Power Doppler imaging is useful to image the stent lumen and the flow transition from the stent into the ICA. Most stents will traverse the external carotid artery origin, but flow through stent interstices is sufficient to retain patency. Recording of pulsed Doppler velocity spectra proximal to, within, and distal to the stent angioplasty site is performed using a "small" sample volume and 60° Doppler angle. Stent diameters are measured for comparison with subsequent postoperative testing.

Stent implantation and balloon angioplasty across an atherosclerotic plaque delivers radial forces to expand the lumen and maintain a larger diameter. After stent delivery, both positive (stent expansion) and negative (wall recoil, myointimal hyperplasia) remodeling occurs with corresponding changes in lumen caliber. Remodeling of the stented ICA is a dynamic process occurring over months and involves a biologic response to the arterial wall injury and the stent.[9-13] For several months after deployment, stent expansion occurs—up to a 40% diameter increase—but this *positive* remodeling may be inhibited by the presence of extensive plaque calcification. Also during this time period, neointimal hyperplasia is also developing within the stent, which is evident on high-resolution B-mode imaging as a homogenous, concentric intimal thickening. Scanning should be performed with a linear array (7–10 MHz) transducer with scanlines perpendicular to the stent to assess the presence of myointimal thickening or stent deformation. Typically, by three months, the anatomic changes

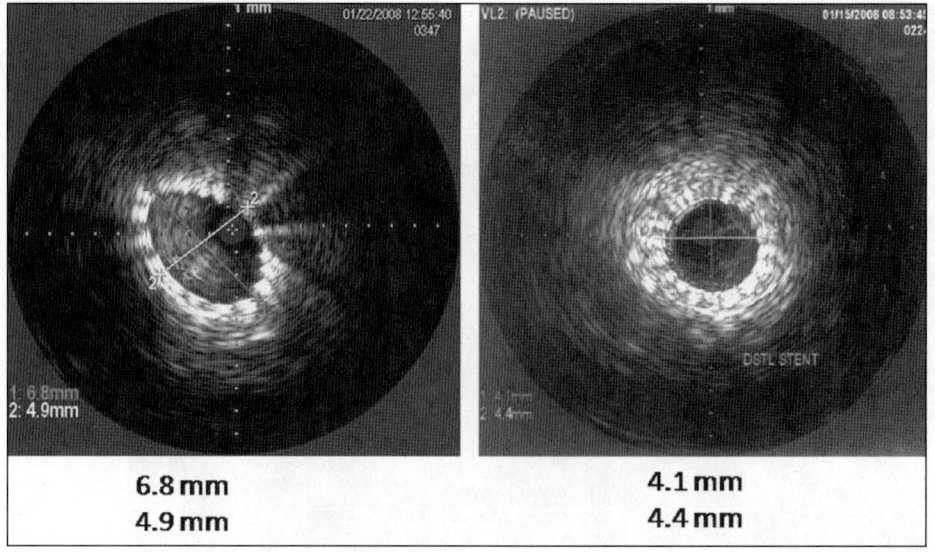

6.8 mm
4.9 mm

4.1 mm
4.4 mm

Figure 20-3. Intravascular ultrasound images following carotid stent deployment and balloon angio-plasty demonstrating elliptical (left) lumen and circular (right) lumen. Completion angiogram was normal (<20% residual stenosis) in both cases.

produced by neointimal hyperplasia exceeds that of stent expansion, yielding the net result of stent lumen reduction and the hemodynamics of an increase in stent PSV with time.[9] The extent and rate of neointimal hyperplasia development varies. Lesions that develop within the first six months after CAS have been observed to regress (i.e., negative remodeling) from a >50% DR to <50% DR stenosis on serial scans. At present, factors associated with in-stent stenosis development are not well understood and no drug therapy has been identified to prevent its formation or induce regression.

Calcified atherosclerotic plaques can inhibit nitinol stent expansion, producing an "eccentric" lumen and PSV elevation. Elliptical stent expansion after balloon angio-plasty has been observed by intravascular ultrasound (Figure 20–3). In some cases, this has been associated with elevated (PSV>150 cm/s) in-stent flow velocity. Similarly, compensatory flow as a result of severe, contralateral ICA stenosis or occlusion can produce PSV elevations, and thus contribute to overclassification of disease if only maximum PSV criteria are used in study interpretation.

After an uncomplicated CAS procedure (i.e., no neurologic events), duplex testing is repeated approximately one month later and then every six months thereafter for one year. Annual testing is recommended beyond the first year if testing documents <50% DR stent and contralateral ICA stenosis. A six-month testing interval is recommended when either ICA has findings of >50% DR stenosis.

DUPLEX SCAN INTERPRETATION

The interpretation criteria used to classify disease (i.e., stenosis severity) following CAS are detailed in Table 20–1. A "normal" CAS site is associated with a smooth, widely patent lumen with nondisturbed flow and a PSV of less than 150 cm/s. The

TABLE 20-1. DUPLEX SCAN CRITERIA FOR GRADING STENOSIS FOLLOWING CAROTID STENT ANGIOPLASTY

Stenosis Category (Diameter Reduction, DR)	PSV (cm/s)	PSV Ratio	EDV (cm/s)	Color/Power Doppler Imaging Findings
<50% (no stent stenosis)	<150	<2	NA	No or minimal lumen reduction
50–75% (mild-moderate stenosis)	>150	>2	<125	Turbulent flow; Stent lumen reduction identified
>75% (severe stenosis)	>300	>4	>125	High-grade stent stenosis imaged; residual lumen <2 mm; damping of distal ICA spectral waveform compared to CCA
Occlusion	NA	NA	NA	No stent flow visualized

PSV, peak systolic velocity
PSV ratio, ratio peak systolic velocity within the stent, or compared to the proximal normal common carotid artery
EDV, end-diastolic velocity
ICA, internal carotid artery
CCA, common carotid artery

PSV$_{STENT}$ ratio along the stent length should be less than 2, as should PSV changes at the proximal and distal stent ends. On transverse imaging, stent should be apposed to the artery wall circumferentially and the lumen patent without anatomic or flow defect. An audit duplex testing of 65 CAS procedures with completion angiograms confirming <20% residual stenosis found duplex-measured mid-stent PSV of 100±27 cm/s (range: 52–145 cm/s) and a stent PSV ratio of 1.19±0.3 (range: 0.8–1.5). The CREST core lab observed the maximum in-stent PSV was <150 cm/sec in 93% of cases one month after the procedure.

The biomechanics of the stented ICA is altered compared to the adjacent non-stented artery, producing a compliance mis-match at the stent ends.[5,9,12] Stent deployment produces a stiffer artery segment (i.e., decreased wall compliance) that theoretically may alter flow hemodynamics and contribute to PSV elevation similar to changes observed in experimental rigid tube flow models. The PSV level in the stent is also related to stent diameter and the angioplasty balloon size used for final dilation after stent deployment. The balloon diameter used for final stent dilation typically varies from 4.5 mm to 6 mm with 5 mm being the most common size used. Residual stent stenosis as a result of incomplete plaque expansion may contribute to an increased PSV$_{STENT}$. In general, completion angiography is considered the "gold standard" for assessing technical success with a <20% residual stenosis as a desired anatomic result. Using intravascular ultrasound to monitor CAS procedures, our vascular group has observed residual stent stenosis not apparent on angiogram in five (7%) of 70 cases, resulting in additional balloon angioplasty. Procedures performed with IVUS monitoring had been associated with a lower mean PSV$_{STENT}$ (94±34cm/s; range: 42–195 cm/s) on initial duplex testing than angiography alone procedures (121±43 cm/s; range: 43–301 cm/s). When a tapered stent is deployed from the distal CCA to the ICA, a progressive increase in PSV along the stent length will be measured due to the decrease in stent diameter. Correlation of "final" balloon diameter with maximum stent PSV on initial duplex testing did not demonstrate a significant difference between <6 mm dia. (111±47 cm/s; range: 52–301) and >6 mm dia (95±34 cm/s; range: 42–251 cm/s) treatment groups.

Interpretation of a maximum stent PSV in the 150 to 200 cm/s range as indicating a >50% DR stenosis is currently a subject of debate. An elevated blood flow velocity in this range is not associated with a pressure gradient and thus would not affect cerebral volume flow, but may influence stent healing and the development of myointimal hyperplasia. A PSV in the 150–200 cm/s range has been observed when completion angiography shows >20% residual stenosis. It is recommended that any stent region that exhibits color or power Doppler features of stenosis be carefully interrogated by B-mode imaging and pulsed Doppler spectral analysis. A focal increase in PSV (ratio >2) and spectra changes of downstream turbulence are reliable duplex criteria for stenosis when an elevated PSV value is recorded. In the absence of an anatomic abnormality, a PSV_{STENT} as high as 200 cm may be measured and not indicate >50% DR stenosis. Incomplete stent dilation and compensatory collateral flow as a result of contralateral ICA occlusion are two conditions associated with elevated stent PSVs. Other ultrasound abnormalities after CAS include incomplete stent apposition to the artery wall with arterial flow imaged outside the stent, stent deformation, and stent migration. Stent deformation may be a result of stent element fracture that should be evaluated by radiograph imaging. Stent migration is typically from distal to proximal due to the longitudinal forces exerted on the stent from a severely calcified plague in the proximal ICA that deforms the stent and pushes it toward the larger diameter CCA.

The reported PSV threshold for >50% diameter-reduction stent stenosis varies in the literature with several vascular groups recommending a higher (150–200 cm/s) value than the 125 cm/s threshold recommended in the University of Washington criteria for carotid bulb atherosclerotic lesions and used in the CREST clinical trial. Our group utilizes multiple criteria when interpreting a >50% DR stent stenosis, including lumen reduction on power Doppler stent imaging, disturbed stent flow with color Doppler aliasing, a PSV value >150 cm/s with spectral broadening, and a PSV_{STENT} ratio >2 (Table 20–1, Figure 20–4). Chahwan et al[10] (Jobst Vascular Institute, Toledo, OH) reported a PSV >150 cm/s and PSV ratio >2.16 correlated with >20% DR stent stenosis while AbuRahma et al[11] reported a PSV >154 cm/s as optimal criteria for >30% stenosis. For >50% DR stenosis, recommended PSV thresholds vary from 170 to 224 cm/s.

There is more uniform agreement regarding the interpretation criteria of high-grade stent stenosis. For severe (>75% DR) stent stenosis, the "combined" hemodynamic criteria of a PSV >300 cm/s, PSV_{STENT} ratio >4, *and* EDV >125 cm/s are used in our vascular laboratory (Figure 20–5). Power Doppler imaging should indicate a <2 mm residual lumen diameter. The absence of standardized velocity criteria for diagnosis of high-grade stent stenosis is related to its infrequent occurrence. The Baylor-Houston vascular group correlated with duplex findings in 11 patients with >70% angiogram-confirmed carotid stent stenosis (18 studies) and found a PSV>300 cm/s, EDV>90 cm/s, and PSV ratio >4 was associated with a positive predictive value of 90%.[13]

CONTRALATERAL CAROTID DISEASE SURVEILLANCE

Bilateral >50% DR carotid bifurcation disease is present in approximately one-half of patients subjected to carotid intervention, including high-grade >75% DR ICA stenosis or occlusion in one-quarter of patients. When patients undergo duplex ultrasound surveillance after ipsilateral carotid intervention, testing will identify stenosis progression

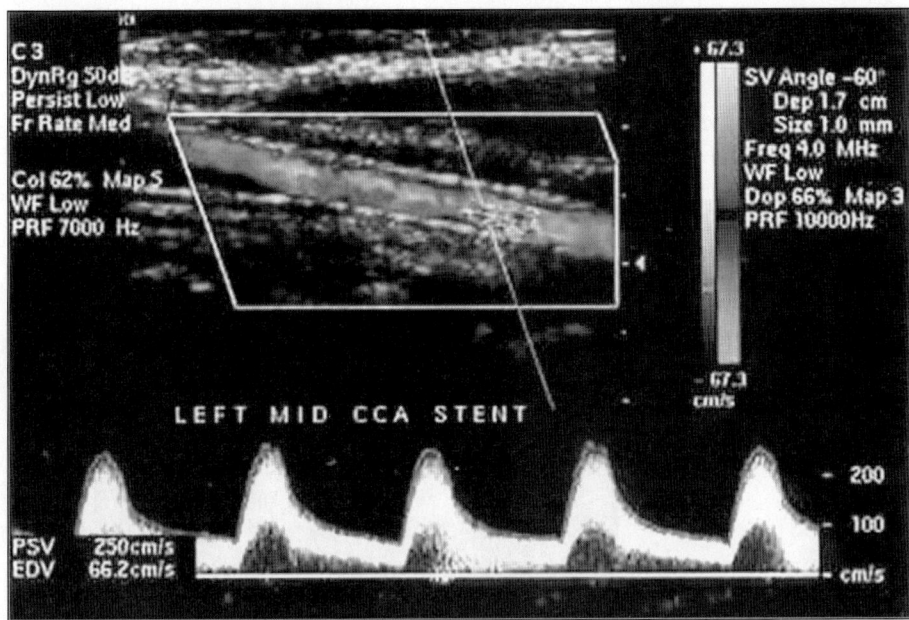

Figure 20-4. Color Doppler image and mid-stent pulsed Doppler velocity recorded after carotid stent angioplasty demonstrating focal stenosis and elevated peak systolic velocity of 250 cm/s; criteria for a 50–75% DR in-stent stenosis.

of the unoperated ICA occurring more commonly (5%/year) than restenosis of the CAS or CEA site (1%/yr).[7] Disease progression for <50% to >50% stenosis is reported to be in the 7–11% ranges and from >50% to >75% stenosis in the 3% range.[2-7] Most clinical reports indicate that stroke after intervention is more commonly associated with contralateral disease progression with neurologic events ipsilateral to the carotid repair infrequent; often despite restenosis to >75% DR.[7-11] These observations support duplex scan surveillance after intervention when a >50% contralateral ICA stenosis is documented. Surveillance programs that identify >75% DR stenosis and performed intervention have reported annual stroke rate of <1%. The low incidence of contralateral disease progression in patients with < 50% stenosis do not justify frequent surveillance after carotid intervention.

UNIVERSITY OF SOUTH FLORIDA EXPERIENCE

Patients undergoing carotid intervention are enrolled in a duplex surveillance program to identify asymptomatic high-grade (>75% DR) stenosis with testing intervals determined by disease severity (Figure 20–6). Disease progression of the unrepaired ICA occurs more frequently than CAS or CEA site restenosis. Surveillance after 242 CEAs in 221 patients demonstrated only one patient (0.5% incidence) developed >75% DR endarterectomy site stenosis compared to a 12% incidence of contralateral ICA disease progression to high-grade stenosis.[7] Overall, the yield of surveillance was approximately 5%; based on carotid testing, intervention was performed on eight patients (CEA-1; contralateral ICA-7). Three patients refused intervention and the

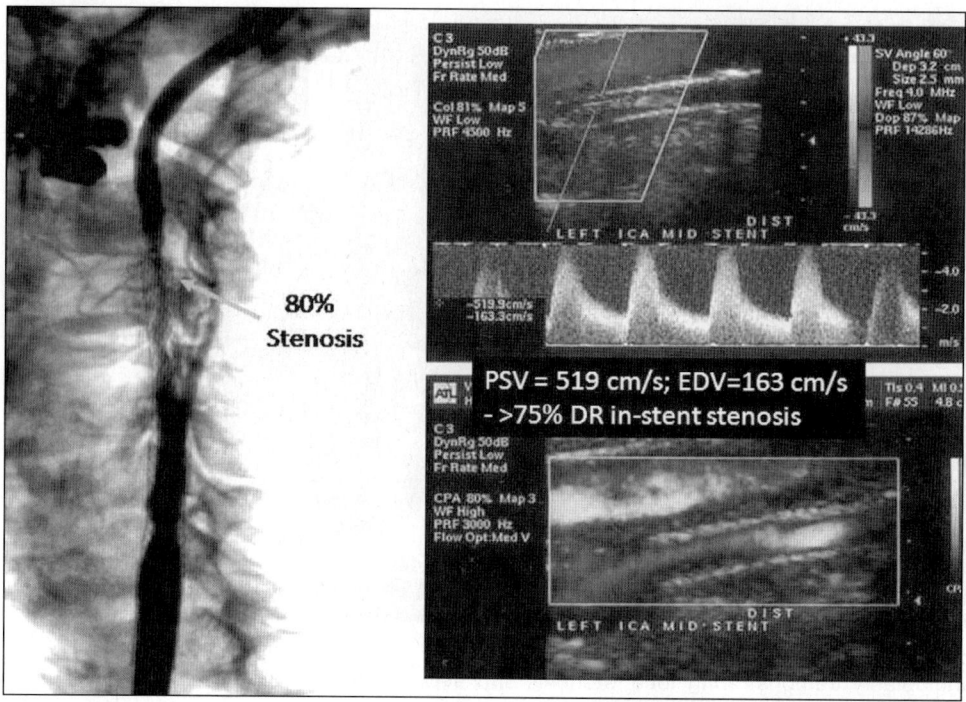

Figure 20-5. Angiogram and duplex ultrasound images of high-grade instent stenosis (arrow) following carotid stent angioplasty. Duplex findings predicted a >75% DR in-stent stenosis based on PSV, EDV, and power Doppler findings.

high-grade ICA stenosis progressed to occlusion with stroke occurring in one patient. During the follow-up period, no disabling strokes occurred ipsilateral to an operated carotid artery, but three strokes occurred in the contralateral cerebral hemisphere.

Duplex surveillance following CAS has yielded similar patient outcomes, but a higher incidence of carotid intervention.[8] A retrospective review of surveillance after 114 CAS procedures (111 patients) demonstrated on both initial and follow-up testing that the majority (>70%) of the stent angioplasty repairs had duplex findings of <50% stenosis. Serial six-month interval testing identified >50% DR in-stent stenosis development in approximately 20% of CAS sites, followed by stenosis regression in nine of 23 sites and disease progression to >75% DR stenosis in six (5%) repairs. During a mean follow-up period of 34 months, all stents remained patent, and six patients, all asymptomatic, who developed a duplex-detected >75% stent stenosis, underwent cerebral angiography that confirmed >70% in-stent stenosis (Figure 20–5). Five of six lesions were managed using endovascular therapy (balloon angioplasty, three; stent angioplasty, three) and the remaining patient had the stent removal, surgical endarectomy, and vein-patch angioplasty. After CAS, three (3%) patients developed nondisabling, reversible ipsilateral neurologic events (30, 45, and 120 days), and duplex testing detected no CAS stenosis in two patients and >50% DR (PSV=185 cm/s) in one patient. Two of the three events were minor involving visual symptoms and one involved contralateral extremity weakness that resolved fully in 72 hours. The yield of duplex surveillance for high-grade CAS stenosis was 5% (six of 114 CAS sites), no stent occlusions. An additional seven patients underwent contralateral carotid intervention for asymptomatic >75% DR ICA stenosis. After 30 days, no patient with >50% CAS stenosis on initial testing or who demonstrated stenosis progression to >50% DR developed ipsilateral neurological symptoms. No CAS or stroke-related deaths were observed during follow-up.

In our experience, duplex surveillance using six-month testing intervals has been sufficient to detect CEA and CAS site stenosis, and follow contralateral >50% DR ICA stenosis for disease progression. The development of >75% stenosis occurred without neurologic symptoms in essentially all patients. Approximately one-quarter of patients with a 50–75% DR ICA stenosis can be expected to progress to >75% DR during a three-year period. Duplex testing within one month of the CAS procedure is useful to exclude stent stenosis and confirm the severity of contralateral ICA disease. Testing at six months after CAS found 10% of sites had developed "new" duplex findings of 50–75% DR stenosis, and decrease in PSV to <150 cm/s in 5% of sites initially classified in the abnormal, >50% residual stent category. Our observations confirmed a dynamic process of stent remodeling and mytointimal hyperplasia does occur within the first six to nine months after CAS. Overall, the yield of surveillance after CAS was higher than after CEA: a 5% reintervention rate for >75% in-stent stenosis and 5% intervention rate for high-grade ICA stenosis.

If duplex testing demonstrates <50% ICA stenosis bilaterally one year after CAS, an annual scan is adequate for monitoring repair site disease progression. The development of hemispheric symptoms in the presence of >50% DR ICA or CAS stenosis, or asymptomatic disease progression to a high-grade stenosis (>75% to 80% DR, end-diastolic velocity >125–140 cm/sec), appears to be appropriate criteria to prompt an evaluation for surgical or endovascular (stent-assisted angioplasty) intervention in

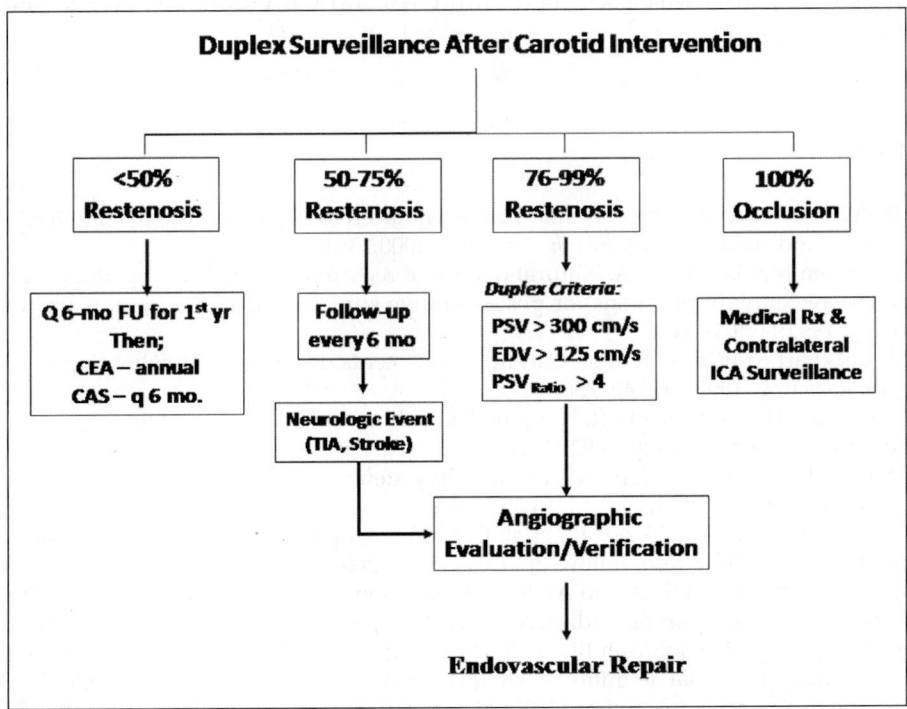

Figure 20-6. Duplex testing protocol and patient management after carotid intervention.

appropriate patients. In our experience, the development of >75% DR stenosis has occurred without neurologic symptoms, and thus angiographic confirmation of disease severity is prudent and recommended.

Both progression and regression of in-stent stenosis was observed on serial testing with the majority (70–80%) of CAS sites demonstrated velocity spectra consistent with <50% DR at postprocedural time intervals ranging from one month to 24 months. Contralateral disease progression remains a risk factor with 5% intervention rate following both CEA and CAS using similar velocity spectra criteria indicating >75% DR stenosis. Our policy of duplex ultrasound surveillance and reintervention for high-grade stenosis was associated with sustained stent patency and infrequent neurologic events. Although the maximum PSV of CAS sites may be increased compared to CEA sites, the development of moderate (50–75%) stenosis is not clinically worrisome, but progression to high-grade (>75%) stenosis may lead to occlusion. At the present time, we recommend angiographic confirmation to those patients who are typically asymptomatic despite the development of a high-grade stent stenosis (EDV >125 cm/s). If angiography confirms the lesion severity and the anatomy is suitable, we have treated these lesions using endovascular therapy.

The yield (i.e., intervention rate for severe stenosis) of duplex surveillance after CEA (3–5%) is less than after CAS (6–10%).[7] The most common abnormality was an asymptomatic myointimal stenosis that progressed in severity on serial duplex scans. Progression of contralateral disease, however, was five times more common. A policy of duplex ultrasound surveillance and reintervention for high-grade stenosis is associated with a low (<1% per year) incidence of ipsilateral hemispheric, disabling stroke. The majority of patients after CEA or CAS have duplex scans indicating bilateral <50% stenosis, and annual follow-up is appropriate. A policy of surveillance and reintervention for high-grade stenosis was associated with CAS and CEA site patency and the absence of disabling stroke.

REFERENCES

1. Hobson II RW. CREST (Carotid Revascularization Endarterectomy versus Stent Trial) background, design, and current status. *Semin Vasc Surg*. 2000;13:139–143.
2. Ricotta JJ, O'Brien MS, Deweese JA. Natural history of recurrent and residual stenosis after carotid endarterectomy: Implications for post-operative surveillance and surgical management. *Surgery*. 1992;112:656–663.
3. Robbin M, Lockhart M, Weber T, et al. Carotid artery stents: Early and late follow-up with Doppler US. *Radiology*. 1997;205:749–756.
4. Ringer AJ, German JW, Guterman LR, Hopkins LN. Follow-up of stented carotid arteries by Doppler ultrasound. *Neurosurgery*. 2002;51:639–643.
5. Lal BK, Hobson RW, Goldstein J, et al. Carotid artery stenting: Is there a need to revise ultrasound velocity criteria? *J Vasc Surg*. 2004;39:58–66.
6. De Borst J, Ackerstaff RGA, de Vries JP, et al. Carotid angioplasty and stenting for postendarterectomy stenosis: Long-term follow-up. *J Vasc Surg*. 2007;45:118–123.
7. Roth SM, Back MR, Bandyk DF, Avino AJ, Riley V, Johnson BL. A rational algorithm for duplex scan surveillance after carotid endarterectomy. *J Vasc Surg*. 1999;30: 453–460.
8. Armstrong PA, Bandyk DF, Johnson BL, et al. Duplex scan surveillance after carotid angioplasty and stenting: A rational definition of stent stenosis. *J Vasc Surg*. 2007;46:460–466.
9. Willfort-Ehringer A, Ahmadi R, Gruber D, et al. Arterial remodling and hemodynamics in carotid stents: A prospective duplex ultrasound study over 2 years. *J Vasc Surg*. 2004;39:728.34.

10. Chahwan S, Miller MT, Pigott JP, et al. Carotid artery characteristics after carotid artery angioplasty and stenting. *J Vasc Surg*. 2007;45:523–526.
11. AbuRahma AF, Abu-Halimah S, Besenhaver J, et al. Optimal carotid duplex velocity criteria for defining the severity of carotid in-stent stenosis. *J Vasc Surg*. 2008
12. Vernhet H, Jean B, Lust S, et al. Wall mechanics of the stented extracranial carotid artery. *Stroke*. 2004;34:e222–224.
13. Zhou W, Felkai DD, Evans M, et al. Ultrasound criteria for severe in-stent stenosis following carotid artery stenting. *J Vasc Surg*. 2008;47:74–80.

Techniques and Outcomes in Carotid Endarterectomy

21

Contemporary Carotid Endarterectomy Results in the United States

Mark W. Fugate, M.D.
Bruce A. Perler, M.D., M.B.A.

Ischemic stroke is one of the most important health care problems in the United States in terms of mortality, morbidity, and cost. Approximately 700,000 new strokes occur each year in the United States: roughly 1,450 new cases per 1,000,000 population. Today, stroke is the third leading cause of death in this country, trailing only heart disease and malignancy, our second leading cause of dementia, and the leading cause of adult disability in America today. There are currently approximately 5.4 million stroke survivors in the United States. One year after experiencing a stroke, two-thirds of the survivors are still left with significant functional limitations. In fact, today, stroke is the leading cause of nursing home admission in America. It is estimated that the direct and indirect health care costs of stroke now exceed $50 billion annually in the United States.[1]

Gowers is credited with first linking extracranial atherosclerotic carotid disease to stroke in 1875. He described a patient with right hemiplegia and blindness in the left eye, and he attributed these symptoms to an occlusion of the left carotid artery.[2] Today, more than 80% of strokes are ischemic, and less than 20% are hemorrhagic. Atherosclerotic cerebrovascular disease is the most common pathophysiologic mechanism for stroke, and atherosclerosis of the cervical carotid artery disease is responsible for 20% to 60% and is, therefore, the most common preventable cause of ischemic stroke. In light of this, it is not surprising that carotid endarterectomy (CEA) has become the most frequently performed peripheral vascular operation in the United States.

Eastcott and colleagues reported the first successful carotid operation in 1954 in which they resected a lesion at the carotid bifurcation and performed a primary anastomosis. This was performed for transient ischemic attacks.[3] The first successful carotid endarterectomy was not performed in this country until 1953 by DeBakey, and this was not reported until 1975.[4] Over the past five decades, this operation has experienced a remarkable evolution, with waxing and waning popularity, largely related to variability in real and perceived outcomes.

EARLY EXPERIENCE IN THE UNITED STATES

After its introduction into clinical practice in the United States in the 1950s, the volume of CEAs performed grew rapidly over the next three decades. By the mid-1980s, more than 100,000 CEAs were performed annually in this country at a cost of $1.2 billion. However, isolated reports, primarily in the medical and neurologic literature, documented unacceptably high rates of perioperative morbidity and mortality, and led to a waning of enthusiasm for CEA with a precipitous decline in referral of patients for operation by the end of the decade

For example, in 1977, Easton and Sherman published a retrospective review of 228 patients who underwent CEA in two 600-bed community hospitals in Illinois that demonstrated an alarmingly high overall stroke and mortality rate of 21.1%.[5] They found a combined stroke and death rate of 18.2% for CEA performed for asymptomatic carotid disease, 21% among patients with transient ischemic attacks (TIAs), and 23% among patients with a previous stroke.[5] Among patients undergoing operation after a severe stroke, the perioperative stroke and death rate was 41.5%. Another important revelation in this study was that operative indications were not standardized or uniform across the population in the series.

Similarly, the landmark RAND Health Services Utilization Study found that 32% of CEAs performed on Medicare patients were performed for inappropriate indications. In this study, the investigators reviewed a random sample of 1,302 Medicare patients undergoing CEA in three different geographic regions. In addition to the 32% of CEAs performed for inappropriate indications, they found 32% performed for equivocal reasons and only 35% for appropriate indications.[6] They also found the 30-day major stroke or death rate to be 9.8% in this patient population.[6] The authors concluded that CEA was overused based on this data and that the risk of the procedure far outweighed the potential benefit. In another analysis of the national Medicare database, Fisher et al analyzed the outcomes of more than 2,000 elderly patients who underwent CEA. They demonstrated a dramatic increase in operative mortality with advancing age, including 3.2% among those in their 70s and 4.7% among octogenarians.[7] Furthermore, they noted that the risk of perioperative mortality was nearly threefold greater when the surgery was performed in low- versus high-volume hospitals.[7]

The common thread of these early reports appeared to be the lack of clear-cut or appropriate indications for the procedure. It was not uncommon for CEA to be performed in the acute setting of major strokes, and thus, with disastrous results. At the other end of the spectrum were procedures performed for asymptomatic, nonsignificant carotid stenoses that conveyed risk to the patient albeit with little to no potential clinical benefit. At this time, the legitimacy of CEA as a means of stroke prevention was seriously questioned. In fact, it was not until completion of broad-based randomized clinical trials that this issue was definitively clarified.

RANDOMIZED TRIALS

In the 1990s, the results of two landmark randomized controlled trials were published, and solidified the role of CEA in the management of symptomatic and asymptomatic carotid disease. In the North American Symptomatic Carotid Endarterectomy Trial (NASCET) in the Unites States and Canada, 659 patients with internal carotid artery stenoses between 70% and 99% with a history of TIA or stroke within three months were randomized to either best medical therapy or CEA and best medical therapy. At two years, a significant reduction in stroke incidence was found in those patients randomized to CEA (9%) versus those randomized to medical therapy (26%).[8] Moreover, the benefit of surgery increased with increasing degrees of stenosis. After the initial NASCET data were published demonstrating the clear benefit of surgery over medical management at two years, these patients continued to be followed, and this benefit persisted for at least eight years of follow-up. In a second limb of the NASCET investigation, CEA was demonstrated to be superior to best medical management in symptomatic patients with a moderate carotid stenosis. Specifically, among 858 patients with a 50–69% stenosis, the five-year stroke risk was 22.2% in the medically managed patients and 15.7% in the CEA cohort. The benefit of CEA over medical management in this patient population has persisted through eight years of continuous follow-up as well.[9–10]

These results were largely validated in another randomized, prospective multicenter trial, the European Carotid Surgery Trial (ECST). In 778 symptomatic patients with a 70–99% internal carotid stenosis, patients undergoing CEA as compared to medical management had a reduction in the incidence of stroke and death from 21.9% to 12.3%.[11]

An even more controversial subset of patients has been those with asymptomatic carotid stenoses. Although in earlier years the majority of CEAs were performed on patients with symptomatic carotid stenosis, that trend has reversed in recent years, at least in the United States, largely due to the results of the NIH-funded Asymptomatic Carotid Atherosclerosis Study (ACAS). This randomized, prospective trial enrolled more than 1,600 patients with at least a 60% carotid stenosis at 39 centers throughout the United States and Canada. The patients were randomized to either aspirin alone or CEA plus aspirin. At five years follow-up, a 53% stroke risk reduction was demonstrated for patients undergoing CEA (11% in the medical group versus 5.1% in the CEA group).[12] More importantly, however, was that CEA was shown to be safe in a large, prospective, randomized and multicenter study. The perioperative stroke and death rate was 2.3% and half of these were related to the preoperative arteriography. The true surgical stroke and death rate was only 1.4%. ACAS proved that CEA was a safe and effective means of stroke prevention in asymptomatic patients with significant carotid stenosis.[12]

After the publication of these landmark studies, the number of CEAs performed in the United States increased substantially from 68,000 in 1990 to 134,000 in 2002. More significant, though, is that the appropriate use of CEA improved dramatically when compared to the findings of the RAND Health Service Utilization Study noted above. The New York Carotid Artery Surgery Study (NYCAS) was a population-based cohort investigaton of all patients undergoing CEA from January 1998 to June 1999 in New York State. Of these 9,588 patients, only 8.6% of operations were performed for inappropriate reasons, as compared to 32% in the RAND study from 1988. Of those deemed inappropriate, the most common reasons were high comorbidity in asymptomatic patients, minimal stenosis, or operating after a major stroke.[13]

CONTEMPORARY USA EXPERIENCE

Institutional Series

Since the publication of the NASCET and ACAS, which proved the safety and efficacy of CEA and its superiority in preventing strokes when compared to best medical management, these findings have been reproduced repeatedly in institutions through-out the United States. For example, in one of the largest individual institutional series reported in this country, surgeons at the Massachusetts General Hospital reported their experience of 2,236 CEAs performed between 1989 and 1999, including only a 5.5% overall perioperative complication rate.[14] The perioperative stroke and death rate was only 1.4%, The most commonly reported complication was neck hematoma (1.7%). At five and 10 years follow-up, actuarial survival was 72.4% and 44.7%, respec-tively, with coronary artery disease, chronic obstructive pulmonary disease, and dia-betes mellitus correlating with decreased longevity. Also shown over this 10-year period was a decrease in resource utilization when comparing the first two years of the study and the last two years. This was realized through decreases in hospital stay and preoperative contrast arteriography over the study period. Analysis of the dura-bility of CEA during a median follow-up of 5.9 years identified a restenosis or occlu-sion rate of 4.5% and a re-operative CEA rate of 3.2%. The excellent results from this study and similar results from other institutions highlight the effectiveness of CEA in stroke prevention, as well as its safety and long-term durability.

Population-based Studies

Although the outcome of CEA as documented in NASCET and ACAS firmly established the role of CEA in the management of symptomatic and asymptomatic pa-tients, respectively, and while the safety of the procedure has been confirmed in indi-vidual institutional series, the safety and efficacy of the procedure has continued to be questioned by some. Specifically, it has been challenged whether the results achieved in randomized clinical trials by highly vetted surgeons, or in individual centers of excellence by high-volume surgeons, truly reflect the outcome of the operation in the surgical community at large. However, multiple population-based analyses have shown equivalent results in larger populations, not exclusive to tertiary referral centers.

Individual State Experience.   In recent years, several population-based analyses have demonstrated excellent results of CEA in community practice, and comparable to the outcomes in tertiary referral centers. For example, a statewide study from North Carolina examined the outcome of all 11,973 CEA operations in 70 of the 157 hospitals in which the procedure was performed between 1988 and 1993 in the state. The perioperative stroke rate for the study period was 1.56% and the death rate was 1.17% for a combined stroke and death rate of 2.62%.[15] Likewise, in a similar analysis of 9,308 CEAs performed by 482 surgeons in 167 hospitals in New York State from 1998 through 1999, the perioperative mortality rate was 1.14% and the nonfatal stroke rate was 2.85% for a combined perioperative stroke and death rate of 3.99%.[16] Another study compared the outcomes of CEA in both Maryland and California. The Maryland Health Services Cost Review Commission (HSCRC) database was retrospectively reviewed and identified 23,237 CEAs performed between 1994 and 2003 by 437 surgeons in 47 nonfederal acute care hospitals in the state, of which only two are university hospitals. Over this 10-year period, the in-hospital stroke rate was 0.73% and the stroke and death rate was 1.3%. The stroke rate also decreased over the time period of the study.[17] Likewise, the California Office of Statewide Health Planning and Development (OSHPD) database was queried for all CEAs performed in that state between 1999 and 2003. During that time, 51,331 CEAs were performed with an in-hospital stroke rate of 0.45% and an overall mortality rate of 0.48%. Also, similar to the Maryland results, the stroke rate in California decreased over the study period.[17] Of note, approximately 85% of the operations in both Maryland and California were performed for asymptomatic carotid disease that may have contributed to the superior results.[17] Another recent study compared the outcomes of CEA performed in Veterans Administration and nonfederal hospitals in Connecticut. Among 7,089 CEAs performed between 1997 and 2002, there were no significant differences in the rates of perioperative stroke (1.4% and 0.3%), death (1.4% and 0.9%), and combined stroke and death (2.8% and 1.2%) among the two hospital groups, respectively.[18]

National Experience: Medicare.   The incidence of stroke increases with advancing age so that elderly patients would appear to potentially most benefit from CEA. However, this is one patient population in which this operation has been particularly controversial due to the perception of increased operative risk. This perception has been based on earlier experiences, as noted above. However, recent population-based evidence suggests that CEA can be safely performed on elderly patients and benefit this patient cohort. For example, a retrospective review of 1,945 CEAs performed on Medicare patients in the state of Georgia in 1993 revealed a 30-day mortality of 1.9% and moderate to severe stroke rate of 1.8%.[19]

It has been argued by some that these large administrative databases underreport subtle strokes, thus minimizing the true surgical morbidity rates. Therefore, it is instructive to focus on operative mortality as a metric in assessing operative risk. Two independent studies involving Medicare patients have shown a progressive decrease in mortality over time for patients undergoing CEA.[20-21] For example, in an analysis of the outcome of CEA performed on more than 3,000 Medicare beneficiaries across the United States from 1990 through 2000, median perioperative mortality declined from 1.87% in 1990 to 1.47% in 1995 and to 0.87% in 2000, reflecting a dramatic improvement in perioperative outcomes.[21]

National Experience.   Other population-based studies have focused on all patients undergoing CEA, not just the elderly. For example, the National Surgical Quality Improvement Program (NSQIP) database was queried for all CEAs performed between 2000 and 2003 at 123 Veterans Affairs and 14 private sector academic medical centers. During the study period, 13,622 CEAs were performed with a combined stroke and death rate of only 3.4%.[22] Similarly, the Nationwide Inpatient Sample (NIS) was recently examined to compare in-hospital stroke and death rates for patients undergoing CEA and carotid artery stenting (CAS). In this analysis of 259,080 carotid revascularization procedures performed in the United States in 2003 and 2004, there was an overall stroke rate of 0.88% for CEA compared to 2.1% with CAS. The mortality rate was also higher for CAS, 1.3%, as compared to 0.39% with CEA.[23] These population-based analyses and others confirm that CEA is being safely performed among the population at large by a wide spectrum of well-trained carotid surgeons in the United States in contemporary practice.

SPECIAL CONSIDERATIONS

One of the ongoing concerns with respect to the outcome of CEA is whether there are specific risk factors or conditions that convey increased operative risk for CEA. This is increasingly important at a time when CAS is being offered as a minimally invasive alternative to CEA.

Age

The prevalence of stroke increases exponentially with advancing age, and the elderly population is the fastest growing segment in our country. Therefore, one would assume that it is the elderly who can most benefit form CEA. In fact, patients aged 80 and older were excluded from NASCET and ACAS, and it has, therefore, been assumed that advanced age represents a high-risk factor for CEA and, therefore, these patients might be optimally treated by CEA. However, compelling evidence accumulated over the past two decades has confirmed the safety of CEA among very elderly individuals. In a recent meta-analysis including more than 20 institutional series and more than 3,000 elderly patients with a minimum age of 75 or 80 who underwent CEA, the perioperative stroke rate was 2.2% and mortality rate was 1.5%.[24] In a population-based analysis of CEA in the state of Maryland from 1990 through 1995, the outcome among octogenarians was the same as younger patient cohorts (perioperative stroke and death rate, 2.6%).[25] In another study, the perioperative mortality rate was higher among nonagenarians than octogenarians, although there was no difference in neurologic outcomes.[26]

Gender

There are conflicting reports on the impact of gender on outcome after CEA. In the ACAS, for example, females received less benefit in terms of stroke prevention than males, having more strokes in both the perioperative period and in long-term follow-up.[11] Other studies have shown no difference in outcomes between males and females.[27] One population-based study examined 14,095 CEAs performed in Virginia between 1997 and 2001, and demonstrated that female gender was not an independent predictor of higher stroke or death rate.[28] Likewise, investigators in Ontario found no difference in perioperative complication rates between males and females in a review of 6,038 CEA patients, 35% of whom were female.[29] Even though female gender has not been shown to increase risk of CEA in large population-based studies such as these, consideration of anatomic (i.e., smaller arteries) and physiologic (i.e., later age at presentation) factors is prudent when performing CEA on females.

Race

Analyses of the impact of race on CEA outcomes have also demonstrated conflicting results. Lucas et al examined national Medicare data to determine postoperative mortality following eight cardiovascular and cancer operations between 1994 and 1999. Black patients in this study had more than 20% higher crude mortality rates in seven of the eight procedures, including CEA. The study suggests multiple reasons for this finding, including more frequent emergent presentation and residence in low-income areas. Additionally, African Americans were more likely to receive care in lower volume hospitals and hospitals with overall higher mortality rates.[30] Likewise, a 2002 meta-analysis demonstrated a 40% greater likelihood of short-term death following CEA for African Americans compared to whites undergoing CEA.[31] In our review of the Maryland HSCRC database, black patients undergoing CEA experienced an increased incidence of in-hospital stroke, longer hospital stays, and higher hospital charges. This research noted that black patients were more likely to undergo CEA in low-volume hospitals and less likely by higher volume surgeons.[32] However, Horner's review of the NSQIP data revealed similarly low stroke and death rates between blacks and white patients in the VA system. Among patients with transient ischemic attack (TIA), though, Hispanic males experienced significantly worse outcomes in terms of stroke and death when compared to white patients.[33] An institutional review from Henry Ford Hospital revealed similar stroke and death rates between black and whites, as well as acceptable protection from ipsilateral stroke without racial variation. African American patients in this study did have a higher incidence of all strokes long-term when compared to white cohorts.[34] The influence of race on the outcome of CEA merits further research. It is not clear at this time whether race, or associated access to care limitations, is the more robust factor influencing outcomes. Nevertheless, there is strong evidence that CEA can be safely performed on African American patients in the United States in contemporary practice.

Hospital/Surgeon Volume

In contemporary practice, many have advocated the regionalization of specialized care and/or high-risk procedures to higher volume centers. In this regard, some have proposed that CEA, like many other high-risk cardiovascular procedures, should be performed exclusively at centers with higher volumes. Likewise, proponents of regionalization of care propose that CEA is performed best by high-volume surgeons. A meta-analysis published in 2007 suggests that the stroke and death rate is significantly lower in high-volume centers, with a critical volume threshold of 79 CEAs per year. Interestingly, this meta-analysis demonstrated that patients undergoing operations performed by lower volume surgeons operating in higher volume centers also experienced lower stroke and death rates, suggesting that hospital infrastructure and available resources rather than surgeon experience was more important in lowering complications.[35] Other population-based studies have shown similar trends of mortality inversely proportional to volume.[36] In California between 1982 and 1994, mortality rates decreased for CEA, lower extremity bypass, and unruptured abdominal aortic aneurysm repair. Higher hospital volume was found to be an important determinant of outcome. However, conflicting data exist regarding volume and outcomes. A retrospective review of CEAs performed in Oregon over a two-year period examined the outcomes between two low-volume (total of 156 CEAs) and one high-volume (total of 404 CEAs) institution. In this study, there was no significant difference in 30-day stroke and death rates between the low- and high-volume centers.[37] This was evident despite the fact that the low-volume centers had significantly older patients, more smokers, and fewer asymptomatic patients.[37] This paper makes a legitimate point that an individual surgeon in a low-volume institution may perform more individual high-risk procedures than another individual surgeon at a higher volume center. Ultimately, it should be recognized that it is surgeons and not hospitals that perform surgery. Further, the ideal break point to define a suitably "high volume" caseload remains to be defined.

High-risk Patients

With the introduction of CAS, there has been a renewed motivation to define the patient deemed "high risk" for undergoing CEA and who, therefore, might be better served by a CAS procedure. However, as previously mentioned, recent literature has repeatedly shown impressively low rates of perioperative stroke and death in large population-based series of patients undergoing CEA, including both high and low risk patients. Some have defined "high risk" as those subgroups excluded from ACAS and NASCET. These exclusion criteria included age >80, prior ipsilateral CEA, previous neck radiation, prior contralateral CEA within four months, and other conditions that could potentially cause symptoms (atrial fibrillation, valvular heart disease, previous stroke with persistent defect), uncontrolled diabetes or hypertension, major organ failure, and significant coronary artery disease.[7,9,11] Gasparis et al reviewed 788 CEAs performed between 1996 and 2001, including 228 (29%) defined as high risk by physiologic or anatomic risk factors similar to those listed above. They found no significant difference in outcomes in patients with significant comorbidities, contralateral carotid occlusions, or anatomically high lesions as compared to "normal risk" patients. Two risk factors associated with higher complication rates were reoperative CEAs and those performed after prior neck radiation.[38] Another study using similar definitions of high-risk patients found only contralateral carotid occlusion to be a significant risk factor for adverse perioperative outcomes.[39] Factors that were not associated with increased risk included age >80, gender, recent ipsilateral hemispheric event, reoperative CEA, recent coronary revascularization, congestive heart failure, or chronic renal failure.[39] One particularly interesting finding in this cohort, however, was the low five-year survival (39%) of patients with two or more of the so-called high-risk factors.[39] This does emphasize the importance of thorough evaluation of risk factors when considering carotid revascularization in asymptomatic patients who may not survive long enough to realize any stroke prevention benefit. Similar conclusions were reached by Nguyen et al. They found no significant difference in perioperative stroke rate in patients with multiple risk factors but 30-day mortality was significantly higher in patients with two or more risk factors.[40]

The definition of the "high risk" patient remains unsettled and hotly debated. One area that cannot be overemphasized is that patients with asymptomatic carotid disease and comorbidities significant enough to limit their life expectancy may not survive long enough to experience the benefit of a stroke preventing intervention such as CEA, even if they can undergo the operation with acceptable perioperative morbidity. In this patient population, modern medical management may be the most prudent option.

CONCLUSIONS

Few surgical procedures have been subjected to the rigorous evaluation applied to CEA. CEA has clearly been established as the "gold standard" for stroke prevention in patients with extracranial symptomatic and asymptomatic carotid artery disease. It seems clear from reported evidence that this procedure has become increasingly safe over the years, and especially during the past decade. While this may reflect, in part, a reduced rate of perioperative complications related to the operation being performed on patients with asymptomatic carotid artery disease, it is also undeniable that the operation is being increasingly performed by well-trained carotid surgeons who perform the procedure on a regular basis, both in academic centers and the community at large.

REFERENCES

1 Goldstein LB, Adams R, Becker K, et al. Primary prevention of ischemic stroke. A statement for healthcare professionals from the stroke council of the American Heart Association. *Stroke*. 2001;32:280–299.

2. Gowers WR. On a case of simultaneous embolism of central retinal and middle cerebral arteries. *Lancet*. 2:794, 1875.

3. Eastcott HHG, Pickering GW, Robb CG: Reconstruction of internal carotid artery in a patient with intermittent attacks of hemiplegia. *Lancet*. 1954;2:994.

4. DeBakey ME. Successful carotid endarterectomy for cerebrovascular insufficiency. *JAMA*. 1975;233:1083–1085.

5. Easton JD and Sherman DG. Stroke and mortality rate in carotid endarterectomy: 228 consecutive operations. *Stroke*. 1977;8:565–568.

6. Winslow CM, Solomon DH, Chassin MR, et al. The appropriateness of carotid endarterectomy. *N Engl J Med*. 1988;318:721–727.

7. Fisher ES, Malenka DJ, Solomon NA, et al. Risk of Carotid Endarterectomy in the Elderly. *Am J Public Health*. 1989;79:1617–1620.

8. North American Symptomatic Carotid Endarterectomy Trial Collaborators. Beneficial effect of carotid endarterectomy in symptomatic patients with high-grade stenosis. *N Engl J Med*. 1991;325:445–453.

9. Barnett HJM, Taylor DW, Eliasziw M, et al. Benefit of carotid endarterectomy in patients with symptomatic moderate or severe stenosis. *N Engl J Med*. 1998;339:1415–1425.

10. Ferguson GG, Eliasziw M, Barr HW, et al. The North American symptomatic carotid endarterectomy trial: surgical results in 1415 patients. *Stroke*. 1999;30:1751–1758.

11. European Carotid Surgery Trialists' Collaborative Group. MRS European carotid surgery trial: interim results for symptomatic patients with severe (70–99%) or mild (0–25%) carotid stenosis. *Lancet*. 1991;337:1235–1243.

12. Executive Committee for the Asymptomatic Carotid Atherosclerosis Study. Endarterectomy for asymptomatic carotid artery stenosis. *JAMA*. 1995;273:1421–1428.

13. Halm EA, Tuhrim S, Wang JJ, et al. Has evidence changed practice? Appropriateness of carotid endarterectomy after the clinical trials. *Neurology*. 2007;68:187–194.

14. LaMuraglia, GM, Brewster DC, Moncure AC, et al. Carotid endarterectomy at the Millennium: what interventional therapy must match. *Ann Surg*. 2004;240:535–546.

15. Maxwell JG, Rutledge R, Covington DL, et al. A statewide, hospital-based analysis of frequency and outcomes in carotid endarterectomy. *Am J Surg*. 1997;174:655–661.

16. Greenstein AJ, Chassin MR, Wang J, et al. Association between minor and major surgical complications after carotid endarterectomy: Results of the New York Carotid Artery Surgery study. *J Vasc Surg*. 2007;46:6:1138–1146.

17. Matsen SL, Chang DC, Perler BA, et al. Trends in the in-hospital stroke rate following carotid endarterectomy in California and Maryland. *J Vasc Surg*. 2006;44: 3:488–493.

18. Weiss JS, Dumas P, Cha C, et al. Safety of carotid endarterectomy in a high-risk population: lessons from the VA and Connecticut. *J Am Coll Surg*, 2006;203:3:277–282.

19. Karp HR, Flanders WD, Shipp CC, et al. carotid endarterectomy among medicare beneficiaries: a statewide evaluation of appropriateness and outcome. *Stroke*. 1998;29:46–52.

20. Goodney PP, Siewers AE, Stukel TA, et al. Is surgery getting safer? National trends in operative mortality. *J Am Coll Surg*. 2002;195:219–227.

21. Sheikh K and Bullock C. Variation and changes in state-specific carotid endarterectomy and 30-day mortality rates, United States, 1991–2000. *J Vasc Surg*. 2003;38:779–784.

22. Stoner MC, Abbott WM, Wong DR, et al. Defining the high-risk patient for carotid endarterectomy: An analysis of the prospective National Surgical Quality Improvement Program database. *J Vasc Surg*. 2006;43:285–296.

23. McPhee JT, Hill JS, Ciocca RG, et al. Carotid endarterectomy was performed with lower stroke and death rates than carotid artery stenting in the United States in 2003 and 2004. *J Vasc Surg*. 2007;46:1112–1118.

24. Narins CR, Illig KA. Patient selection for carotid stenting versus endarterectomy: a systematic review. *J Vasc Surg*. 2006;44:661–672.
25. Perler BA, Dardik A, Burleyson GP, Gordon TA, Williams GM. The influence of age and hospital volume on the outcome of carotid endarterectomy. *J Vasc Surg*. 1998;27: 25–31.
26. Teso D, Edwards RE, Frattini JC, et al. safety of carotid endarterectomy in 2,443 elderly patients: lessons from nonagenarians - are we pushing the limit? *J Am Coll Surg*. 2005;200(5): 734–741.
27. Sternbach Y, Perler BA. The influence of female gender on the outcomes of carotid endarterectomy: a challenge to the ACAS findings. *Surgery*. 2000;127:272–275.
28. Harthun NL, Kongable GL, Baglioni AJ, et al. Examination of sex as an independent risk factor for adverse events after carotid endarterectomy. *J Vasc Surg*. 2005;41:223–230.
29. Kapral MK, Wang H, Austin PC, et al. Sex differences in carotid endarterectomy outcomes: results from the ontario carotid endarterectomy registry. *Stroke*. 2003;34:1120–1125.
30. Lucas FL, Stukel TA, Morris AM, et al. Race and surgical mortality in the United States. *Ann Surg*. 2006;243:281–286.
31. Kennedy BS. Does race predict short-term mortality after carotid surgery? The results of a meta-analysis. *J Natl Med Assoc*. 2002;94:25–30.
32. Dardik A, Bowman HM, Gordon TA, et al. impact of race on the outcome of carotid endarterectomy: a population-based analysis of 9,842 recent elective procedures. *Ann Surg*. 2000;232:704–709.
33. Horner RD, Oddone EZ, Stechuchak KM, et al. Racial variations in postoperative outcomes of carotid endarterectomy: evidence from the veterans affairs national surgical quality improvement program. *Med Care*. 2002;40:35–43.
33. Conrad MF, Shepard AD, Pandurangi K, et al. Outcome of carotid endarterectomy in African Americans: Is race a factor? *J Vasc Surg*. 2003;38:129–137.
34. Holt PJE, Poloniecki JD, Loftus IM , et al. Meta-analysis and systematic review of the relationship between hospital volume and outcome following carotid endarterectomy. *Eur J Vasc Endovasc Surg*. 2007;33:645–651.
35. Manheim LM, Sohn M, Feinglass J, et al. Hospital vascular surgery volume and procedure mortality rates in California, 1982–1994. *J Vasc Surg*. 1998;28:45–58.
36. Peck C, Peck J, Peck A. Comparison of carotid endarterectomy at high- and low-volume hospitals. *Am J Surg*. 2001;181:450–453.
37. Gasparis AP, Ricotta L, Cuadra SA, et al. High-risk carotid endarterectomy: Fact or fiction. *J Vasc Surg*. 2003;37:40–46.
38. Reed AB, Gaccione P, Belkin M, et al. Preoperative risk factors for carotid endarterectomy: Defining the patient at high risk. *J Vasc Surg*. 2003;37:1191–1199.
39. Nguyen LL, Conte MS, Reed AB et al. Carotid Endarterectomy: Who is the High-Risk Patient? *Semin Vasc Surg*. 2004;17:219–223.
40. Yadav JS, Wholey MH, Kuntz RE, et al. Protected carotid-artery stenting versus endarterectomy in high-risk patients. *N Engl J Med*. 2004;351:1493–1501.

22

Performance Measurement for Carotid Endarterectomy

Timothy F. Kresowik, M.D.

PERFORMANCE MEASUREMENT

Performance measures of quality in health care can be classified as outcome measures, process measures, structural measures, and surrogate measures (Table 22-1). Outcome measures include measures of treatment success as well as complication (morbidity/mortality) rates. Process measures examine whether or not certain diagnostic or therapeutic interventions are performed. Good process measures utilize processes that have an evidence-based relationship to improved outcomes. Structural and surrogate measures are indirect indicators of the quality of care. Structural measures indicate whether or not a "structure" exists that is thought to be associated with better quality (e.g., the institutional availability of certain specialists or procedures that might be necessary to treat complications associated with a procedure). Surrogate measures are designed to indicate training or experience. Board certification status or annual procedural volumes are examples of surrogate measures.

The purpose of performance measurement is important in determining the necessary specifications of the measures (Table 22-2). Performance measures can be used primarily for two purposes: quality improvement or accountability/judgment. Measurement for quality improvement generally implies confidential feedback of data. This could involve a voluntary registry or be part of the maintenance of certification process for board certification. Comparisons to other physicians is provided primarily to identify areas where there is likely to be room for improvement and thus to focus quality improvement efforts. Measurement for accountability/judgment purposes includes programs that involve public reporting of data. Another example of accountability measurement is the strong push in health care by government and other payers to theoretically reward higher quality by utilizing "pay for performance" strategies. Performance measurement for accountability/judgment should have more stringent specification requirements than measurement for quality improvement. Outcome measures used for accountability/judgment must be risk adjusted and process measures should have specifications that incorporate appropriate

TABLE 22-1. TYPES OF PERFORMANCE MEASURES/CEA EXAMPLES

Measure Type	Example for CEA	Need for Adjustment Criteria	Potential for Perverse Incentive
Outcome	Stroke or death rate	Adjust for patient risk	Avoid high risk patients
Process	Perioperative antiplatelet administration	Adjust for contraindications	No
Structural	Participation in ACS/NSQIP	No	No
Surrogate	CEA volume/year	No	Increase unnecessary procedures

CEA-Carotid endarterectomy, ACS-NSQIP-American College of Surgeons National Quality Improvement Program

TABLE 22-2. USE OF PERFORMANCE MEASURES

Use	Examples	Statistical Significance	Perverse Incentives
Quality improvement only	Voluntary registry Maintenance of certification	Not essential	No
Accountability/Judgment	Public reporting Pay for performance	Very important	Avoid high risk or noncompliant patients

exclusions. Sample sizes and statistical significance also become very important considerations when the performance measures are used for accountability/judgment purposes.

The failure to include valid risk adjustment and/or exclusions in accountability measurement not only may be fundamentally unfair to the physicians being measured, but also it has the potential to have adverse consequences for patients. Unadjusted measures can have the unintended consequence of creating a disincentive to caring for patients who are likely to have poor outcomes or cannot comply with care processes because of their lack of appropriate resources. This perverse incentive may increase the financial disadvantage to providers of health care for these disadvantaged populations and exacerbate the health care access difficulties these populations already experience.

OUTCOME MEASURES

Outcome measures have the most face validity with both clinicians and the public. The combined event rate for stroke and mortality following CEA is often considered the "gold standard" indicator of surgical quality for the procedure. Unfortunately, this "gold standard" is reported in many different ways that do not come close to standardized. Although mortality is as hard an endpoint as exists, the time period for postoperative reporting influences the validity of comparisons. The randomized trials utilized a 30-day postoperative period for morbidity/mortality assessment.[1-7] Some

CEA outcome reports utilize administrative (billing) data associated with the hospitalization. Comparing in-hospital mortality for a procedure, that often has only a one-day hospital stay associated with it, to a 30-day mortality rate is obviously invalid. Perioperative cardiac events, a common cause of CEA associated mortality, can occur days after a seemingly uncomplicated procedure.

The measurement of perioperative stroke rates presents even more problems for valid comparison. The diagnosis of stroke can depend on the aggressiveness of the assessment. Most of the randomized trials incorporated a routine preoperative and postoperative neurologic exam by an independent physician. A subtle change in neurologic status is certainly more likely to be picked up by this approach. Even with standardized assessment, the definition of stroke will influence the reported incidence. The North American randomized trials utilized as a definition of stroke any new or worsened neurologic deficit that persisted beyond 24 hours following the onset.[1-4] The European symptomatic trial included as strokes only deficits that persisted for one week.[5] The source of data for retrospective data collection also has a profound influence on the validity of reported perioperative stroke incidence. Administrative data may underreport complications that have no influence on reimbursement. Comorbidities and complications can be confused in administrative datasets.

Valid outcome comparison necessitates risk adjustment. The most important risk factor for perioperative stroke or death following CEA is the preoperative symptom status of the patient. The randomized trial data from the North American Symptomatic Carotid Endarterectomy Trial (NASCET) and the Asymptomatic Carotid Atherosclerosis Study (ACAS) suggest that the risk of perioperative stroke or death following CEA is up to 4 times higher in patients with ipsilateral hemispheric symptoms than in patients who have never had ipsilateral symptoms[6,7] (Table 22-3). In large retrospective reviews incorporating individual medical record (hospital chart) abstraction of over 20,000 Medicare patients undergoing CEA, we consistently demonstrated that CEA outcomes should be stratified by at least three preoperative symptom status levels.[8,9] The three categories we used were *asymptomatic, symptomatic* (recent ipsilateral hemispheric or ocular TIA or stroke) and *nonspecific* (contralateral, vertebrobasilar, or remote ipsilateral symptoms). The nonspecific category accounts for approximately 40% of the patients undergoing CEA. The failure to use the third category will mean that these "nonspecific" patients, who have an intermediate risk between the NASCET definition of symptomatic and asymptomatic patients, will be variably incorporated into symptomatic or asymptomatic groups, which can result in invalid comparisons.

TABLE 22-3. SUGGESTED BENCHMARK OUTCOMES FOR CEA COMPARISON

Study	Population	Study Period	Number of Procedures Procedures	Mortality (%)	Combined Event Rate** (%)
North American Carotid Endarterectomy Trial (NASCET)7	Symptomatic*	1987–1996	1415	1.1	6.5
Asymptomatic Carotid Atherosclerosis Study (ACAS)6	Asymptomatic	1987–1993	721	0.1	1.5

*Ipsilateral carotid territory stroke or TIA within 120 days prior to procedure

**Stroke or death at 30 days

Other outcome measures for CEA such as cardiac morbidity or cranial nerve injuries also present significant barriers to valid comparisons. If one wanted to compare cardiac morbidity following CEA, it would be important to adjust for baseline cardiac risk and to have a standard protocol for assessing perioperative cardiac complications. There are a number of clinical risk factors and a multitude of screening studies that may be used to assess cardiac risk. Clinical risk factor documentation and the use of cardiac risk screening studies are highly variable among institutions and physicians. The aggressiveness of perioperative surveillance (e.g., troponin measurement performed routinely vs. performed only in patients who develop clinical symptoms) will profoundly influence the observed myocardial infarction rate. Valid comparison of cardiac complications is not feasible for community-wide retrospective comparisons because of the variability in both risk assessment and perioperative surveillance for events. Documentation of other complications of CEA (e.g., cranial nerve injuries) are also dependent on the aggressiveness of surveillance.[10] Superior laryngeal and even vagal injuries can have subtle clinical manifestations. Hoarseness due to cranial nerve injury could be attributed to "endotracheal tube trauma" if a laryngeal exam is not performed.

In addition to the problem of risk adjustment, annual case volumes adequate for valid statistical differentiation of outcomes at the individual surgeon or even institutional level are often not achieved. Sample size considerations are especially important for procedures like CEA with infrequent adverse outcome occurrence rates. Stroke and death following CEA are infrequent events. If one was comparing two surgeons with reported combined event rates (stroke or death) of 2% and 4% respectively, it appears that one surgeon has one-half the adverse outcome rate of the other and an informed patient should choose the surgeon with the 2% rate. If the reported rate of 2% actually represents one adverse event in 50 patients performed over the last year and the 4% rate two adverse events in 50 patients performed over the last year, it is obvious that the rate differences are not statistically significant even without consideration of risk adjustment. Fifty CEA procedures per year is at the higher end of the typical individual volume spectrum for surgeons. The comparison becomes even more problematic if the adverse events are not of equal severity. If one attempts to stratify adverse events by categories such as death, disabling permanent stroke, temporary stroke, ipsilateral stroke, and the like, the sample size issue becomes even more critical.

Complete risk adjustment and adequate case volumes to achieve statistical significance are less critical if performance measurement is used only for quality improvement purposes. Many surgeons underestimate their complication rates unless measurement is performed. Every surgeon should have an adverse outcome monitoring process in place that includes calculation of outcomes for comparison. Comparisons to national benchmarks can indicate the need for quality improvement and provide information for valid informed consent discussions with patients. Risk vs. benefit discussions should be based on the surgeon's own outcome data whenever possible.

PROCESS MEASURES

Process measures are generally better suited than outcome measurement for accountability/judgment measurement because of the aforementioned limitations of outcome measures. Process measures are not as dependent on patient risk status and thus more directly measure the performance of the physician. As long as process measures have adjustments for medical contraindications and patient decisions, the potential for a perverse incentive should not exist. Process measures are more clearly actionable than outcome measures. Documenting that a surgeon is an outlier with respect to higher adverse outcomes does not help to determine if or how the outcomes can be improved. On the other hand, performance on process measures can often be improved by a systematic approach such as standing orders or other protocols. Improvement on some processes (e.g., perioperative antiplatelet drug administration for CEA) will lead to better outcomes.

Good process measures have an evidence-based linkage to outcomes. If the process in question lacks that linkage, it will not be accepted as valid by the clinician and could even potentially be harmful. In the area of CEA, many care processes lack a clear association with superior outcomes. It would be inappropriate to use measures such as type of anesthesia (local vs. general), reversal of heparin, or method of cerebral perfusion monitoring as indicators of quality since the linkage between these processes and outcomes is variable in the literature. Other processes such as perioperative administration of antiplatelet therapy, use of heparin anticoagulation, and patching have clear linkage to improved outcomes.[8,11-14] In an analysis of the data from the multistate CEA project, the preoperative administration of aspirin or ticlopidine (30% risk reduction), intraoperative use of heparin (51% risk reduction), and patching (27% risk reduction) were all associated with significantly lower adverse event rates.[8] Significant variation in processes from state to state was also demonstrated in this project. Not all processes that have an evidence link to better outcomes are ideal performance measures. Since utilization of heparin is almost universal, there is no significant gap in care. Use of a process measure with near 100% performance creates a burden of collection without much potential benefit. Both the perioperative use of antiplatelet drugs and patching rates show both variable performance and room for improvement. These two measures would meet the criteria for process measures useful in an accountability setting.

Other process measures that have been proposed for CEA as well as other surgical procedures are in the areas of prophylactic antibiotic administration and beta blocker administration for prevention of perioperative cardiac morbidity. Although it is clear that use of a prophylactic antibiotic is appropriate if prosthetic material is used for CEA patching, the overall rate of infection is extremely low. The impact of process measures for proper antibiotic choice and timing are thus less likely to have an overall impact on the outcomes of CEA patients than for other surgical procedures (e.g., "clean contaminated" procedures). On the other hand, it still may be useful to make sure that perioperative antibiotics are given appropriately in all CEA cases with prosthetic patching since the consequences of patch infection can be catastrophic.

A measure focused on perioperative beta blocker administration has characteristics that are attractive as a process measure since cardiac complications are an important cause of perioperative morbidity and mortality in patients undergoing CEA. Unfortunately, the evidence supporting efficacy as a routine process in all patients is lacking and there is potential for harm. Current recommendations from the American Heart Association/American College of Cardiology evidence-based guideline support beta blocker use in patients with evidence of cardiac ischemia on preoperative testing and in those patients who are chronically on beta blockers.[15] It is difficult to construct valid process measures from all guideline statements. Because of the variability in cardiac assessment and testing in practice, and thus the documentation of "ischemia on preoperative testing," it is problematic to construct a measure that will define a measure denominator that will be homogenous across different settings. It would also be inappropriate to suggest that all patients undergoing CEA should undergo preoperative cardiac ischemia testing just in order to make a decision about beta blocker use. Patients chronically on beta blockers are easier to capture for measurement purposes across settings.

STRUCTURAL MEASURES

There are currently no structural measures being used for CEA although certain structural elements are essential for the safe performance of CEA. Having the capability of continuous postoperative blood pressure monitoring and intravenous vasoactive drug administration is obviously necessary. A hospital at which CEA is performed must also have 24 hour emergent surgical capability for the evacuation of neck hematoma or treatment of carotid thrombosis. There is no evidence that CEA is being performed at institutions without these capabilities. There is also no evidence that having the capability of more sophisticated procedures (e.g., intra-arterial cerebral thrombolytic administration) will result in better outcomes of CEA.

One structural measure that has potential is the participation in a validated outcomes collection and reporting program such as the Veterans Administration (VA) or American College of Surgeons (ACS) National Surgical Quality Improvement Program (NSQIP).[16] Using outcomes assessment and comparison for confidential quality improvement avoids some of the perverse incentives associated with public reporting of outcomes. The participation in the program of outcome assessment becomes the public reported structural measure as opposed to publicly reporting the outcomes.

SURROGATE MEASURES

One of the consequences of the lack of available measures for public accountability was the call for use of surrogate measures (e.g., the Leapfrog group initiative).[17] In the absence of other measures the Leapfrog group suggested using hospital procedural volume parameters as a surrogate measure of quality. Although it is hard to argue with the concept that experience is important in procedures, the evidence base for a specific volume threshold for CEA is lacking.[18-20] The observed volume outcome relationships observed for CEA are confounded by the fact that high volume is generally associated with a higher percentage of asymptomatic and thus lower risk patients.[19-20] The Leapfrog group eventually backed away from their initial recommendation regarding a hospital threshold for CEA volume.

Carotid endarterectomy does not require the interaction of a multidisciplinary team to the same degree as a procedure like coronary artery bypass grafting. This makes it harder to accept the importance of hospital experience as opposed to individual surgeon experience. It seems intuitively obvious that a hospital with 20 different surgeons performing an average of five CEA procedures each per year would not necessarily be superior to a hospital with a single surgeon performing 75 procedures per year. Annual procedure rates also do not take into account the overall experience of a surgeon. A surgeon who has performed 25 procedures per year for 10 years would likely have accumulated a superior experience to one who is in his or her first year of practice, regardless of the overall hospital volume of the institution where that physician practices.

Of even greater concern are the potential unintended consequences of using volume alone as a surrogate measure of quality. The only real area for growth in performing carotid intervention is in the asymptomatic population. If the message to physicians is that one should only be performing carotid intervention if one has high volumes, the pressure to perform more procedures is obvious. If that pressure translates into more asymptomatic patients undergoing procedures, especially those with comorbidities who might otherwise be recommended for observation, the potential for more harm than good exists. If the increased volume in the asymptomatic population is not accompanied by a low procedural adverse outcome rate, the overall population stroke morbidity may be increased. This issue becomes of critical importance with carotid stenting, seen by some as a minimally invasive procedure, as more and more physicians want to "get into the game" and consider applying the procedure to older and sicker neurologically asymptomatic patients.

Board certification, specifically added qualifications in vascular surgery, is another surrogate measure of quality. Board certification does indicate at least a minimum level of experience as a trainee with a procedure. Some studies have suggested an improvement in outcomes associated with surgeons who are certificate holders.[19] Board certification obviously does not necessarily indicate continued experience and/or good outcomes with a procedure. The concerns about using board certification as a surrogate measure of quality are political. Traditionally, many trainees in surgery, neurosurgery, and thoracic surgery did have experience with CEA. Currently, especially with the growth of carotid stenting, many trainees in these disciplines may have little or no exposure to CEA. Although using board certification as a surrogate measure can have negative implications for some surgeons, the perverse incentive associated with a volume measure and thus the potential negative implications for patients do not exist.

QUALITY IMPROVEMENT

Performance measurement is an important component of quality improvement. Measurement of one's own performance and comparison to others is useful for identifying areas for improvement. Outcome and process measurements can both be useful for quality improvement purposes. An important concept in performance measure comparison is benchmarking. The term benchmark is sometimes used in different ways. The term benchmark should not be seen as synonymous with the average, but rather seen as the highest reasonably achievable performance. Maximal quality improvement does not occur if average performers are satisfied and do not seek to achieve the performance of those at the top of the curve. Perfect performance (e.g., a 0% adverse event rate) is not a reasonably achievable goal for a procedure such as CEA. Performance equal to that achieved in the randomized controlled trials (6.5% combined stroke/ mortality rate for patients presenting with recent ipsilateral stroke or TIA and a 1.5% combined event rate for asymptomatic patients) is a reasonable outcome benchmark for CEA[6,7] (see Table 22-3). On the other hand, 100% performance is achievable and thus a suitable benchmark for many process measures (e.g., perioperative antiplatelet therapy) if exclusion criteria are used.

Quality improvement also requires understanding of the concept of system change. System change can have varying meanings depending on the situation. The system can be seen as the whole care system (e.g., the interaction of the patient with multiple physicians, other health care professionals, and ancillary staff). A system may also represent the practice of an individual surgeon. Optimal performance in either concept of system is often not achieved without a protocol for delivery of care. Many operating room procedures use formal protocols to optimize care and prevent errors. An example of a system change that has been recommended for the operating room is the preoperative marking of the operative site by the responsible surgeon in order to reduce the possibility of wrong side procedures. In addition to preventing errors of commission, the use of protocols decreases the likelihood that an important component of the care process would be inadvertently overlooked (errors of omission).

One example of the importance of system thinking specific for CEA is in the area of preoperative administration of antiplatelet therapy. Even if the surgeon is committed to 100% performance for this process measure, the lack of a formal protocol makes 100% performance unlikely. Even though many patients presenting for CEA are taking antiplatelet agents, some are not and may "slip through the cracks" unless the therapy is part of a protocol or care plan. The "system" can even work against the surgeons' expressed wishes. In one institution, patients were being instructed as part of the preoperative anesthesia evaluation to stop all antiplatelet medication at least seven days prior to CEA. This recommendation originated from surgeons performing nonvascular procedures because of their concerns about hemorrhage. A formal CEA protocol that included clear instructions about preoperative antiplatelet therapy is more likely to achieve optimal results.

In previous work in the state of Iowa, we demonstrated that multi-institution performance monitoring and confidential feedback can improve the outcomes of CEA.[21] We promoted the use of a common data collection tool for CEA processes and outcomes. Hospitals in Iowa accounting for 75% of the procedures performed in Iowa participated in ongoing data collection. Hospitals received regular comparison data without identification of other institutions. We demonstrated improvement in process measures, including patching and antiplatelet therapy. We also demonstrated significant overall improvements in outcomes.

CURRENT PERFORMANCE MEASUREMENT EFFORTS

Surgeons desiring to participate in nationally standardized outcomes assessment can elect to participate in the carotid intervention (CEA and CAS) registry available through the Society for Vascular Surgery (SVS)[22] (Table 22-4). Voluntary registries have some limitations with regard to comparisons because of the lack of formal training regarding data collection and oversight of the data abstraction process. Nonetheless, some formal outcome assessment is inherently superior to relying on estimates based on surgeon recall alone. The NSQIP begun in the VA system and now available in the private sector through the ACS has a tested risk adjustment methodology and a formal data abstraction training program.[23] Some process measures are beginning to be incorporated into the ACS/NSQIP. However, the NSQIP was designed to collect outcomes for a wide variety of surgical procedures. Some risk variables and outcomes pertinent for CEA are not part of the program.

TABLE 22-4. PERFORMANCE MEASUREMENT INFORMATION

American College of Surgeons/National Surgical Care Improvement Program.
    https://acsnsqip.org
Centers for Medicare & Medicaid Services: Physician Voluntary Reporting Program.
    http://www.cms.hhs.gov/PVRP/
Physician Consortium for Performance Improvement.
    http://www.physicanconsortium.org
Surgical Care Improvement Program.
    http://www.medqic.org/scip/
Vascular Registry - Carotid Stenting and Endarterectomy.
    http://www.vascularweb.org

There are currently no CEA specific process measures being utilized in Centers for Medicare and Medicaid Services (CMS) performance measurement programs. CEA procedures would be included in the proposed beta blocker measure in the Surgical Care Improvement Program (SCIP).[24] The Physician Consortium for Performance Improvement is developing performance measures relating to preoperative cardiac risk assessment, perioperative cardiac protection, prophylactic antibiotics, and DVT prophylaxis.[25] The measures related to preoperative cardiac risk assessment and perioperative cardiac protection will include CEA procedures in the denominator. The SVS proposed several measures as part of the CMS call for specialty specific measures to be included in the Physician Voluntary Reporting Program (PVRP).[26] Perioperative antiplatelet therapy and heparin administration for CEA were included as proposed process measures. None of the measures have to date been selected for inclusion in this program.

SUMMARY

Performance measurement in medicine has received a great deal of attention recently with the introduction of the concept of "pay for performance." Surgeons should be aware of the differences and limitations of outcome, process, structural, and surrogate measures. Measurement for quality improvement only or measurement for accountability/judgment have distinct purposes that have important implications with regard to the specification of measures, need for risk adjustment, and sample size/statistical significance requirements. Surgical volume should not be used as a surrogate measure for quality. Outcome measurement in CEA should include risk adjustment for the type of and indication for the procedure using standard definitions. It seems unlikely that there will be adequate statistical power at an individual surgeon or hospital level to use outcomes of CEA as valid performance measures for public reporting or pay for performance. In addition, the use of outcomes measures in accountability/judgment programs can create perverse incentives. However, documented participation in standardized confidential outcome monitoring may be suitable as a publicly reported quality measure. Some process measures such as perioperative use of antiplatelet therapy and patching may have potential as accountability/judgment measures (e.g., suitable for public reporting/pay for performance) as well as for quality improvement. Individual surgeons should adopt protocols that include cardiac risk assessment and protection, pre- and postoperative use of aspirin, prophylactic antibiotics if prosthetic patches are used, and routine patching for CEA. This should lead to not only better results on performance measures, but more importantly, better outcomes for patients.

REFERENCES

1. North American Symptomatic Carotid Endarterectomy Trial Collaborators. Beneficial effect of carotid endarterectomy in symptomatic patients with high-grade carotid stenosis. *N Engl J Med*.1991;325:445–453.
2. Mayberg MR, Wilson SE, Yatsu F, et al, for the Veterans Affairs Cooperative Studies Program 309Trialist Group. Carotid endarterectomy and prevention of cerebral ischemia in symptomatic carotid stenosis. *JAMA*. 1991;266:3289–3294.
3. Executive Committee for the Asymptomatic Carotid Atherosclerosis Study. Endarterectomy for asymptomatic carotid artery stenosis. *JAMA*. 1995;273:1421–1428.
4. Barnett HJM, Taylor DW, Eliasziw M, et al. Benefit of carotid endarterectomy in patients with symptomatic moderate or severe stenosis. *N Engl J Med*. 1998;339:1415–1425.
5. European Carotid Surgery Trialists' Collaborative Group. Randomised trial of endarterectomy for recently symptomatic carotid stenosis: final results of the MRC European Carotid Surgery Trial (ECST). *Lancet*. 1998;351:1379–1387.
6. Young B, Moore WS, Robertson JT, et al. An Analysis of Perioperative Surgical Mortality and Morbidity in the Asymptomatic Carotid Atherosclerosis Study. *Stroke*. 1996;27:2216–2224.
7. Ferguson GG, Eliasziw, M, Barr HW, et al. The North American Symptomatic Carotid Endarterectomy Trial: Surgical results in 1415 patients. *Stroke*. 1999;30:1751–1758.
8. Kresowik TF, Bratzler DW, Karp HR, et al. Multistate utilization, processes and outcomes of carotid endarterectomy. *J Vasc Surg*. 2001;33:227–235.
9. Kresowik TF, Bratzler DW, Kresowik RA, et al. Multistate improvement in process and outcomes of carotid endarterectomy. *J Vasc Surg*. 2004;39:372–380.
10. Hertzer NR, Feldman BJ, Beven EG, Tucker HM. A prospective study of the incidence of injury to the cranial nerves during carotid endarterectomy. *Surg Gynecol Obstet*. 1980;151: 781–4.
11. Kretschmer G, Pratschner T, Prager M, et al. Antiplatelet treatment prolongs survival after carotid bifurcation endarterectomy: analysis of the clinical series followed by a controlled trial. *Ann Surg*. 1990;211:317–322.
12. Lindlblad B, Persson NH, Takolander R, et al. Does low-dose acetylsalicylic acid prevent stroke after carotid surgery? A double-blind, placebo-controlled randomized trial. *Stroke*. 1993;24:1125–1128.
13. Abu Rahma AF, Khan JH, Robinson PA, et al. Prospective randomized trial of carotid endarterectomy with primary closure and patch angioplasty with saphenous vein, jugular vein, and polytetrafluoroethylene: Perioperative (30-day) results. *J Vasc Surg*. 1996;24: 998–1007.
14. Jackson MR, Clagett GP. Use of Vein or Synthetic Patches in Carotid Endarterectomy. In: Loftus, CM, Kresowik, TF. *Carotid Artery Surgery*. 1st Ed. New York: Thieme Medical Publishers, Inc; 2000:281–290.
15. American College of Cardiology; American Heart Association Task Force on Practice Guidelines (Writing Committee to Update the 2002 Guidelines on Perioperative Cardiovascular Evaluation for Noncardiac Surgery); American Society of Echocardiography; American Society of Nuclear Cardiology; Heart Rhythm Society; Society of Cardiovascular Anesthesiologists; Society for Cardiovascular Angiography and Interventions; Society for Vascular Medicine and Biology; Fleisher LA, Beckman JA, Brown KA, et al. ACC/AHA 2006 guideline update on perioperative cardiovascular evaluation for noncardiac surgery: focused update on perioperative beta-blocker therapy. *J Am Coll Cardiol*. 2006;47:2343–2355

16. Khuri SF. The NSQIP: a new frontier in surgery. *Surgery*. 2005;38:837–843.
17. Birkmeyer JD, Finlayson EV, Birkmeyer CM. Volume standards for high-risk surgical procedures: potential benefits of the Leapfrog initiative. *Surgery*. 2001;130:415–422.
18. Cebul RD, Snow RJ, Pine R, et al. Indications, outcomes, and provider volumes for carotid endarterectomy. *JAMA*. 1998;279:1282–1287.
19. Pearce WH, Parker MA, Feinglass J, et al. The importance of surgeon volume and training in outcomes for vascular surgical procedures. *J Vasc Surg*. 1999;29:768–776.
20. Birkmeyer JD, Siewers AE, Finlayson EV, et al. Hospital volume and surgical mortality in the United States. *N Engl J Med*. 2002;346:1128–1137.
21. Kresowik TF, Hemann RA, Grund SL, et al. Improving the outcomes of carotid endarterectomy: Results of a statewide quality improvement project. *J Vasc Surg*. 2000:31:918–926.
22. Vascular Registry - Carotid Stenting and Endarterectomy. http://www.vascularweb.org
23. American College of Surgeons/National Surgical Care Improvement Program. https://acsnsqip.org
24. Surgical Care Improvement Program. http://www.medqic.org/scip/
25. Physician Consortium for Performance Improvement. http://www.physican consortium.org
26. Centers for Medicare & Medicaid Services: Physician Voluntary Reporting Program. http://www.cms.hhs.gov/PVRP/

23

Effect of Statins on Carotid Endarterectomy

Benjamin S. Brooke, M.D. and
Bruce A. Perler, M.D., M.B.A.

At a time when vascular surgeons are treating an increasingly elderly patient population with extensive comorbidities, providing optimal medical management during the perioperative period is critical to minimize the rate of complications and ensure that patients achieve superior benefit following vascular interventions. Over the past decade, agents such as beta-blockers, aspirin, or other antiplatelet medications have proven to reduce adverse postoperative outcomes, and have rightfully assumed a place in our overall therapeutic armamentarium. Most recently, several studies have also demonstrated dramatic improvements in the postoperative outcomes for patients taking a statin medication at the time of cardiovascular surgery. It appears that statins may be the next protective medication prescribed to the majority of patients undergoing major vascular surgery. While the beneficial effect of statins applies to individuals undergoing a variety of peripheral vascular interventions, some of the most significant and exciting overall results occur among patients undergoing carotid endarterectomy (CEA).

STATINS

Statins belong to a class of drugs known to inhibit 3-hydroxy 3-methylglutaryl coenzyme A (HMG CoA) reductase. This enzyme converts HMG-CoA into mevalonic acid, a cholesterol precursor, which is the rate-limiting step in hepatic cholesterol synthesis (Figure 23-1). Statins inhibit this enzymatic pathway within hepatocytes, as well as endothelial cells, vascular smooth muscle cells, and inflammatory cells.[1] In addition to inhibiting endogenous cholesterol synthesis in the liver, statins also increase the uptake and degradation of low density lipoproteins (LDL), inhibit the secretion of lipoproteins, inhibit LDL oxidation, and inhibit the expression of scavenger receptors.[2] The clinical result is a 25% to 50% reduction in circulating low-density lipoprotein

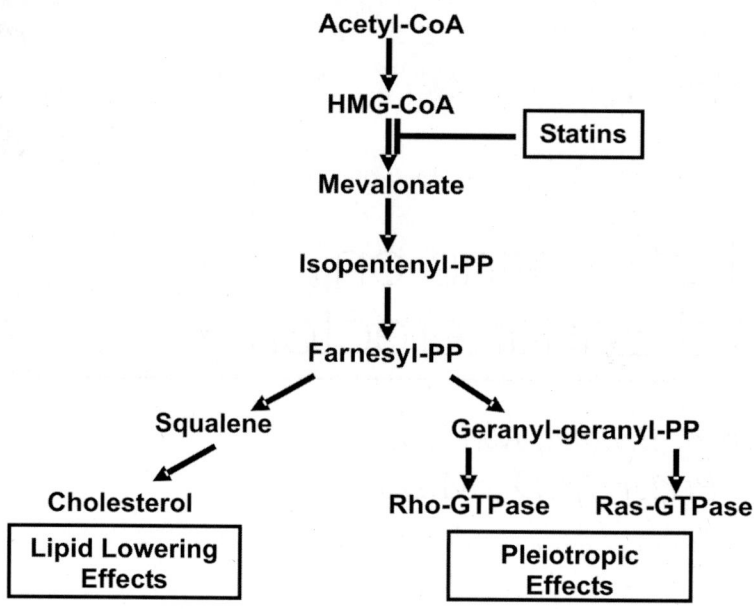

Figure 23-1.

(LDL) cholesterol, as well as markedly lower levels of total serum cholesterol and triglycerides.

The effectiveness of statin therapy has led to a significant demand for these medications. Since the initial statin was approved by the Food and Drug Administration (FDA) in 1987, these agents quickly became the gold standard for the treatment of hypercholesterolemia. This was encouraged by numerous randomized clinical trials demonstrating that reductions in serum lipid levels produced by statins correlated with a decrease in adverse cardiovascular events including myocardial infarctions (MIs) and cardiac related deaths, as well as increased long-term survival.[3-9] These improvements in morbidity and mortality were demonstrated in a broad range of high-risk medical patients including those admitted with acute coronary syndrome, acute myocardial infarctions, impaired left ventricular function, diabetes, and patients with both normal and abnormal lipid levels. And these findings were also supported by numerous reports showing a dose-dependent relationship between statin therapy and the progression of atherosclerosis.[10,11] Recent studies indicate that high-dose statin therapy may even regress the size of atheromatous plaques over time.[12] Interestingly, similar improvements in outcomes have not been shown in clinical trials of non-HMG CoA reductase lipid-lowering medications. In light of this, and in view of the prevalence of coronary artery disease in the western world, it is not surprising that statin drug sales totaled $15.5 billion in the United States in 2004, or roughly 6.6% of all prescription drug sales.[13]

STATINS AND CARDIOVASCULR SURGERY

Patients undergoing major vascular surgery are known to be at increased risk for adverse cardiac events during the perioperative period. Myocardial infarction continues to be the most important cause of perioperative morbidity and mortality after vascular surgery.[14] Given the findings in nonsurgical patients, it was hypothesized that statin therapy might reduce adverse cardiac outcomes during the perioperative period in this population. Some of the first encouraging results were demonstrated in patients on perioperative statin therapy undergoing coronary artery bypass graft (CABG) surgery. Dotani et al. reported the initial study, which demonstrated a significant reduction in mortality and adverse cardiac events at both 60 days and at one year following CABG.[15] This was confirmed by a follow-up study by Pan et al. in which statin use was associated with a significant reduction in the 30-day all-cause mortality (3.8% vs. 1.8%; $P<0.05$).[16] Similar results were also observed in patients on statins undergoing percutaneous coronary angioplasty or stenting procedures.[17]

These findings were followed by several observational studies that showed that statin therapy was associated with a lower incidence of perioperative mortality and adverse cardiac events in patients undergoing major noncardiac vascular surgery. A study reported by Kertai et al. showed a dramatic reduction in all-cause and cardiac-related mortality for patients on statin therapy undergoing elective AAA repair.[18] Several other retrospective studies have examined the effect of statin therapy in patients undergoing any major vascular surgery. Lindenauer et al. performed a large retrospective review of 77,000 patients on statin therapy undergoing major noncardiac vascular surgery at hospitals across the United States, and found a 38% lower risk of mortality (OR: 0.62; 95% CI: 0.58-0.67) among patients treated at the time of their operation.[19] Similarly, Poldermans et al. performed a case-control study showing that statins were associated with a lower rate of vascular-related death, including fatal MI or stroke, when compared to controls (8% vs. 25%; $P<0.001$).[20] O'Neil-Callahan et al. demonstrated a reduction in 30-day combined all-complication rate associated with statin therapy, but interestingly, did not find a reduction in mortality.[21]

There have been two small prospective studies that have examined the efficacy of perioperative statin therapy in patients undergoing major vascular surgery. The first study carried out by Durazzo et al. randomized patients undergoing AAA repair, LE revascularization, or CEA to receive a statin or placebo 30 days prior to their operation.[22] Patients taking statins in this trial were found to have a three-fold decrease (8% vs. 26%; $P = 0.031$) in the rate of combined cardiovascular events including acute MI, ischemic stroke, unstable angina, and death from cardiac causes at six months. The second prospective nonrandomized clinical trial by Schouten et al. administered statin therapy to patients for 40 days prior to their elective vascular procedure, and continued the medication when patients resumed oral intake in the postoperative period.[23] This study showed that statin therapy significantly reduced the composite end-point of perioperative death and myocardial infarction (8.8% vs. 14.7%; $P<0.01$). Moreover, this prospective study showed that perioperative statin therapy was not associated with increased side effects such as postoperative myopathy or rhabdomyolosis.

The benefits of statin therapy in the vascular surgery population appear to extend beyond cardiac morbidity in the perioperative period. For example, Abbruzzee et al. found that patients on statin therapy undergoing autogenous infrainguinal bypass procedures experienced higher primary-revised (94% vs. 83%; $P<0.02$) and secondary (97% vs. 87%; $P<0.02$) graft patency rates at two-years.[24] This study, however, did not show any statistically significant improvement in primary patency, limb salvage, or survival. In another recent report by LaMuraglia, et al., including 2,127 CEA procedures, statin use was independently associated with decreased long-term incidence of restenosis.[25]

STATINS AND STROKE

Each year, approximately 700,000 individuals in the United States experience a stroke. Cerebrovascular events are the third leading cause of death and the leading cause of disability among adults in the western world today.[23] Although it is well established that hypercholesterolemia is a significant risk factor for coronary artery disease and its ischemic complications, the relationship between hypercholesterolemia and stroke has been more equivocal.[24] Large epidemiological studies have shown that the link between serum cholesterol levels and stroke is not as strong as the association between cholesterol levels and coronary artery disease.[25] Nevertheless, an increasing number of clinical trials have clearly demonstrated that statin drugs are highly effective in primary and secondary stroke prevention.

Over 26 randomized clinical trials to date have assessed the efficacy of statin therapy for the reduction of stroke as a primary or secondary outcome in nonsurgical patients.[9] While these trials have been somewhat heterogeneous, assessing different statin agents and varying doses, they have come to similar conclusions. In the 4S trial, simvastatin therapy resulted in a significant reduction in long-term stroke incidence, while pravastatin resulted in a 31% reduction in stroke incidence in the Cholesterol and Recurrent Events Trial (CARE).[4,6] A 19% risk reduction for stroke was reported in the Long-Term Intervention with Pravastatin in Ischaemic Disease (LIPID) study, while the Myocardial Ischemia Reduction with Aggressive Cholesterol Lowering (MIRACL) study demonstrated a significant reduction in stroke incidence with statin therapy.[7,8] The Heart Protection Study was the largest single trial comprising over 20,000 patients, and showed that statin therapy significantly reduced the number of patients experiencing strokes and TIAs, as well as the subsequent requirement for CEA or angioplasty.[5] A recent meta-analysis of all these randomized trials, including more than 90,000 patients, found a pooled 21% risk reduction for stroke that correlated with reductions in levels of LDL cholesterol.[9] These findings are supported by several reports showing that statin therapy significantly reduces carotid intima-media thickness. However, it is of interest that patients in several of these studies with normal lipid levels also received the benefit of stroke reduction with statin therapy. This extensive experience clearly indicates that statins are highly effective in the long-term prevention of stroke, and suggests that this benefit may be partially independent of the cholesterol-lowering effect of the drugs.

STATINS AND CAROTID ENDARTERECTOMY

CEA is the most frequently performed peripheral vascular operation in this country and remains the "gold standard" treatment for carotid atherosclerotic disease. The safety and efficacy of this procedure, as well as its superiority when compared to the best medical management of carotid artery disease, was clearly established for symptomatic and asymptomatic patients by the NASCET and ACAS trials, respectively.[26] Over the past two decades, there has been a remarkable reduction in the rate of perioperative stroke and death among patients undergoing CEA.[27] Nevertheless, even when this procedure is performed in centers with superior outcomes, a small fraction of patients undergoing CEA will experience perioperative ischemic complications. These may result from dislodged embolic plaque during vessel manipulation intraoperatively, watershed ischemia during arterial cross-clamping, or perioperative clot formation and embolization. Although the benefit of statins in the long-term reduction of stroke among high-risk medical patents at risk was established, no investigation had examined the potential influence of statins on reducing cerebrovascular complications among patients undergoing CEA. In view of this, the authors recently undertook an analysis of the outcome of CEA performed at the Johns Hopkins Medical Institutions over a 10-year period, with particular emphasis on the influence of statin medications.[28]

Carotid endarterectomy was performed on 1,566 patients at the Johns Hopkins Hospital or Johns Hopkins Bayview Medical Center between 1994 and 2004, including 126 (8%) patients who underwent a combined CEA/CABG procedure. The operations were performed by 13 attending surgeons, including 10 vascular and three neurosurgeons, and residents in training. There were 987 (63%) male and 579 (37%) female patients, with a mean age of 72.2 + 9.9 years, and included 1,408 (90%) Caucasian, 142 (9%) African-American, 14 (1%) Asian, and two (0.1%) Hispanic individuals. Comorbidities included hypertension in 1,247 (80%), hyperlipidemia 787 (50%), coronary artery disease in 765 (49%), diabetes mellitus in 407 (26%), smoking in 372 (24%), history of MI in 296 (17%), history of CABG in 268 (17%), history of atrial fibrillation in 153 (10%), congestive heart failure in 128 (8%), and chronic renal insufficiency in 87 (6%) patients. In every case, the operated stenosis was greater than 50%, and it was greater than 70% in 94.8% and greater than 80% in 83.8% of cases. An ulcerated plaque was noted in 215 (19%) of the cases.

The indication for operation was symptomatic disease in 660 (42%) patients, including a history of prior stroke in 226 (14%) and transient ischemic attacks in 434 (28%); and asymptomatic stenoses in 906 (58%) cases. The technical details of the operation varied with surgeon preference. Intraluminal shunts were used in 1,195 (76.3%) and patch closure was performed in 860 (54.9%) cases. The operation was performed under general anesthesia in 1,447 (92.4 %) and under cervical block in 119 (7.6%) cases.

At the time of operation, 657 (42%) patients were taking an HMG-CoA reductase inhibitor (statin) drug. The agents utilized included atorvastatin in 332 patients (mean dose: 20 ± 10 mg/day), simvastatin in 189 patients (mean: 20 ± 10 mg/day), pravastatin in 91 patients (mean: 30 ± 20 mg/day), lovastatin in 32 patients (mean: 30 ± 10 mg/day), and fluvastatin in 13 patients (mean: 30 ± 10 mg/day). Patients taking statins were significantly younger, more often male, and more frequently had hyperlipidemia, coronary artery disease, hypertension, and a history of smoking. Chronic renal insufficiency, symptomatic carotid disease, and the use of a carotid patch were more frequent in the patients not taking statins. Among all cases, including combined CEA/CABG, there were 21 (1.3%) perioperative deaths and 49 (3.1%) perioperative strokes. Among the 1,440 patients undergoing isolated CEA, the 30-day stroke and death rates were 2.5% and 0.8%, respectively. Myocardial infarctions occurred in 25 (1.6%) cases. The mean length of stay was three days.

Statin use was associated with reduction in perioperative strokes (1.2% vs. 4.5% [$p<0.01$]); mortality (0.3% vs. 2.1% [$p<0.01$]); and median (interquartile range) length of hospitalization (2[2-5] vs. 3[2-7] days [$p<0.05$]). Likely confounders were adjusted for using multiple logistic regression analysis including beta-blocker use, symptomatic status, hyperlipidemia, atrial fibrillation, chronic renal insufficiency, and combined CABG/CEA procedures. With this regression model, perioperative statin use was found to independently reduce the odds of stroke threefold (OR[95%CI]; 0.35 [0.15-0.85], $p<0.05$) and death fivefold (OR[95%CI]; 0.20 [0.04-0.99], $p<0.05$) (Table 23-1). The decreased perioperative stroke rate observed with statin use persisted regardless of the year of surgery (Figure 23-2). Finally, the 30-day incidence of perioperative myocardial infarction trended lower in the statin group (1.2% vs. 2.1%; $p = 0.191$), although the low number of cardiac events in this study likely precluded this from having the power to reach statistical significance.

In another study utilizing an administrative database, Kennedy et al. reviewed 3,360 CEAs performed at multiple hospitals throughout western Canada. This series included 1,480 (44%) patients who were taking a statin at the time of surgery.[29] When patients were stratified by presence or absence of symptoms at presentation, statin use

TABLE 23-1. COMPARISON OF OBSERVATIONAL STUDIES EVALUATING STATIN USE DURING CEA WITH ADJUSTED ODDS RATIOS FOR IN-HOSPITAL STROKE AND MORTALITY.

Outcome	McGirt et al. (N = 1,566) Odds Ratio (95% CI)	Kennedy et al. (N = 2,031)* Odds Ratio (95% CI)
Stroke	0.41 (0.18-0.93)	Not Reported
Stroke or Death	Not Reported	0.55 (0.31-0.97)
Mortality	0.21 (0.05-0.96)	0.24 (0.06-0.91)

*Only evaluated patients that were symptomatic at presentation

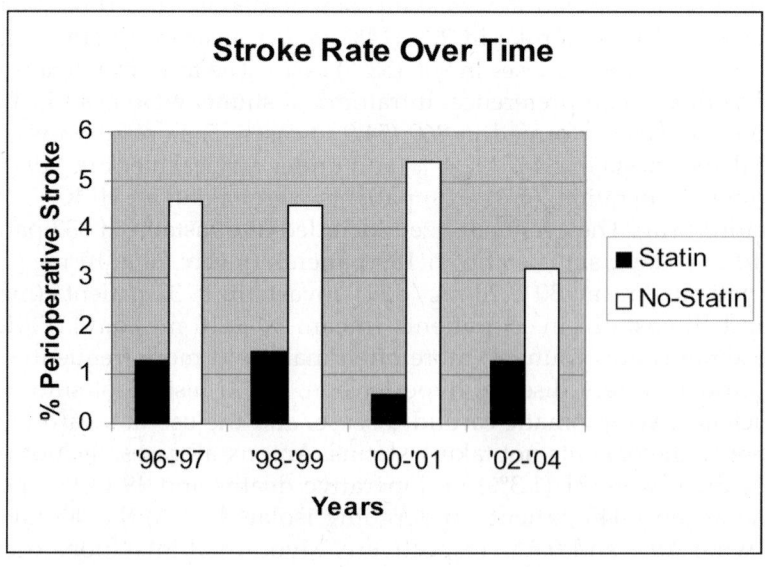

Figure 23-2.

by symptomatic patients was found to be associated with a lower in-hospital mortality rate (0.4% vs. 1.2%; $P = 0.052$) and a lower rate for the composite outcome of ischemic stroke or death (2.5% vs. 4.1%; $P = 0.045$), compared to symptomatic patients not taking a statin. After adjusting for confounders using regression analysis, the authors found that statin use was independently associated with a 75% reduction (OR: 0.25; 95%CI: 0.07-0.90) in the odds of death and 45% reduction (OR: 0.55; 95% CI: 0.32-0.95) in the odds of ischemic stroke or death among symptomatic patients (Table 23-1). However, no statistically significant difference in mortality or stroke was found for statin use in asymptomatic patients.

Together, these data suggest that statins have a significant acute neuroprotective benefit during the perioperative period for the majority of patients undergoing CEA. While there are several potential mechanisms for the observed reductions of cerebrovascular events, it seems intuitive that the major benefit of statin therapy in the acute setting is unrelated to its cholesterol-lowering ability. Rather, it is more likely that one of several lipid-independent, so-called pleiotropic, effects of statins may be responsible for the reduction in stroke (Table 23-2).

PLEIOTROPIC EFFECTS OF STATINS

The benefit of statin therapy during CEA appears to derive from several different mechanisms. While a reduction in serum lipids certainly may improve outcomes over the long term, there is a growing body of data suggesting that the acute protective effects of statins during the perioperative period are independent of lipid-lowering. These nonlipid-mediated or pleiotropic functions of statins include diverse cellular effects including increased endothelial nitric oxide synthase (eNOS) expression, reduced production of endothelin-1 and reactive oxygen species, reduction in inflammatory molecules including, cytokines, chemokines, adhesion molecules and C-reactive protein, reduction of intravascular thrombosis, and regulation of vascular smooth muscle

TABLE 23-2. PLEIOTROPIC MECHANISMS BY WHICH STATINS MAY PROTECT DURING THE CEA PERIOPERATIVE PERIOD.

Mechanism	Clinical benefit of Statins	Cellular & Molecular Effects of Statins
Endothelial function	Flow-mediated vasodilation	↑ eNOS & NO bioavailability
		↓ Adhesion molecule expression (ICAM-1, E-Selectin)
Inflammation	Plaque Stabilization	↓ Activation of macrophages/monocytes
		↓ Production of chemoattractants (MCP-1)
		↓ Release of cytokines (IFN-γ, IL-6, TNF-α, IL-1, IL-8)
		↓ Release of proteolytic enzymes (MMP-1, MMP-2, MMP-9)
		↑ Release of anti-inflammatory cytokines (IL-4, IL-10)
Coagulation	Inhibition of thrombosis	↓ Tissue Factor
		↓ PAI-1
		↓ vWF
		↑ tPA
		↓ Factors V, VII, XIII, prothrombin

cell migration and proliferation.[2,29,30] Statins produce these pleiotropic effects by depleting intermediates in the cholesterol synthesis pathway called isoprenoids, which serve as important lipid attachment molecules for the posttranslational modification of Rho, Ras, and their associated G-protein signaling pathways (Figure 23-1). Once activated, Rho and Ras costimulate nuclear transcription factors that promote an increase in numerous inflammatory processes such as cytokine production and adhesion molecule expression, as well as promote cellular processes that induce thrombosis and reduce vasodilation.

The clinical benefit of these pleiotropic effects during the CEA perioperative period may derive through several specific mechanisms (Table 23-2). For one, statins improve flow-mediated vasodilation through inhibition of the Ras pathway with the resulting upregulation of eNOS. This rapid increase in NO bioavailability helps control vasomotor tone, inhibit leukocyte and platelet adhesion, and maintain a thromboresistant interface between the bloodstream and the vessel wall.[31,32] These effects on the vascular endothelium may protect the brain and heart during the operation by improving collateral blood flow and enhancing arterial vasodilation during states of compromised blood flow. In addition, these mechanisms help prevent thrombosis and embolism during the postoperative period. This is supported by several animal models of ischemic stroke, which showed that statin therapy reduces infarct size by up to 46% through upregulating eNOS and improving cerebral blood flow.[33]

The stabilization of carotid atheromatous plaques is another potential source of cerebral and cardiac protection attributable to statin pleiotrophy during the CEA perioperative period (Table 23-2). Numerous in vitro and in vivo data have shown that statin therapy suppresses numerous inflammatory processes that degrade extracellular matrix, promote thrombosis, and lead to plaque disruption.[2,30-32] This includes reducing inflammatory cell activation (particularly macrophages and monocytes), adhesion, and activation at potentially vulnerable sites along the vessel wall. Statin therapy taken during the preoperative period may, therefore, stabilize atheromatous plaques that would otherwise be disrupted, embolize, and lead to a perioperative stroke or MI. Several recent studies support this conclusion by showing that carotid plaques taken from patients following CEA had significantly lower levels of MMP-1, MMP-2, MMP-9, and IL-6, along with fewer macrophages and higher collagen contents if they were taking a statin medication preoperatively.[34,35] These inflammatory processes are also associated with the progression of vascular aneurysm disease, which may also be suppressed by statin therapy.

A third pleiotropic mechanism by which statins may protect during the perioperative period is through inhibition of local and systemic pathways that promote thrombosis and coagulation (Table 23-2). By way of Rho inhibition, statins down-regulate tissue factor on the endothelial surface that promotes thrombosis, as well as activate protein C, which stimulates the intrinsic anticoagulation cascade. In addition to these effects mediated at the vessel wall, statins also reduce the activation of systemic coagulation factors including factor VII, factor V, factor XIII, and prothrombin. Collectively, these effects appear to reduce acute thrombosis and clot formation during the perioperative period.

STATINS DURING THE PERIOPERATIVE PERIOD

These data support the preoperative administration of statin therapy among patients undergoing major vascular surgery. While an increasing percentage of patients who present for peripheral vascular intervention are already on these drugs, it begs asking whether one should initiate statin therapy among patients who are not, even if they present with normal lipid levels. The demonstrated safety and efficacy of these medications suggests that all patients should at least be offered the choice of starting statin therapy before their surgery.

Our experience with CEA at Johns Hopkins, and other work, raises other important questions. For example, how long should patients be taking statin medications before their operation in order to receive a therapeutic benefit? In most observational studies that demonstrated a reduction of adverse postoperative outcomes, it was assumed that patients were on long-term statin therapy prior to surgery, but the exact duration was usually not known. In the two prospective studies, beneficial effects were observed for patients started on statins roughly a month prior to their surgery. Given that statins appear to provide benefit during the perioperative period through both pleiotropic and lipid-lowering mechanisms, it would make sense to start patients as early as possible before their operation. Further, optimal dosing regimens are yet to be determined. Another crucial issue is how long statin therapy can be stopped during the postoperative period before the drug's effectiveness is lost. Some studies in medical patients suggest that the benefit of long-term statin administration for acute coronary events may be lost as early as 72 hours following statin withdrawal.[36] As the majority of patients undergoing vascular surgery can resume oral intake within 24 hours, a reasonable approach might be to restart statin therapy at this time and continue indefinitely unless contraindicated.

Statin therapy may represent a major breakthrough in the medical management of vascular surgery patients for the reduction of adverse cardiovascular and cerebrovascular outcomes. The collective experience reported over the past several years shows that statin therapy is beneficial during the perioperative period, particularly in regard to reducing mortality, stroke, and cardiovascular morbidity. Recent work from Johns Hopkins and elsewhere indicate that statins may make CEA, already a very safe and effective operation, even safer. Future clinical trials and investigation will be helpful to determine the optimal timing and dosing regimen of statin therapy so that vascular surgery patients may achieve the maximum benefit of these medications during the perioperative period.

REFERENCES

1. Stancu C, Sima A. Statins: mechanism of action and effects. *J Cell Mol Med*. 2001;5:378–387.
2. Bellosta S, Ferri N, Bernini F, et al. Non-lipid-related effects of statins. *Ann Med*. 2000;32:164–176.
3. Shepherd J, Cobe Sm, Ford I, et al., the West of Scotland Coronary Prevention Study Group. Prevention of coronary heart disease with pravastatin in men with hypercholesterolemia. *N Engl J Med*. 1995;333:1301–1307.
4. Scandinavian Simvastatin Survival Group. Randomised trial of cholesterol lowering in 4,444 patients with coronary heart disease: the Scandinavian Simvastatin Survival Study (4S). *Lancet*. 1994;344:1383–1389.
5. Heart Protection Study Collaborative Group. The MRC/BHF Heart Protection Study of cholesterol lowering with simvastatin in 20,536 high risk individuals: a randomized placebo-controlled trial. *Lancet*. 2002;360:7–22.
6. Sacks FM, Pfeffer MA, Moye LA, et al. for the Cholesterol and Recurrent Events Trial investigators. The effect of pravastatin on coronary events after myocardial infarction in patients with average cholesterol levels. *N Engl J Med*. 1996;335:1001–1009.

7. White HD, Hines RJ, Anderson NE, et al. Pravastatin therapy and the risk of stroke. *N Engl J Med*. 2000;243:317–326.

8. Waters D, Schwart GG, Olsson AG, et al. for the MIRACL Study investigators. Effects of atorvastatin on stroke in patients with unstable angina or non-Q wave myocardial infarction: a Myocardial Ischemia Reduction with Aggressive Cholesterol Lowering (MIRACL) substudy. *Circulation*. 2002; 106:1690–1695.

9. Amarenco P, Labreuche J, Lavallee P, Touboul PJ. Statins in stroke prevention and carotid atherosclerosis: systematic review and up-to-date meta-analysis. *Stroke*. 2004;35:2902–2909.

10. Prospective Studies Collaboration. Cholesterol, diastolic blood pressure and stroke: 13,000 strokes in 450,000 people in 45 prospective cohorts. *Lancet*. 1995;346:1647–1653.

11. Crouse JR III, Byington RP, Bond MG, et al. Pravastatin, lipids, and atherosclerosis in the carotid arteries (PLAC-II). *Am J Cardiol*. 1995;75:455–459.

12. Nissen SE, Nicholls SJ, Sipahi I MD, et al. Effect of Very High-Intensity Statin Therapy on Regression of Coronary Atherosclerosis. *JAMA*. 2006;295:1556–1565.

13. Consumer Reports: Best Buy Drugs. The Statin Drugs. Available at: www.crbestbuy drugs.org. Assessed April 10, 2006.

14. Mangano DT, Layug EL, Walace A, Tateo I. The Multicenter Study of Perioperative Ischemia Research Group. Effect of atenolol on mortality and cardiovascular morbidity after noncardiac surgery. *N Engl J Med*. 1996;335:1713–1720.

15. Dotani MI, Elnicki DM, Jain AC, Gibson CM. Effect of preoperative statin therapy and cardiac outcomes after coronary artery bypass grafting. *Am J Cardiol*. 2000;86:1128–1130.

16. Pan W, Pintar T, Anton J, et al. Statins are associated with a reduced incidence of perioperative mortality after coronary artery bypass graft surgery. *Circulation*. 2004;110(suppl II):II45–II49.

17. Chan AW, Bhatt DL, Chew DP, et al. Early and sustained survival benefit associated with statin therapy at the time of percutaneous coronary intervention. *Circulation*. 2002;105: 691–696.

18. Kertai MD, Boersma E, Westerhout CM, et al. Association between long-term statin use and mortality after successful abdominal aortic aneurysm surgery. *Am J Med*. 2004;116:96–103.

19. Poldermans D, Bax JJ, Kertai MD, et al. Statins are associated with a reduced incidence of perioperative mortality in patients undergoing major noncardiac vascular surgery. *Circulation*. 2003;107:1848–1851.

20. Lindenauer PK, Pekow P, Wang K, et al. Lipid-lowering therapy and in-hospital mortality following major noncardiac surgery. *JAMA*. 2004;291:2092–2099.

21. O'Neil-Callahan K, Katsimaglis G, Tepper MR, et al. Statins decrease perioperative cardiac complications in patients undergoing noncardiac vascular surgery. The Statins for Risk Reduction in Surgery (StaRRS) Study. *J Am Coll Cardiol*. 2005;45:336–342.

22. Durazzo AE, Machado FS, Ikeoka DT, et al. Reduction in cardiovascular events after vascular surgery with atorvastatin: a randomized trial. *J Vasc Surg*. 2004;39:967–976.

23. Schouten O, Kertai MD, Bax JJ, et al. Safety of perioperative statin use in high-risk patients undergoing major vascular surgery. *Am J Cardiol*. 2005;95:658–660.

24. Abbruzzese TA, Havens J, Belkin M, et al. Statin therapy is associated with improved patency of autogenous infrainguinal bypass grafts. *J Vasc Surg*. 2004;39:1178–1185.

25. LaMuraglia GM, Stoner MC, Brewster DC, et al. Determinants of carotid endarterectomy anatomic durability: Effects of serum lipids and lipid-lowering drugs. *J Vasc Surg*. 2005;41: 762–768.

26. North American Symptomatic Carotid Endarterectomy Trial Collaborators. Beneficial effect of carotid endarterectomy in symptomatic patients with high-grade carotid stenosis. *N Engl J Med*. 1991;325:445–53.

27. Matsen SL, Chang DC, Perler BA, et al. Trends in the in-hospital stroke rate following carotid endarterectomy in California and Maryland. *J Vasc Surg*.(in press).

28. McGirt MJ, Perler BA, Brooke BS, et al. 3-hydroxy-3-methylglutaryl coenzyme A reductase inhibitors reduce the risk of perioperative stroke and mortality after carotid endarterectomy. *J Vasc Surg*. 2005;42:829–836.

29. Kennedy J, Quan H, Buchan AM, et al. Statins are associated with better outcomes after carotid endarterectomy in symptomatic patients. *Stroke*. 2005;36:2072–2076.
30. Schonbeck U, Libby P. Inflammation, immunity, and HMG-CoA reductase inhibitors: statins as anti-inflammatory agents? *Circulation*. 2004;109(suppl II):II18–II26.
31. Vaughn CJ. Prevention of Stroke and Dementia with statins: Effects beyond lipid lowering. *Am J Cardiol* 2003;91 (Suppl): 23B–29B.
32. Koh KK. Effects of statins on vascular wall: vasomotor function, inflammation, and plaque stability. *Cardiovasc Res*. 2000;47(4):648–657.
33. Sironi L, Cimino M, Guerrini U, et al. Treatment with statins after induction of focal ischemia in rats reduces the extent of brain damage. *Arterioscl Thromb Vasc Biol*. 2003; 23: 322–327.
34. Crisby M, Nordin-Fredriksson G, Shah PK, Yano J, Zhu J, Nilsson J. Pravastatin treatment increases collagen content and decreases lipid content, inflammation, metalloproteinases, and cell death in human carotid plaques: implications for plaque stabilization. *Circulation*. 2001;103:926–33
35. Molloy KJ, Thompson MM, Schwalbe EC, Bell PRF, Naylor R, Loftus IM. Comparison of levels of matrix metalloproteinases, tissue inhibitor of metalloproteinases, interleukins, and tissue necrosis factor in carotid endarterectomy specimens from patients on versus not on statins preoperatively. *Am J Cardiol*. 2004;94:144–146.
36. Heeschen C, Hamm CW, Laufs U, et al. Withdrawal of statins in patients with acute coronary syndromes. *Circulation*. 2003;107:27.

24

Surgery for Coils/Kinks and Radiation-Injured Carotid Artery

Dhiraj M. Shah, M.D.

Coiling of the carotid artery has been noted for many years. Since the introduction of duplex ultrasound and angiography of the carotid artery for extracranial disease, associated coils/kinks and redundancy of the carotid artery has been observed; however, its relationship to symptoms of extracranial carotid artery disease has not been established. Kink may cause hemodynamic disturbance when acute. Two groups of patients show these findings from two different etiologies. Young adults or children have been shown to have carotid artery kink/coil or redundancy due to developmental causes. These are found usually at autopsy or during unrelated investigation of the cerebrovascular tree. At times, this type of coil or kink may be inadvertently injured during oropharyngeal surgical operations. The incidence of carotid artery coiling or kink unassociated with atherosclerosis is unknown. However, all vascular surgeons have seen and dealt with carotid artery coil and kinking at the time of carotid endarterectomy due to atherosclerosis. The acquired type of carotid artery kinking or coiling is produced by a mechanism similar to elongation of the artery due to atherosclerosis or hypertension. Since the carotid artery is fixed between the base of the skull and the aortic arch, hypertension/atherosclerosis may elongate the artery, which could be liable to redundancy, or kinking or coiling in coronal, sagittal, or transverse plane.[1]

The symptoms of carotid artery coil and kink when produced are similar to those produced by extracranial carotid artery disease due to atherosclerosis. Isolated coiling or kinking producing symptoms is rare, although occasionally, when all other causes are ruled out documentation of carotid artery kinking with production of symptoms by rotation or changing of the neck may necessitate treatment of carotid artery kink or coil alone. At the time of carotid endarterectomy, almost all carotid arteries will show some amount of redundancy without any hemodynamic significance, and is usually corrected with carotid endarterectomy. However, significant kinking, coiling, or redundancy may need extra steps in the performance of carotid endarterectomy. Although exact incidence of coiling and kinking is unknown, it is reported to be somewhere between 1.1% up to 30%. In our database, we found 112 patients with significant carotid artery kinking or coiling requiring extra steps at the time of eversion carotid endarterectomy in 7,377 patients.

SURGICAL TREATMENT

Historically, coil/kink of the carotid artery has been treated by arteriopexy or fixation of the internal carotid artery to the sternocleidomastoid muscle with external suture placement. Other procedures include 1) resection of the internal carotid artery and reanastomosis, 2) resection of the common carotid artery and elongated internal carotid artery and reanastomosis, 3) bypass to the internal carotid artery beyond the kink, 4) long patch angioplasty, 5) caudad ICA reimplantation into the common carotid artery, 6) plication, and 7) eversion endarterectomy with correction of the kink or coil. Integral to all surgical techniques is complete mobilization of the common, external, and internal carotid arteries, release of all fibrous bands adherent to the coil and kinking, and exposure of the internal carotid artery up to the base of the skull beyond the disease. Care should be taken to avoid fracture of the artery because of eccentric dilation and medial thinning. Some suggest general anesthesia should be used because of the extensive dissection, but the operation can be done under regional/cervical block anesthesia.

The carotid artery should be mobilized in all planes and straightened out. There could be tethering by eccentric fibrous bands that should be dissected carefully in order for the artery to be straightened out. Our preferred method for treatment of kink/coil and redundant carotid artery is the use of the eversion technique, and then caudad elongation of the internal carotid artery and reanastomosis of the internal carotid artery obliquely to the common carotid artery, with or without excision of the excess internal carotid artery.

Standard incision is made along the anterior border of the sternocleidomastoid muscle obliquely. After lateral mobilization of the sternocleidomastoid muscle, the carotid bifurcation is exposed. The common, internal, and external carotid arteries are mobilized. The internal carotid artery is completely mobilized beyond the kink/coil along with the atherosclerotic lesion. The patient is usually heparinized with 30 u/k body weight.[2] After clamping of the internal, common, and external carotid arteries, the internal carotid artery is divided off the common carotid artery in an oblique fashion, taking a patch of the common carotid artery; the stoma is usually one and a half times the diameter of the common carotid artery (Figure 24–1). The endarterectomy of the internal carotid artery is done by the eversion technique in the usual fashion; all the debris is removed under direct vision and flushed out (Figure 24–2). Similarly, endarterectomies of the common and external carotid arteries are also done, and all the atheroma is removed. After this, the redundancy of the internal carotid artery is assessed. If the redundancy is moderate, it can be treated by opening the internal carotid artery longitudinally along its medial border and lengthening the incision of the common carotid artery, then performing a long anastomosis (Figure 24–3). If the redundancy is excessive, then the internal carotid artery is excised for appropriate length, is tailored to reach the stoma of the common carotid artery, and then reanastomosis is performed. Depending on the amount of coiling and redundancy, any modification between the two extremes can be tailored to suit the patient.

Most operations are done under cervical block anesthesia and shunt is utilized on demand in approximately 3% to 4% of cases overall. We usually use a Javid type of

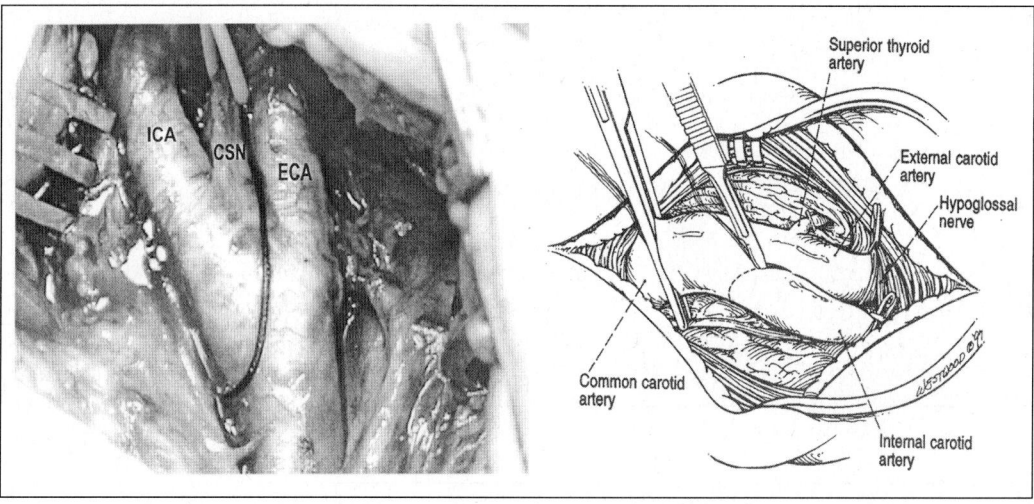

Figure 24-1. Anatomy for eversion carotid endarterectomy. (Line drawing with permission. William B. Westwood. Westwood Medical Communications)

shunt. When a shunt is needed, it should be carefully introduced into the internal carotid artery beyond the disease and the kink/coil and secured there with a shunt clamp (Figure 24–4). Then the proximal end of the shunt is introduced into the common carotid artery. After the introduction of the shunt, endarterectomy is completed and redundancy is assessed. The reanastomosis is then done around the shunt in the

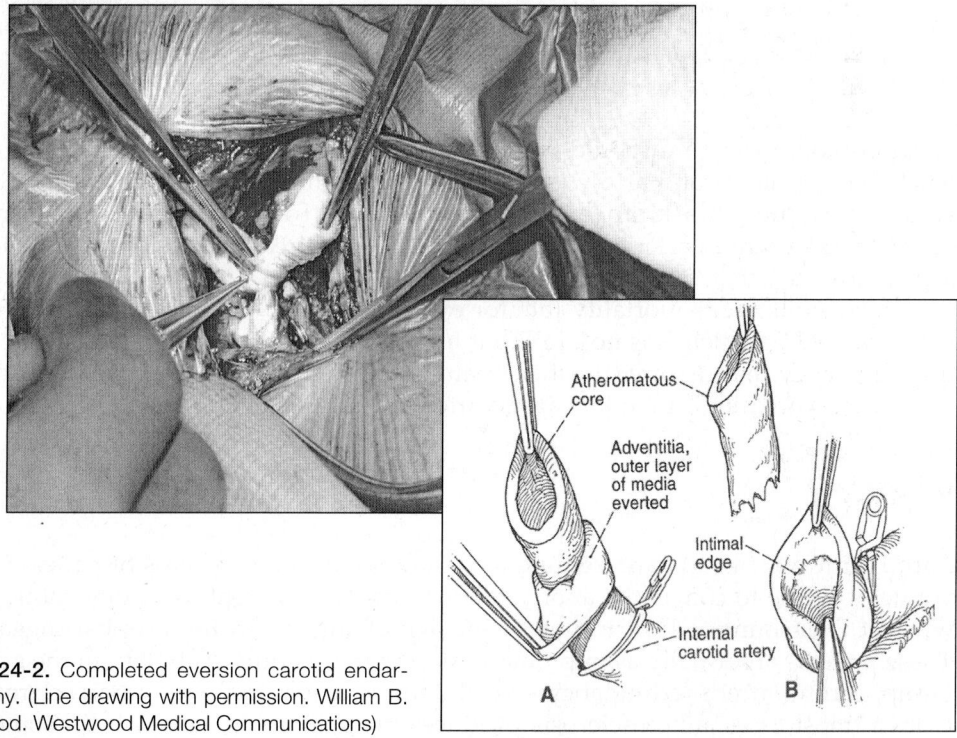

Figure 24-2. Completed eversion carotid endarterectomy. (Line drawing with permission. William B. Westwood. Westwood Medical Communications)

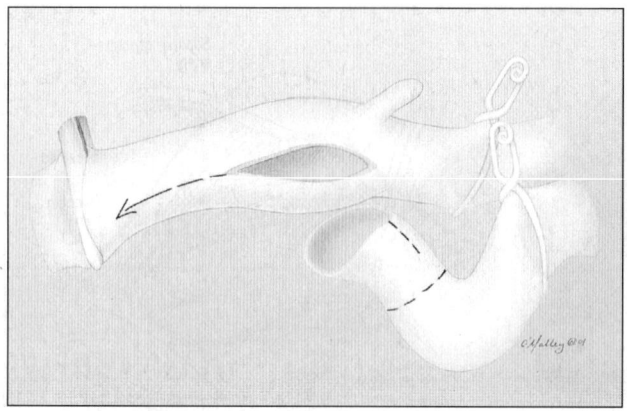

Figure 24-3. Technique to treat coil/kink with eversion endarterectomy (Line drawing with permission. Jilliam O'Malley)

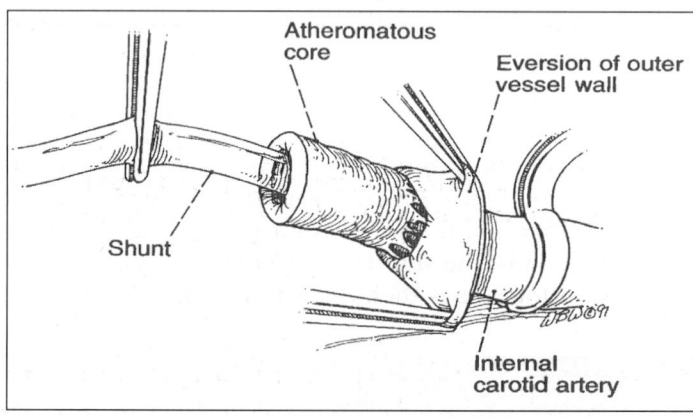

Figure 24-4. Use of shunt with eversion endarterectomy. (Wth permission. William B. Westwood. Westwood Medical Communications)

usual fashion. Extra care should be taken to avoid torsion of the ICA over the shunt. Since the internal carotid artery is divided off the common carotid artery in the eversion technique, this is an excellent technique for treatment of redundant, coiled/kinked carotid arteries because it does not require any extra step, procedure, or anastomosis to correct the redundancy.

The overall stroke mortality rate for eversion carotid endarterectomy in 7,377 patients was 1.7%, which was not different for the 112 patients who had associated kink or redundancy that required further treatment. Carotid artery coil/kink/redundancy is a relative contraindication for carotid artery stenting.

SUMMARY

Carotid artery kink/coil and redundancy may occur in two groups of patients. In the young, it is due to congential anomaly and is usually thought to be innocuous except when it is encountered during other incidental surgery in the oropharyngeal area. These patients are usually asymptomatic and do not require treatment. In the acquired group, carotid artery redundancy or coil/kink is associated with atherosclerotic disease. In most cases, atherosclerosis produces the symptoms; however, in some cases after exclusion of all other causes, the kink itself may cause the symptoms and should be corrected. Various surgical procedures have been suggested for the treatment of coil/kinked carotid artery. Our preference is to treat this condition in association with eversion carotid endarterectomy, which produces durable and excellent results.

RADIATION-INJURED CAROTID ARTERY

Radiation injury to the large blood vessel has been well documented. Radiation to the neck for cervical cancer treatment with acceleration of atherosclerosis in the carotid artery producing symptoms is also recognized. The mechanism of injury to the carotid artery is similar due to injury to the endothelium, increased permeability involving cytokine/monocytes/platelets/growth factor, and acceleration of degenerative or atherosclerotic process. It also causes increased fibrosis and reaction around the carotid artery. The actual incidence of irradiated carotid artery disease is unknown as it is frequently accompanied by de novo atherosclerotic disease and usually not separately entered into the registry.[3]

A 22% prevalence producing greater than 70% carotid stenosis in patients with previous neck radiation therapy has been reported. Generally, carotid endarterectomy in these patients is thought to be of high risk because of the reaction around the carotid artery, encagement of cranial nerves associated with the carotid artery in the process, and frequently associated previous scar or radical neck surgery. Therefore, stenting as an alternate treatment of choice was suggested. Although carotid stenting showed initial acceptable results in irradiated carotid artery disease, it has been shown that the restenosis rate is much higher in the irradiated stent group compared to the control stent group for de novo atherosclerotic disease. Similarly, stent patency is much lower. As a result, it is suggested that surgical treatment should be preferred.[4]

In spite of the speculation that surgery could be difficult, many series have shown equivalent surgical result in terms of stroke/mortality, complications, and durability in irradiated atherosclerotic carotid disease. Various surgical treatment options are available including longitudinal endarterectomy with patch because usually the artery is small, a bypass to the internal carotid artery beyond the disease, and eversion carotid endarterectomy. In our experience, eversion endarterectomy is possible in radiation-injured carotid artery disease. There are subtle differences; that is, increased fibrosis and reaction around the carotid artery requiring careful dissection to avoid injury to cranial and recurrent laryngeal nerve, especially the internal carotid artery up to the base of the skull. Irradiated internal carotid artery does not become redundant; therefore, when it is divided off the common carotid artery, one should be careful to develop an exact flap of the common carotid artery. A caudad mobilization and tailoring may not be possible. Shunt can be used in the usual fashion.

In performing the eversion carotid endarterectomy, there is some difference in the radiation-injured artery. Usually, the adventitia is thick and the atheroma is more adherent to the wall of the carotid artery. Therefore, the stoma of the internal carotid artery should be larger than usual. A plane should be developed at the apex of the divided internal carotid artery and gradually moved cephalad. Because of the thickness of the adventitia, it may be difficult to evert the adventitia over the atheroma. Nonetheless, it can be done. Since the plaque is more adherent, the distal intima may occasionally need to be incised off. However, because of the nature of the increased adherence, the chance of distal dissection of the intima is very small. Closure and healing of the carotid artery and neck has not shown added risk. Overall outcome of surgical treatment of irradiated carotid artery is similar to that of carotid endarterectomy at large.

SUMMARY

Radiation-injured accelerated atherosclerotic carotid artery disease is well known. Its clinical presentation and treatment options are similar to those of extracranial carotid artery disease. Surgical treatment offers durable results. Carotid artery stenting shows increased restenosis and lower patency rates.

REFERENCES

1. Busuttil RW, Memsic L, Thomas DS. Coiling and kinking of the carotid artery. In: Rutherford RB, ed. *Vascular Surgery, 4th Ed*, Vol.II. Philadelphia: W.B. Saunders. 1995: 1588–1593.
2. Darling RC III, Mehta M, Roddy SP, et al. Eversion carotid endarterectomy: A technical alternative that may obviate patch closure in women. *Cardiovasc Surg*. 2003;11(5):347–352.
3. Abayomi OK. Neck irradiation, carotid injury and its consequences. *Oral Oncol*. 2004; 40:872–878.
4. Protack CD, Bakken AM, Saad WA, et al. Radiation arteritis: A contraindication to carotid stenting? *J Vasc Surg*. 2007;45:110–7.

25

Durability of Redo Carotid Operations

Daniel J. Reddy, M.D. and Jae-Sung Cho, M.D.

Endarterectomy or reconstruction of the carotid bifurcation for atherosclerotic occlusive disease has been performed for 50 years.[1] Over this half century, this procedure has been employed in clinical practice for stroke prevention with increasing frequency. Over the last 25 years, it has become one of the most commonly performed hospital procedures[2] (Figures 25–1 and 25–2). Of crucial value to this operation is the actual removal or unburdening of the carotid bifurcation of atherosclerotic plaque. Additionally, techniques developed for such treatment of atherosclerotic disease of the carotid artery have been effectively employed in treatment of other pathologic entities including carotid aneurysm, carotid body tumors, carotid dissection, and recurrent carotid stenosis (RCS)

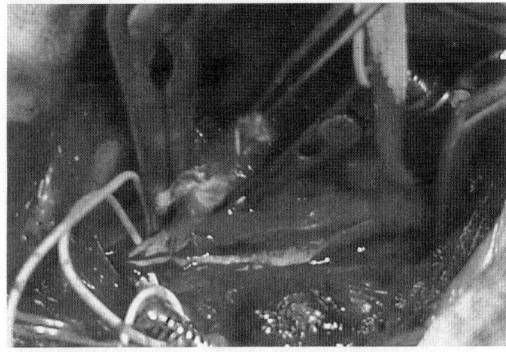

Figure 25-1. Appearance of the potential benefit of unburdening the carotid bifurcation of the carotid atheroma by carotid endarterectomy followed by autogenous vein patch angioplasty in a 49-year-old woman who continues to smoke cigarettes. With permission: Rosenthal D, Archie JP Jr., Avila MH, et al. Secondary recurrent carotis stenosis. *J Vasc Surg.* 1996;24(3):424–428.

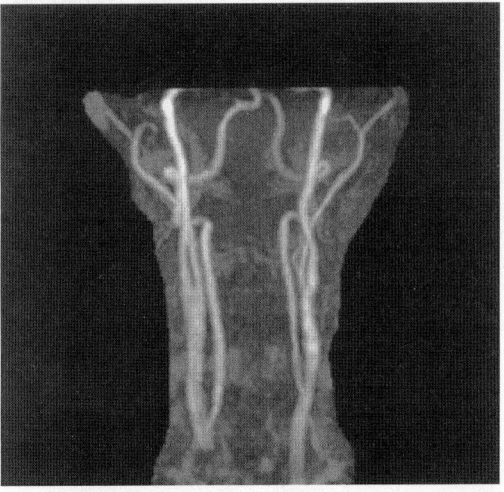

Figure 25-2. Two-year post operative surveillance magnetic resonance of the right carotid artery in the patient from Figure 25–1.

(Figures 25–3 and 25–4). Though successful in the vast majority of patients, carotid endarterectomy provokes a paradoxical response in some patients resulting in carotid restenosis. Interested vascular surgery centers such as the Henry Ford Hospital have identified small cohorts of patients developing recurrent carotid stenosis following carotid endarterectomy. Moreover, the vascular surgeon's commitment to patient surveillance by diligent and ongoing postoperative follow-up is designed to understand and report on the natural history of the operative treatment of arterial disease. Crucial to an understanding of the natural history of the reoperative treatment of carotid disease is an understanding of durability of such treatment permitting prudent patient selection for retreatment. As practice patterns evolve and vascular surgeons search for the indications for carotid angioplasty and stenting in both primary and reoperative applications, the durability of redo carotid operation is an essential datum point against which these new treatment modalities can be measured (Figures 25–5 and 25–6).

BACKGROUND

Although RCS was first reported by Stoney and String in 1976[3], a consensus opinion regarding an optimum management algorithm for secondary operations for RCS has not emerged. Evidence on which consensus could be based has yet to emerge owing to five disparate facts which have identified.

1. Even though redo carotid operations (RCO) for recurrent stenosis can be performed with very low combined stroke and mortality rates, comparable to primary carotid operations, overall morbidity rates are increased.

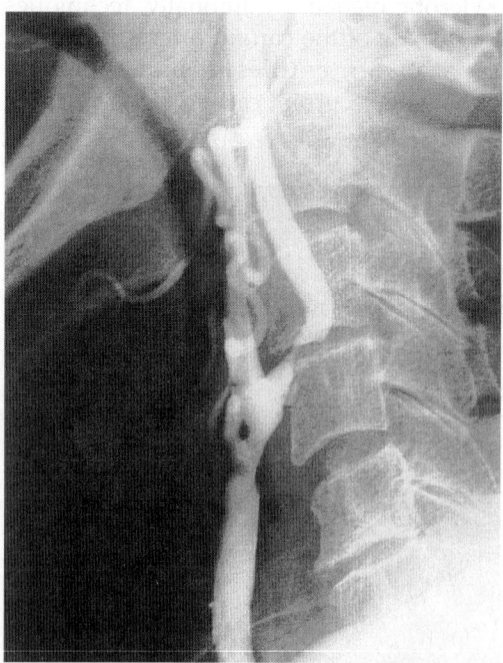

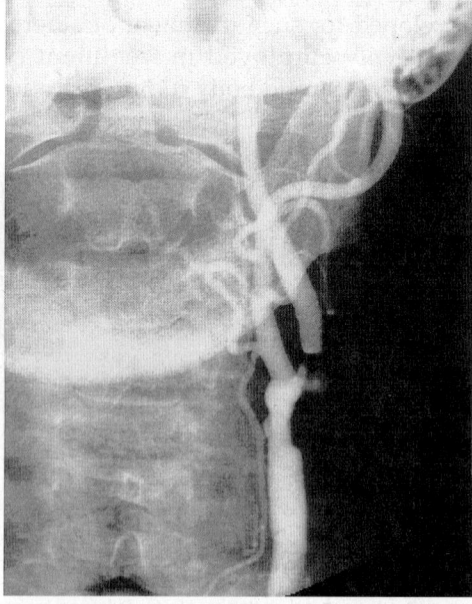

Figure 25-3. Arteriogram of asymptomatic recurrent left carotid bifurcation stenosis from recurrent atherosclerosis 16 years after carotid endarterectomy.

Figure 25-4. Anterior-posterior (AP) image of the late follow recurrent pre-occlusive stenosis described in Figure 25–3. Successful redo carotid endarterectomy and patch angioplasty was performed and the patient reentered post-operative surveillance.

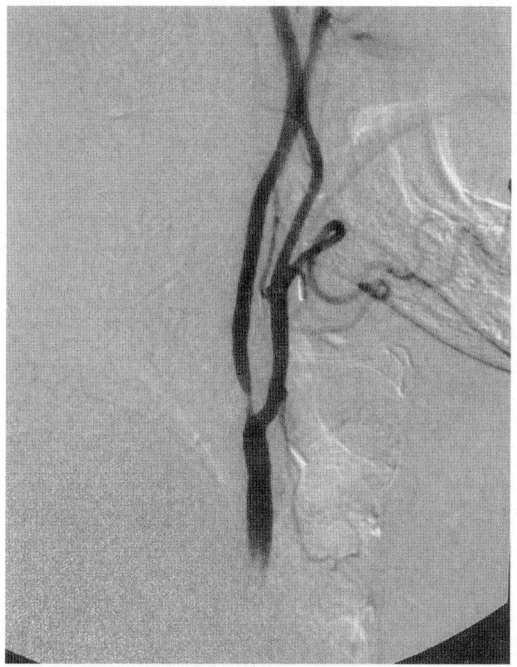

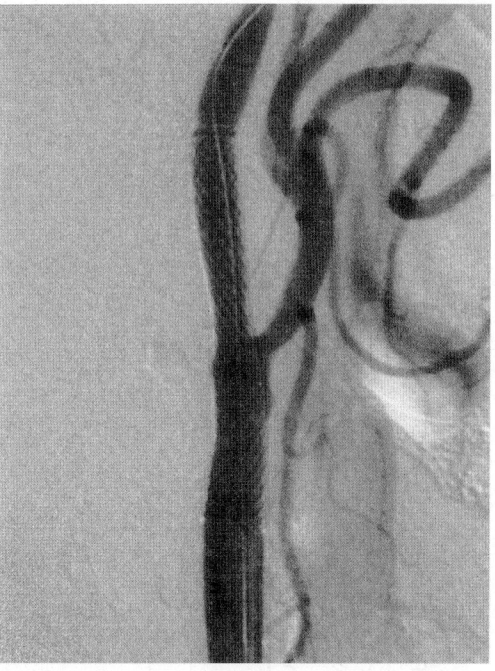

Figure 25-5. Recurrent carotid stenosis one year following carotid endarterectomy and patch angioplasty. The presumed etiology for restenosis was intimal hyperplasia.

Figure 25-6. Immediate results for carotid angioplasty and stenting of the lesion described in Figure 25–5 are satisfactory. Long term follow-up for angioplasty/ stenting comparable to long term follow-up for redo carotid operations are unknown.

2. Asymptomatic RCS usually runs a benign course and may regress, particularly when it occurs in the early postoperative period.
3. The pathogenesis of RCS is not uniform and mirrors the bimodal distribution of early and late recurrences.
4. Patients with severe or preocclusive RCS experience sudden, unheralded, catastrophic stoke from carotid occlusion at a higher rate than patients with primary preocclusive stenoses.
5. In the most recent era, emerging endovascular devices and technologies may have been employed for benign RCS based on an overstatement of indication or on the faulty premise that RCO for significant RCS is "high risk" and to be avoided at all costs.[2-8]

INCIDENCE OF RECURRENT CAROTID STENOSIS

Many series, including ours at Henry Ford Hospital have demonstrated that redo carotid operations can be performed safely and effectively, are not properly classified as "high risk" per se (Table 25–1). Although reported series have documented that redo carotid operations (RCO) can be performed with stroke morbidity and mortality rates similar to those of primary carotid endarterectomy (CEA)[4, 5, 9], the cranial nerve injury rates for RCO are generally considered higher than those for primary CEA.[6-15]

TABLE 25–1. INCIDENCE AND OUTCOME FOR REDO CAROTID OPERATIONS FOR RECURRENT CAROTID STENOSIS. SELECTED REVIEW OF RECENT LITERATURE FROM A VARIETY OF VASCULAR CENTERS AND INVESTIGATORS

Center	Sudy period	# pts/ # arteries	Indi- cations	Stroke	TIA	Death	30-day stroke & death	MI	Cranial nerve injury	Mean follow- up	Stroke- free survival	Freedom from restenosis (>80%)
Ochsner Clinic 19	1/84-8/95	67/74	Sx 65% Asx 35%	1.4%	NA	1.4%	2.8%	NA	2.7%	48.2 mos	93.6% @ 5 yrs (ipsilateral)	NA
NYU 21	1/80-12/96	74/83	Sx 41.5% Asx 35.3%	3.7%	NA	0	3.7%	0%	1.2%	35 mos	83.5% with veins; 93.9% with prosthetics @ 3 yrs	NA
Raleigh 20	1/81/=12/99	66/69	Sx 48% Asx 52%	1.4%	1.4%	0	2.9%	0%	4.3%	50 mos	90% @ 5 yrs (cumulative) 86% @ 10 yrs	88.2% @ 5 yrs (>50%)
Charleston W. VA. 9	10/91-10/98	124/124	Sx 78% Asx 22%	4.8%	4%	0	4.8%	0	17%	49 mos	82% @ 5 yrs (cumulative)	95% @ 5 yrs. (>50%)
Cleveland Clinic 7	1/89-12/99	199/206	Sx 43% Asx 57%	3.4%	NA	1.0%	5.3%	1.0%	1.0%	47 mos	92% @ 5 yrs	89% @ 5 yrs
Stanford 6	9/93-3/98	40/40	Sx 50% Asx 50%	0%	0%	0	0%	2.5%	10%	14 mos	NA	NA
Loyola 4	8/76-8/96	69/82	Sx 66% Asx 34%	4.8%	1%	0	4.8%	2%	7.3%	NA	92.3% @ 5 yrs	92.3% @ 5 yrs
Henry Ford 8	1/90-12/2000	64/66	Sx 48% Asx 52%	3%	3%	0	3%	5%	6%	52 mos	93% @ 5 yrs (ipsilateral)	96% @ 5 yrs

Sx = symptomatic; Asx = Asymptomatic; NA = not available

With permission from The Society for Vascular Surgey and The Association for Vascular Surgery Reference 8.

Recurrent stenosis that develop within the first two years usually result from neointimal hyperplasia and seem less likely to cause symptoms as compared to late atherosclerotic lesions.[1-15] Particularly vulnerable torecurrent carotid stenosis are female patients who continue to smoke and have their initial operation prior to age 50 years (Figure 25–1).[16]

The incidence rate of RCS ranges from 1.2–36%;[1-14] however, hemodynamically significant lesions develop in only 1–8% of patients.[4, 5] It generally is indicated for symptomatic lesions[11, 13, 16, 17] and for asymptomatic lesions with >80% stenosis.[18]

MORBIDITY OF RECURRENT CAROTID OPERATIONS

There are many large series in the literature reporting excellent early results with RCO that are comparable to those with primary CEA.[4, 6, 14, 19-21] It is beyond dispute that RCO is intrinsically more challenging than primary CEA with respect to the intraoperative management of the recurrent lesion and to the risk of cranial nerve injuries. AbuRahma,[7] in a review of personal series of 124 RCOs compared to 265 primary CEAs, reported significantly higher perioperative stroke (4.8% versus 0.8%) and cranial nerve injury rates (17% versus 5.3%) for secondary CEA than primary CEA. The Mayo Clinic series, based on 82 patients treated for RCS, reported a combined morbidity and morality rate of 10.8%, five times the risk of a primary CEA at the same institution.[22]

For the most part, the adverse outcomes result from cranial nerve injuries that have been reported to be as high as occurring in 48% of cases.[4, 9, 10, 20, 23-25] Clinically important nerve injuries are far fewer (Table 25–1). In general, these injuries result from difficult dissections owing to postoperative tissue reaction that obscures the normal planes of dissection with scar[4,10] (Figures 25–7, 25–8, 25–9, 25–10, and 25–11). Despite the experience that most injuries involving cranial nerves X (vagus), XII (hypoglossal), IX (glossopharyngeal), VII (facial), XI (spinal accessory), and the superior laryngeal nerve are transient[2, 7, 8, 24], these injuries may be clinically disabling and require prolonged recovery time, often many months, prior to full recovery. Some are permanent (Table 25–2).

TABLE 25-2. COMPLICATIONS

	Number of patients (%)
Stroke	2 (3)
TIA	2 (3)
Cardiac	3 (5)
CN injury	
Partial transaction CN XII	1 (1.5)
Permanent vocal cord paralysis	1 (1.5)
Transient CN X palsy	1 (1.5)
Transient CN XI	1 (1.5)
Transient mandibular nerve palsy	2 (3)
Brachial artery thrombosis	1 (1.5)
Neck hematoma requiring evacuation	2 (3)

TIA, transient ischemic attack; CN, cranial nerve (some patients had more than one complication). With permission: Cho JS, Pandurangi K, Conrad M F, et al. Safety and durability of redo carotid operation: An 11-year experience. *J Vasc Surg.* 2004;39:155–161.

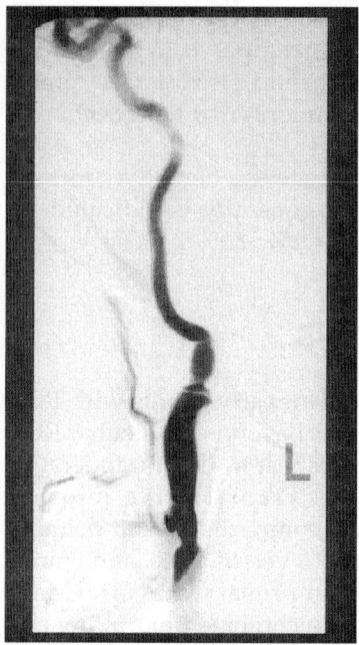

Figure 25-7. Angiogram 12 years following left carotid endarterectomy and Dacron patch angioplasty obtained for the physical finding of a symptomatic, expanding pulsatile mass. Demonstrated is a false aneurysm at the proximal end of the Dacron patch. Redo carotid operation was required to prevent rupture, thrombosis or embolization.

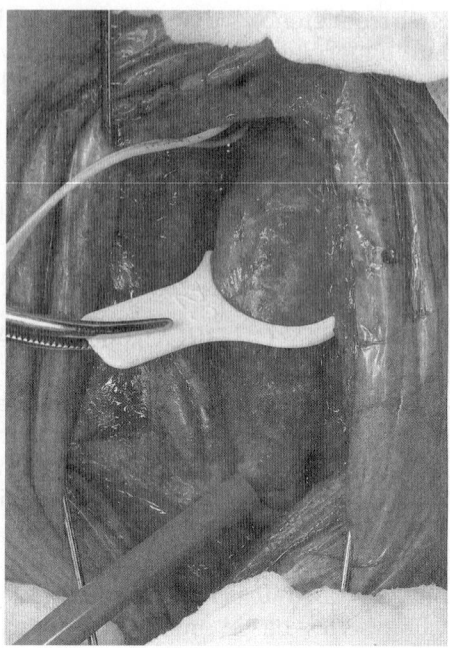

Figure 25- 8. Operative photo of the false aneurysm depicted in Figure 25–7 measuring 20mm diameter.

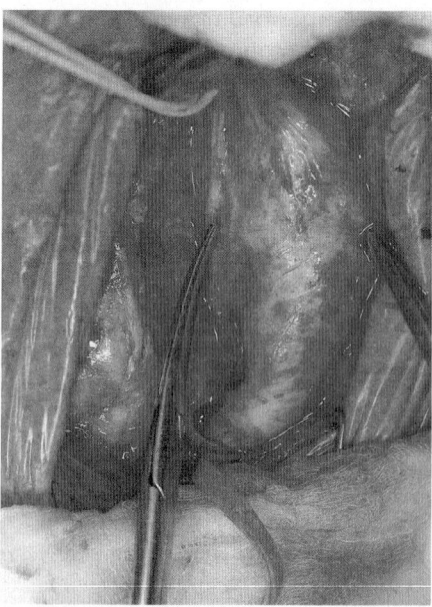

Figure 25-9. Operative photo of the false aneurysm demonstrating the adherent vagus (Xth) cranial nerve which can be safely dissected free of the mass.

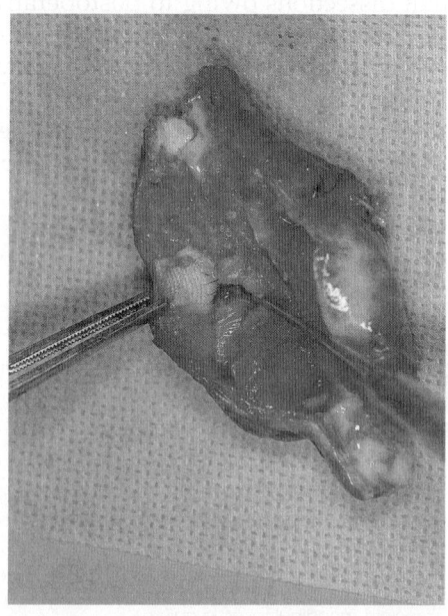

Figure 25- 10. Operative photo of the resected specimen demonstrating the Dacron patch and the false aneurysm originating at the disrupted sutured line threatening rupture. The false aneurysm is laden with large amounts of laminated chronic thrombus threatening carotid thrombosis or embolization.

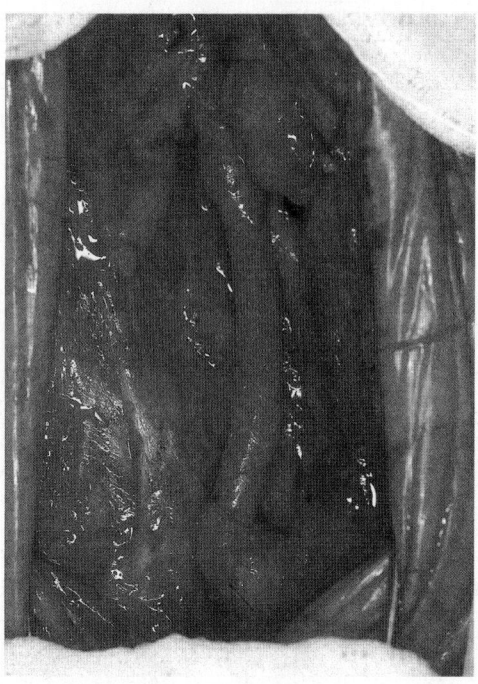

Figure 25-11. Operative photo of the completed interposition vein graft reestablishing arterial continuity following resection of the false aneurysm requiring redo carotid operation.

The continuous efforts to improve therapeutic options in all areas of vascular surgery, and for the *bona fide* high-risk patients in particular, the contemporaneous emergence of carotid artery balloon angioplasty and stenting (CAS) have applied this new treatment modality for RCS carotid disease.[25-32] Long-term follow-up data regarding this alternative treatment modality are, however, not yet possible. When available, these results will need to be compared with those achieved by redo carotid operations.

DURABITY OF REDO CAROTID OPERATIONS

In the authors' series of 66 RCOs performed between 1990 and 2000 at the Henry Ford Hospital, there were no perioperative deaths, two strokes (3%), and four cranial nerve injuries (6%).[8] These results are comparable to those of the authors' combined stroke and death rate of 3.9% for 1,045 primary CEAs performed between 1990 and 1999,[3] and other reports in the literature (Table 25–3). With respect to long-term efficacy of RCO, the cumulative five-year and 10-year ipsilateral stroke-free survival rates were 93% and 75%, respectively (Figures 25–12 and 25–13). These results are, again, comparable to those for primary CEA, 93% at five years and 75% at 10 years.[33] Other investigators have also reported similar results (Table 25–1). When stratified by symptom status, the results of RCO for asymptomatic patients were comparable to those for primary CEA[33] and to those of Asymptomatic Carotid Atherosclerotic Study (ACAS).[34] Similarly, for symptomatic patients, the five-year and nine-year estimates for ipsilateral stroke-free survival were both 84%, comparable to the primary CEA results[33] and to North American Symptomatic Carotid Endarterectomy Trial data.[35] Patients without

TABLE 25-3. COMPARISON OF COMPLICATIONS BETWEEN RCO AND PRIMARY CEA

	RCO(%)	Primary CEA	*p* value
Stroke	3	3	.99
Death	0	0.9	.5
TIA	3	0.5	.02
CN injury	6	2.5	.08
Cervical hematoma	3	1.7	.6
MI	3	1.1	.2
Death, stroke, TIA	6	4	.5
Death, stroke, TIA, MI	9	5	.2
TIA, CN injury, cervical hematoma	12	5	.01
All combined	18	10	.03

RCO, Redo carotid operation; CEA, carotid endarterectomy, TIA, transient ischemic attack; CN, cranial nerve; MI, myocardial infarction. With permission: Cho JS, Pandurangi K, Conrad M F, et al. Safety and durability of redo carotid operation: An 11-year experience. *J Vasc Surg.* 2004;39:155–161.

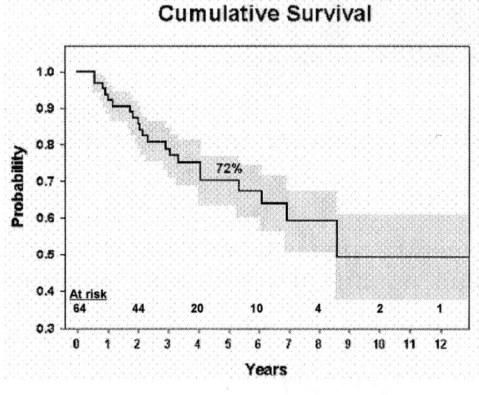

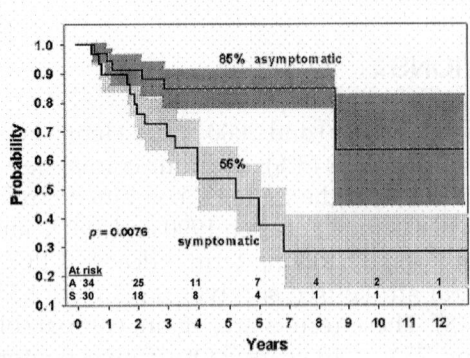

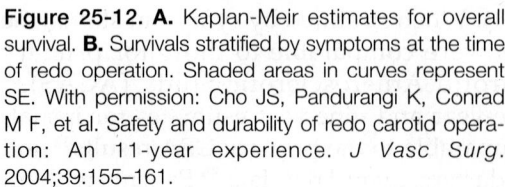

Figure 25-12. A. Kaplan-Meir estimates for overall survival. **B.** Survivals stratified by symptoms at the time of redo operation. Shaded areas in curves represent SE. With permission: Cho JS, Pandurangi K, Conrad M F, et al. Safety and durability of redo carotid operation: An 11-year experience. *J Vasc Surg.* 2004;39:155–161.

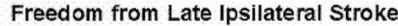

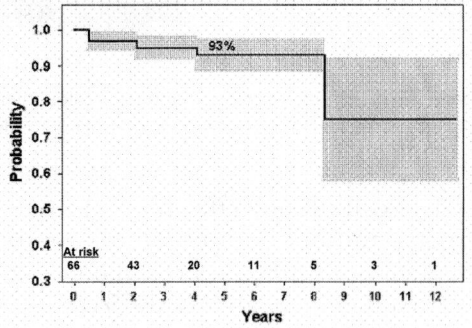

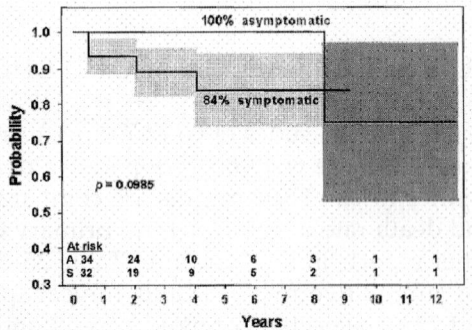

Figure 25-13. A. Kaplan-Meir estimates for freedom from late ipsilateral stroke. **B.** Survival stratified by symptoms (below) at the time of redo operation. Shaded areas in curves represent SE. With permission: Cho JS, Pandurangi K, Conrad M F, et al. Safety and durability of redo carotid operation: An 11-year experience. *J Vasc Surg.* 2004;39:155–161.

symptoms appeared to enjoy a higher degree of ipsilateral stroke prevention than did those with symptoms, although statistical significance was not achieved. Late survival, however, was increased in patients who presented without symptoms. These results confirm that RCO is as effective as primary CEA is in stroke prevention.

FREEDOM FROM SECONDARY RESTENOSIS

An evaluation of the durability of RCO showed that the freedom from >80% secondary restenosis was 96% at five years.[8] The ACAS and other prospective surveillance programs have observed late recurrence rates ranging from 4.9–21% at seven years.[15, 17, 36] The rate of late symptomatic recurrence or significant restenosis following RCO was 19.5% in one series.[21] In the authors' series, only one patient developed an ipsilateral stroke that was specific to secondary recurrent carotid stenosis.[8] These findings reaffirm that RCO is an effective and durable means of stroke prevention with comparable efficacy to that of primary CEA (Figure 25–14). This is an area of possible durability limitation for carotid angioplasty and stenting, and established a performance profile of redo carotid operations to be matched by CAS in all but the *bona fide* "high-risk" patient group.

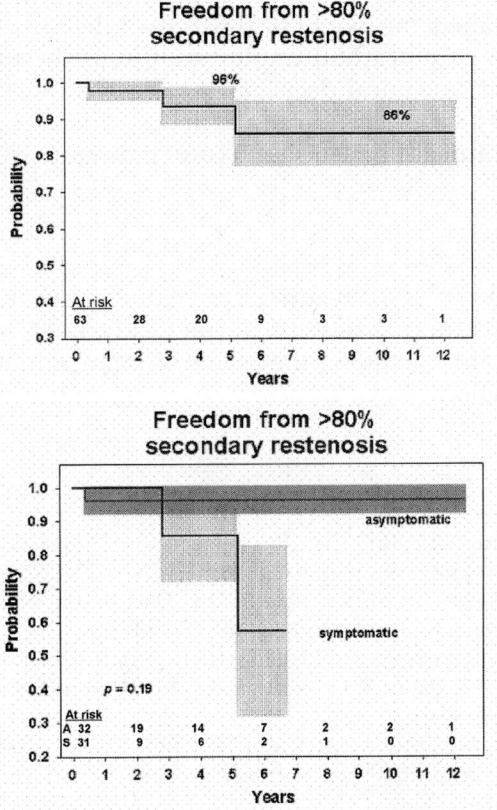

Figure 25-14. A. Kaplan-Meir estimates for freedom from >80 secondary restenosis. **B.** Survivals stratified by symptoms at the time of redo operation. Shaded areas in curves represent SE. With permission: Cho JS, Pandurangi K, Conrad M F, et al. Safety and durability of redo carotid operation: An 11-year experience. *J Vasc Surg.* 2004;39:155–161.

LATE RESULTS AFTER CAS

Although there has been some speculation that CAS for RCS may stimulate already activated neointimal hyperplasia and lead to higher rates of recurrent stenosis than that for primary atherosclerosis, the available data are conflicting. Leger et al, on the other hand, observed >60% secondary RCS in six of eight (75%) patients treated with CAS for RCS at a mean follow-up of 20 months; the two patients without recurrences had the shortest follow-up interval at 12 months.[37] Lal et al in their series of 122 CASs, of which 66% were done for RCS, reported the five-year probability of (80% recurrent stenosis was 6.4% and that of (60% recurrent stenosis was 16.4%.[38] No differences were noted in the cumulative recurrent stenosis-free rates between recurrent or primary carotid stenosis. On the contrary, AbuRahma et al compared 58 RCOs with 25 CASs for RCS and noted a significant difference in the probability of freedom from >50% secondary restenosis at three years: 100% with RCO versus 44% with CAS.[5] In a subset of patients who underwent treatment for early (<24 months) RCS, four-year probability of stroke-free survival was 88% after RCO and 63% after RCS (p = 0.067), while freedom from >50% secondary restenosis was 100% and 52%, respectively (p<0.0001).[39] Rockman et al also observed, in their short follow-up (13.9 months) of 18 CAS for RCS, a higher incidence of >50% recurrent stenosis with CAS, although statistical significance was not achieved.[40] Lal et al have recently noted that the very presence of a carotid stent alters the biophysical nature of the carotid bifurcation and even the basic follow-up tool, the carotid duplex scan, must be re-evaluated and recalibrated to provide reliable clinical decisions-making.[41] It is evident that both future data will be required by vascular surgeons to make evidence-based decisions for their patients and that the future for patients with carotid disease will likely improve.

CONCLUSION

Secondary carotid operations for recurrent carotid stenosis and other related indications are being performed safely and effectively with long-term durability. Alternatives methods are expanding the potential treatment armamentarium and require continued evaluation.

REFERENCES

1. Eastcott HH, Pichering GW, Rob CG. Reconstruction of internal carotid artery in a patient with intermittent attacks of hemiplegia. *Lancet.* 1954 Nov 13; 267(6846) 994–996.
2. Cronenwett J. *The Dartmouth Atlas of Health Care.* Dartmouth, NH: Center for the Evalative Clinical Sciences at Dartmouth Medical School, 200 ed.
3. Stoney RJ, String ST. Recurrent carotid stenosis. *Surgery.* 1976;80:705–710.
4. Mansour MA, Kang SS, Baker WH, et al. Carotid endarterectomy for recurrent stenosis. *J Vasc Surg.* 1997;25:877–883.
5. AbuRama AF, Bates MC, Stone PA, Wulu JT. Comparative study of operative treatment and percutaneous transluminal angioplasty/stenting for recurrent carotid disease. *J Vasc Surg.* 2001;34:831–838.
6. Hill BB, Olcott C, Dalman RL,et al. Reoprations for carotid stenosis is as safe as primary carotid endarterectomy. *J Vasc Surg.* 1999;30:26–35.
7. O'Hara PJ, Hertzer NR, Karafa MT, et al. Reoperation for recurrent carotid stenosis: Early results and late outcome in 199 patients. *J Vasc Surg.* 2001;34:5–12.

8. Cho JS, Pandurangi K, Conrad M F, et al. Safety and durability of redo carotid operation: An 11-year experience. *J Vasc Surg*. 2004;39:155–161.

9. AbuRahma AF, Jennings TG, Wulu JT, et al. Redo carotid endarterectomy versus primary carotid endarterectomy. *Stroke*. 2001;32:2787–2792.

10. Nitzberg RS, Mackey WC, Prendiville E, et al. Long-term follow-up of patients operated on for recurrent stenosis. *J Vasc Surg*. 1991;13:121–127.

11. Das MB, Hertzer NR, Ratliff NB et al. Recurrent carotid stenosis: a five-year series of 65 re-operations. *Ann Surg*. 1985;202:28–35.

12. Piepgras DG, Sundt TM, Jr., Fode NC, Mussman LA. Recurrent carotid stenosis: Results and complications of 57 operations. *Ann Surg*. 1986;203:205–213.

13. Washburn WK, Mackey WC, Belkin M, O'Donnell TF, Jr. Late stroke after carotid endarterectomy: The role of recurrent stenosis. *J Vasc Surg*. 1992;15:1032–1037.

14. Lattimer CR, Burnand KG. Recurrent carotid stenosis after carotid endarterectomy. *Br J Surg*. 1997;84:1206–1219.

15. Healy DA, Zierler RE, Nicholls SC, et al. Long-term follow-up and clinical outcome of carotid restenosis. *J Vasc Surg*. 1989;10:662–669.

16. Rosenthal D, Archie JP Jr., Avila MH, et al. Secondary recurrent carotis stenosis. *J Vasc Surg*. 1996;24(3):424–428.

17. Treiman GS, Jenkins JM, Edwards Sr. WH, et al. The evolving surgical management of recurrent carotid stenosis. *J Vasc Surg*. 1992;16:354–363.

18. O'Donnell TF, Jr., Rodrigues AA, Fortunato JE, et al. Management of recurrent carotid stenosis: should asymptomatic lesions be treated surgically? *J Vasc Surg*. 1996;24:207–212.

19. Ballinger BA, Money SR, Chatman DM, et al. Sites of recurrence and long-term results of redo surgery. *Ann Surg*. 1997;225:512–517.

20. Archie JA Jr. Reoperations for carotid artery stenosis: role of primary and secondary reconstructions. *J Vasc Surg*. 2001;33:495–503.

21. Rockman CB, Riles TS, Landis R, et al. Redo carotid surgery: an analysis of materials and configurations used in carotid reoperations and their influence on perioperative stroke and subsequent recurrent stenosis. *J Vasc Surg*. 1999;29:72–81.

22. Meyer FB, Piepgras DG, Fode NC. Surgical treatment of recurrent carotid artery stenosis. *J Neurosurg*. 1994;80:781–787.

23. Bartlett FF, Rapp JH, Goldstone J, et al. Recurrent carotid stenosis: Operative strategy and late results. *J Vasc Surg*. 1987;5:452–456.

24. AbuRahma AF, Choueiri MA. Cranial and cervical nerve injuries after repeat carotid endarterectomy. *J Vasc Surg*. 2000;32:649–654.

25. Gagne PJ, Riles TS, Jacobowitz GR, et al. Long-term follow-up of patients undergoing reoperation for recurrent carotid artery disease. *J Vasc Surg*. 1993;18:991–1001.

26. Ricotta JJ, O'Brien-Irr MS. Conservative management of residual and recurrent lesions after carotid endarterectomy: long-term results. *J Vasc Surg*. 1997;26:963–972.

27. Lanzino G, Mericle RA, Lopes DK,et al. Percutaneous transluminal angioplasty and stent placement for recurrent carotid artery stenosis. *J Neurosurg*. 1999;90:688–694.

28. Hobson II. RW, Goldstein JE, Jamil Z, et al. Carotid restenosis: Operative and endovascular management. *J Vasc Surg*. 1999;29:228–235.

29. Diethrich EB, Nidaye M, Reid DB. Stenting in the carotid artery: initial experience in 110 patients. *J Endovasc Surg*. 1996;3:42–62.

30 Henry M, Amor M, Masson I, et al. Angioplasty and stenting of the extracranial carotid arteries. *J Endovasc Surg*. 1998;5:293–304.

31 Yadav JS, Roubin GS, Iyer S, et al. Elective stenting of the extracranial carotid arteries. *Circulation*. 1997;95:376–381.

32 Bergeron P, Becquemin JP, Jausseran JM, et al. Percutaneous stenting of the internal carotid artery: the European CAST I study. *J Endovasc Surg*. 1999;6:155–159.

33 Conrad MF, Shepard AD, Pandurangi K, et al. Outcome of carotid endarterectomy in African Americans: Is race a factor? *J Vasc Surg*. 2003;38:129–137.

34 Executive Committee for the Asymptomatic Carotid Atherosclerosis Study. Endarterectomy for asymptomatic carotid stenosis. *JAMA*.1995;273:1428.

35 North American Symptomatic Carotid Endarterectomy Trial Collaborators. Beneficial effect of carotid endarterectomy in symptomatic patients with high-grade stenosis. *N Engl J Med*. 1991;325:445–453.

36 Johnson CA, Tollefson DFJ, lsen SB, et al. The natural history of early recurrent carotid artery stenosis. *Am J Surg*. 1999;177:433–436.

37 Leger AR, Neale M, Harris JP. Poor durability of carotid angioplasty and stenting for treatment of recurrent artery stenosis after carotid endarterectomy: An institutional experience. *J Vasc Surg*. 2001;33:1008–1014.

38 Lal BK, Hobson II.RW, Goldstein J, et al. In-stent recurrent stenosis after carotid artery stenting: Life table analysis and clinical relevance. *J Vasc Surg*. 2003;38:1162–1169.

39 AbuRahma AF, Bates MC, Wulu JT, Stone PA. Early postsurgical carotid restenosis: Redo surgery versus angioplasty/stenting. *J Endovasc Ther*. 2002;5:566–572.

40 Rockman CB, Bajakian D, Jacobowitz GR, et al. Impact of carotid artery angioplasty and stenting on management of recurrent carotid artery stenosis. *Ann Vasc Surg*. 2004;2:151–157

41 Lal BK, Hobson RW II, Goldstein J. Carotid artery senting is here a need to revise ultrasound velocity criteria? *Ann Vasc Surg*. 2004;1:58–66.

Cerebrovascular Revascularization Procedures

26

Complex Carotid and Vertebral Revascularizations

Ramon Berguer, M.D., PH.D.

The procedures and approaches described below are not necessarily complex, but they all differ in some substantial manner from the standard approaches used to access the carotid and vertebral arteries and the supraaortic trunks. The techniques described here either simplify a particular traditional exposure or they offer access to an arterial segment not reachable through the established approaches. I will mention under each heading how I came about these techniques.

DIRECT APPROACH TO THE ASCENDING AORTA AND SUPRAAORTIC TRUNKS BY UPPER MIDSTERNOTOMY

The direct approach to the supraaortic trunks is best made by means of an upper midsternotomy.[1] The traditional full splitting sternal incision is unnecessary and carries substantial associated morbidity. My experience with upper midsternotomy started when a fellow, in the process of opening a sternum through the midline, lost control of the oscillating saw that exited the sternum laterally at the level of T4. While wondering what to do with this awkward incision, I inserted a pediatric sternal retractor in the incision and spread it. It was obvious that the exposure obtained sufficed to access the ascending aorta, and the origin of the innominate and left carotid arteries.

This limited approach is appealing in that the continuity—and hence stability—of the chest cage is maintained from T4 down, and the pain and respiratory problems that attend mobility of the two halves of the sternum are avoided. This is basically a cervical incision extended through part of the sternum.

The midline incision that divides the sternum is carried through the upper three or four segments of the latter with an oscillating saw. At the level of T4, the saw is turned into a right angle. This will result in a subperiostial fracture when both sides of the sternum are retracted. The incision is spread slowly over a period of five minutes using a pediatric sternal retractor. Spreading the edges too rapidly may result in

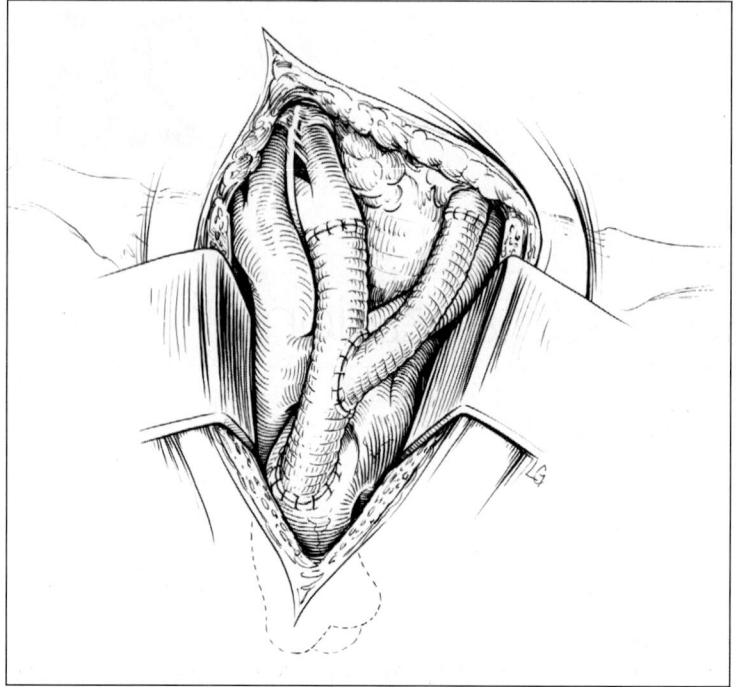

Figure 26-1. Bypass from the ascending aorta to the innominate and left common carotid arteries through a partial upper hemisternotomy.

tearing or avulsion of the brachycephalic vein. The pericardium is incised exposing the ascending aorta (Figure 26–1). The innominate artery bifurcation is exposed through the neck part of this incision contiguous with the upper sternotomy. Pericardial stay sutures will keep the medial edges of the lungs out of the field. The segment of ascending aorta that will be used for exclusion clamping is selected.

The innominate artery bifurcation is isolated in the upper third of the incision. Care is taken to avoid damage to the recurrent nerve, either when dissecting the proximal subclavian or the back of the proximal segment of the common carotid artery. While surgeons are well aware of the trajectory of the recurrent nerve under the proximal right subclavian, it is not always realized how close the right recurrent nerve courses to the posterior wall of the first inch of the common carotid artery. If a branch is to be extended from the main graft (ascending aorta to innominate) to the left common carotid artery, the latter is isolated close to the midline behind the sternum (Figure 26–2). The anastomoses for the reconstruction proceed along the usual steps.[2] Closing of the incision requires three or four wire loops.

CROSSING THE NECK THROUGH THE RETROPHARYNGEAL TUNNEL

We have advocated crossing the neck through the retropharyngeal space instead of using the traditional pretracheal route.[3-4] The retropharyngeal tunnel is short, about 5 cm, and does not interfere with a future midsternotomy or tracheotomy as a pretracheal tunnel. Given the natural distribution of atherosclerotic disease in the supra-

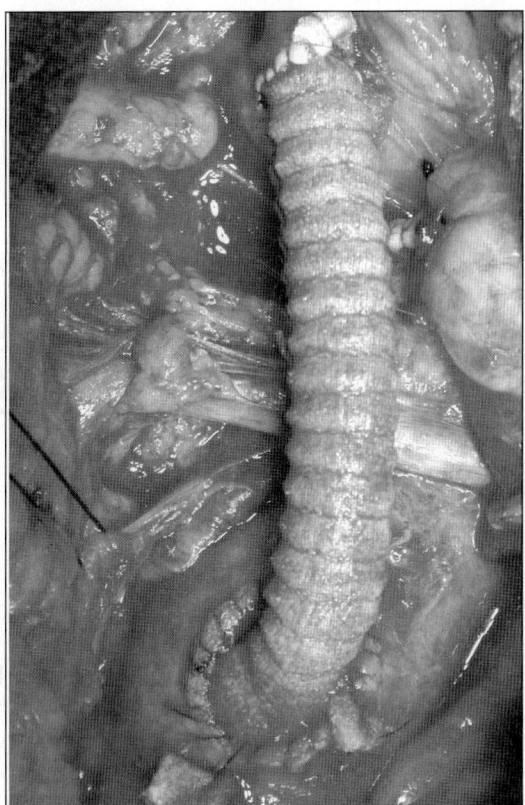

Figure 26-2. Operative photograph. Bypass from the ascending aorta to the distal innominate bifurcation through an upper mid-sternotomy. The flattened brachiocephalic vein can be seen crossing behind the bypass.

aortic trunks, the most frequent indication to cross the neck with a bypass is to bring blood supply to a left carotid bifurcation, or rarely, to a contralateral subclavian artery (Figure 26–3). With the advent of thoracic endografting, there is often a need to cover the origin of the left subclavian, and sometimes, the left common carotid artery origin, and this can be accomplished by supplying the left carotid system from the right side (right carotid or subclavian arteries).

The idea for the retropharyngeal pathway arose from dog experiments where we needed to supply both carotids with a constructed Y-shaped vein graft[5] to study the influence of flow rate in the development of intimal hyperplasia in vein grafts of the same caliber. Once both carotid systems had been exposed in the neck of the dogs, it was obvious that lifting the pharynx and crossing in front of the vertebra provided a much shorter pathway between both carotids for the limited length of vein graft available.

The draping of the neck requires the endotracheal tube be fixed to the forehead so that the neck may be turned from side to side as the anastomoses are done in each side (Figure 26–4). Exposure of the recipient common carotid artery is, as usual, anterior to the internal jugular vein. Once the common carotid is isolated, dissection proceeds posterior to it and medial to the sympathetic chain, which runs immediately behind the common carotid artery. We enter the retropharyngeal space by palpating the vertebrae and sliding the pulp of the finger on top of the lamina prevertebralis with the pharynx on top of the finger. The prevertebral tunnel opens with minimal resistance. As the finger crosses the vertebral bodies, the lips of the cervical vertebrae are felt. The other half of the tunnel is accessed through the opposite side of the neck. Once the tunnel is

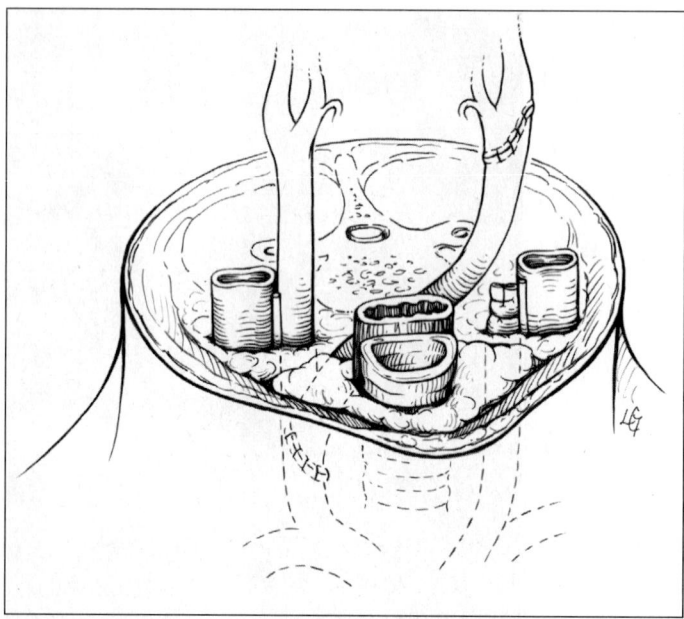

Figure 26-3. The retropharyngeal bypass. The bypass crosses the midline in front of the lamina prevertebralis and behind the pharynx.

achieved, we place a Penrose drain through it that will be used to guide the bypass graft that will eventually be placed there. The sites for the donor anastomoses are chosen as low as possible so that the bypass graft will cross the midline in an oblique course. This will facilitate a proper layout for the distal (contralateral) anastomosis that will be made to the base of the carotid bifurcation, perhaps extending into the bulb and combining it with an internal carotid endarterectomy (Figure 26–5). The size of the bypass graft will be 7-8 mm, depending on the size of the common carotid artery (Figure 26–6). For bypasses in this location, we have preferred PTFE material to any other, including vein grafts.

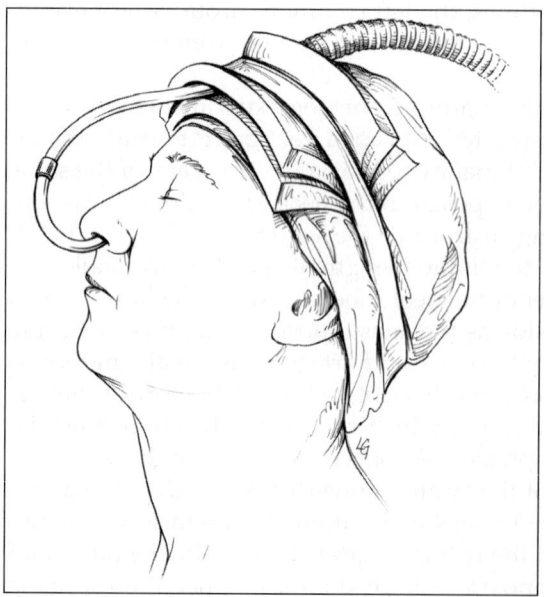

Figure 26-4. Nasopharyngeal intubation with the endotracheal tube.

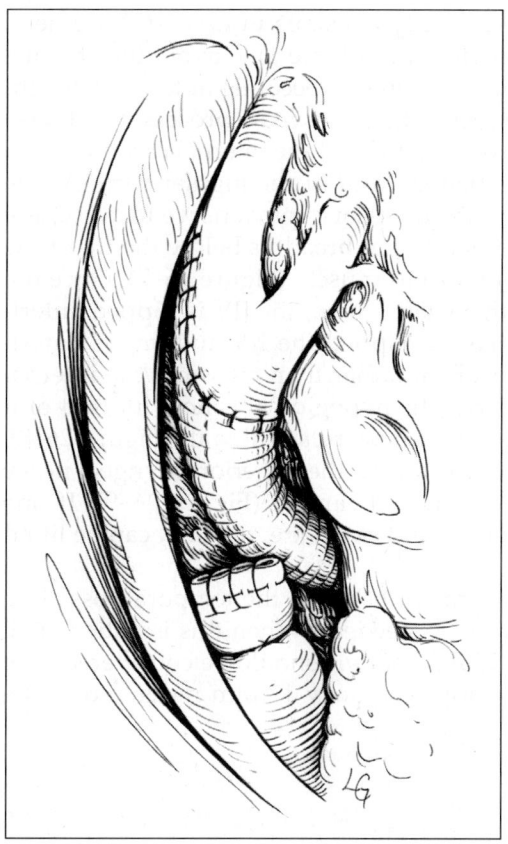

Figure 26-5. The bypass graft emerging from behind the pharynx is anastomosed to the carotid bifurcation. In this patient, as is often the case, the recipient carotid bifurcation has been cleaned of plaque by an eversion endarterectomy.

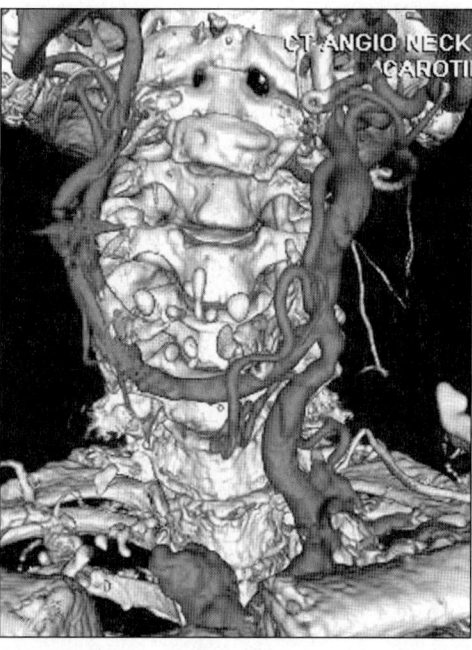

Figure 26-6. Post operative CT angio of a left carotid to right carotid bypass in a patient with a single source of brain supply in his left carotid.

I have not seen any space occupying problems with a graft in this retropharyngeal position in the 74 cases where I have used it. Although I have not observed any obstruction dysphagia because of the mass effect of a graft in the retropharyngeal space last year, I had a patient with temporary dysphagia that required feedings through a percutaneous gastrostomy for four weeks. The patient postoperatively had an abnormality of motion of the larynx. I do not know if the problem in this patient had to do with the trauma of developing the tunnel by blunt retropharyngeal fingering or with glossopharyngeal nerve stretching when doing the distal anastomosis to the high cervical internal carotid artery above the bulb.

APPROACH TO THE HIGH CERVICAL INTERNAL CAROTID ARTERY

I approach lesions at the C1-C2 level of the cervical internal carotid artery (ICA) through the retrojugular space.[6] I saw the advantages of approaching the distal cervical ICA through a *retrojugular approach* while dissecting the distal vertebral artery to do a distal (C2-C1) bypass:[7] the internal carotid was easily available in its C1-C2 segment. The two advantages provided by the retrojugular approach are 1) to avoid the obstruction caused by the trajectory of the internal jugular vein that becomes anterior to the internal carotid artery and covers it as it approaches the transverse process of C1, and 2) to avoid the obstacle of the hypoglossal crossing in front of the internal carotid.

For this approach, we go behind rather than in front of the jugular vein. As we start the dissection, the first step is identifying the accessory spinal nerve to avoid any damage to it. This nerve is located two and a half finger breadths below the tip of the mastoid along the anterior edge of the sternomastoid muscle (Figure 26–7). Once the accessory spinal is identified and tagged with a silastic loop, the IJV is flipped anteriorly with the vagus. The ICA is dissected, having flipped the IJV and vagus anteriorly. This leaves the hypoglossal nerve anterior to, rather than crossing, the internal carotid artery. With the vagus flipped anteriorly, the hypoglossal is now in front of it and the internal carotid can be dissected along its posterolateral wall (Figure 26–8). The dissection proceeds unobstructed by any nerve until the superior laryngeal nerve (SLN) exits the vagus and loops around the internal carotid (Figure 26–9). If one needs to obtain an additional 5 mm of internal carotid exposure, the SLN can be lifted and the ICA dissected under it.

For internal carotid artery lesions in the segment between the temporal fossa and the transverse process of C1, an *anterior approach* is needed.[8] When this is anticipated, unilateral subluxation of the ipsilateral mandibular condyle should be considered. The subluxated joint will result in an overbite of approximately 12 mm measured at the

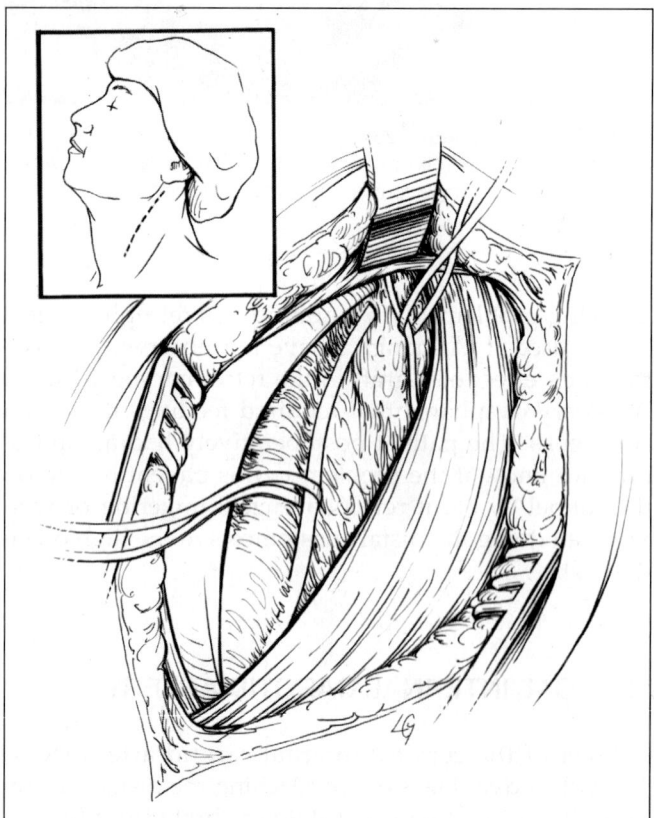

Figure 26-7. Retrojugular approach to the mid-cervical carotid artery. The first steps are the same for this operation and for distal vertebral bypass. The vagus nerve is moved anteriorly. The accessory spinal nerve has been identified at the top of the dissection and retracted gently with the Silastic loop.

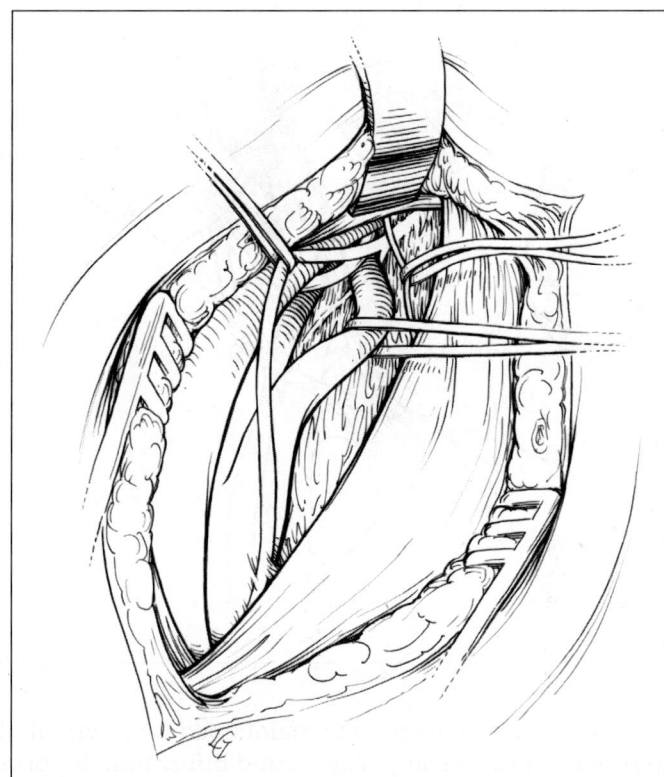

Figure 26-8. Dissecting the mid-cervical carotid through the retrojugular space shows the superior laryngeal nerve crossing the posterolateral wall of the internal carotid artery of the level of C2.

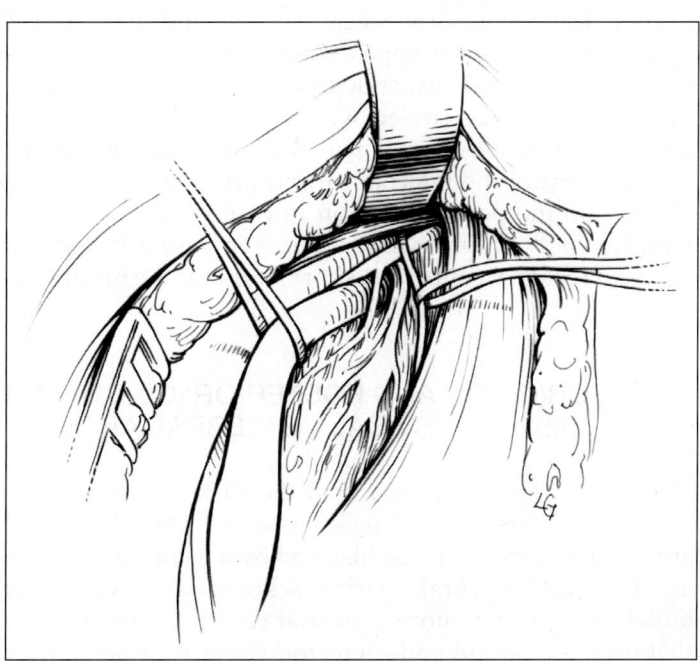

Figure 26-9. The mid-cervical ICA is dissected. The SLN is seen crossing the ICA in front of the superior cervical cervical ganglion.

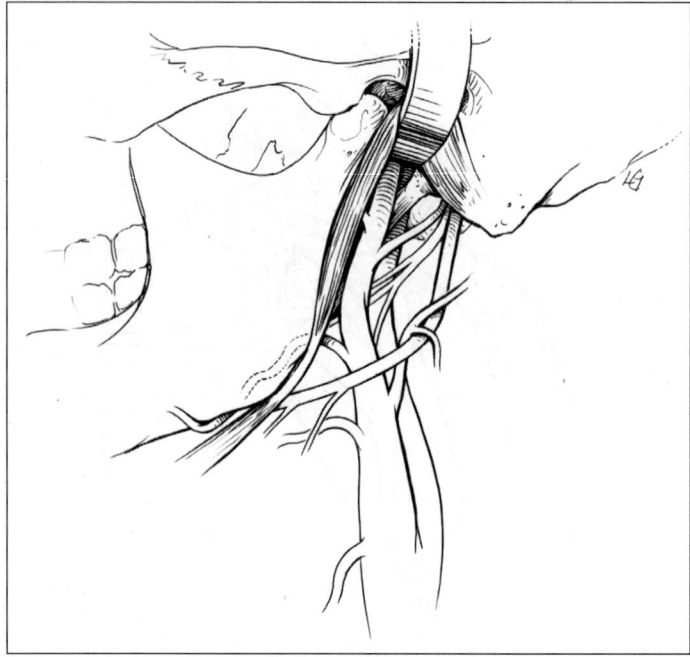

Figure 26-10. Elements in the anterior approach to the infratemporal carotid. The glossopharyngeal nerve beneath the external and above the internal carotid arteries. The digastric muscle is usually cut rather than retracted as shown. The styloglossal muscle is seen above the ICA.

incisives. The subluxation is maintained by a wire that circles the mandible and goes through the nasal spine. The carotid bifurcation is approached in the standard manner. Its exposure is continued by division of the digastric muscle and the occipital artery that courses transversely beneath it. The ICA is isolated above the hypoglossal nerve (Figure 26–10). Dissection cranially over the ICA identifies the single or double trunk of the glossopharyngeal nerve crossing the ICA and coursing posterior to the external carotid. The styloid process can be palpated. Its removal and that of the styloglossus apparatus is done if it appears that it will increase exposure of the roof of the dissection tunnel. Sometimes, styloidectomy does not increase exposure. The infrapetrosal carotid can now be circled with a silastic loop and accessed for arteriotomy and/or anastomosis of a bypass. I use a small detachable clamp (Schwartz, Heifitz) to temporarily control the internal carotid artery before advancing a #2 balloon catheter occluder into the petrous portion to control backflow. The arterial edges are anchored with two 6-0 polypropylene sutures in case a balloon fails or is punctured, and one needs to regain access of the short stump of the infrapetrosal carotid artery.

ANTERIOR(C2-C1) AND POSTERIOR (C0-C1) APPROACH TO THE DISTAL CERVICAL VERTEBRAL ARTERY

The most common approach to the distal vertebral artery at the C1, C2 segment is through an *anterolateral* neck incision.[7] The approach to this segment through an antero-lateral incision was inspired by a technique described by Henry[9] in order to ligate the distal vertebral artery (backflow) at this level for hemorrhage control after a bullet injury of the more proximal cervical vertebral artery. The incision is similar to that used for carotid endarterectomy and is prolonged by a further centimeter toward

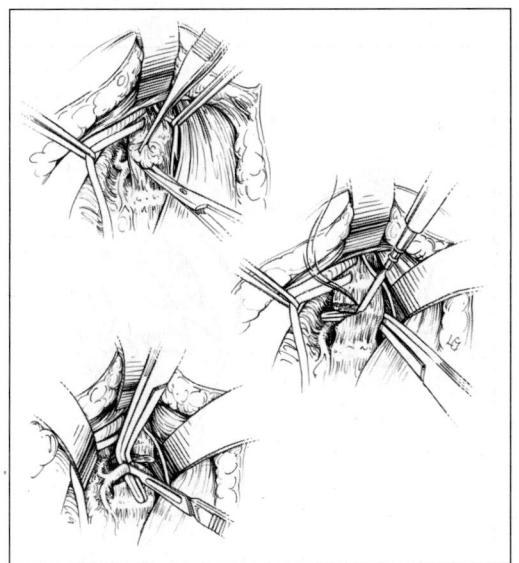

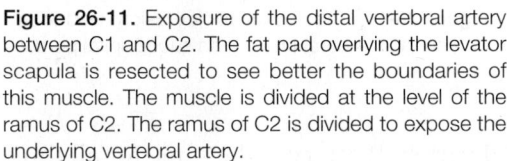

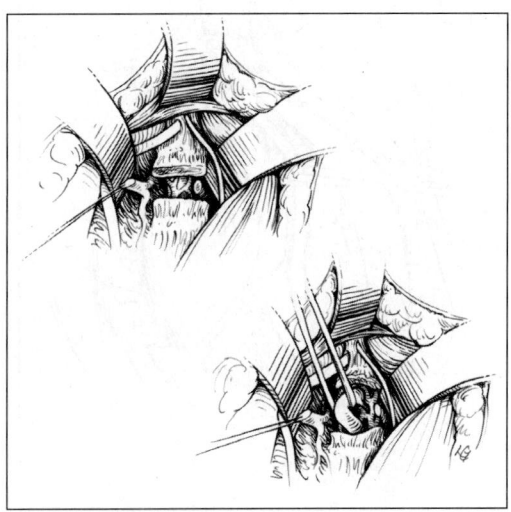

Figure 26-11. Exposure of the distal vertebral artery between C1 and C2. The fat pad overlying the levator scapula is resected to see better the boundaries of this muscle. The muscle is divided at the level of the ramus of C2. The ramus of C2 is divided to expose the underlying vertebral artery.

Figure 26-12. With the ramus divided and held by stay sutures the vertebral artery is seen crossing underneath and covered by a plexus of veins. The artery is freed from the surrounding veins and prepared for anastomosis.

the mastoid tip. It is not uncommon to have to divide the external auricular branch of the occipital nerve (Figure 26–10).

The first landmark to identify is the accessory spinal nerve (XI), which is found between the internal jugular and the sternomastoid two and a half finger breadths below the tip of the mastoid (Figure 26–7). The nerve is followed distally. As we dissect the XI nerve with the help of a silastic loop around it, the digastric muscle is usually divided to provide added exposure. The nerve is dissected past the transverse process of C1. The characteristic bony prominence of the latter can be easily felt by sliding the finger over the nerve cranially. At this level, the nerve is on top of the internal jugular vein as the latter rests on the transverse process of C1. The fibro-fatty layer overlying the scalenus anticus is removed (Figure 26–11). The next step is the location of the ramus of C2 as it merges under the anterior edge of the levator scapula. The muscle is divided over the C2 ramus and the musculotendinous insertion of this muscle on the transverse process is cleared from the bony process itself to increase exposure (Figure 26–11). Once the levator muscle is divided, the artery can be seen bulging behind the ramus as it crosses beneath it. After dividing the ramus and holding its ends apart with two stay sutures the distal VA is exposed and the paravertebral venous plexus is dissected away and cauterized (Figure 26–12). The artery is lifted by a silastic loop between C1 and C2. There is redundancy in the course of the artery, which at this intervertebral segment allows for the exposure of a length of VA sufficient to construct the distal anastomosis of a graft to it.

The reconstruction of the VA at this level is usually done by means of a common carotid-to-distal VA vein graft (Figure 26–13). It may also be done by transposing the external carotid to the distal VA, or in special circumstances, by transposing the VA to

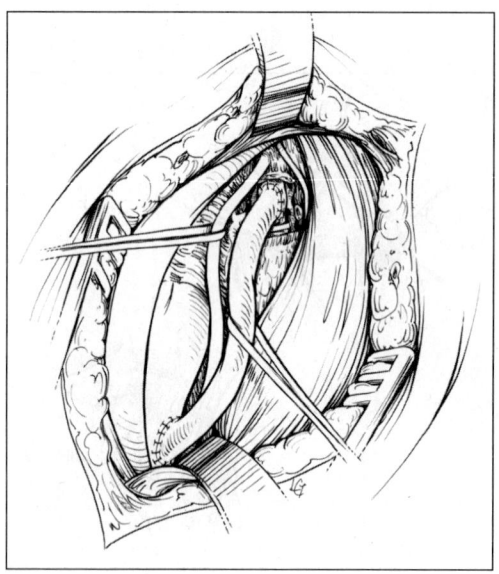

Figure 26-13. A completed common carotid to distal vertebral bypass.

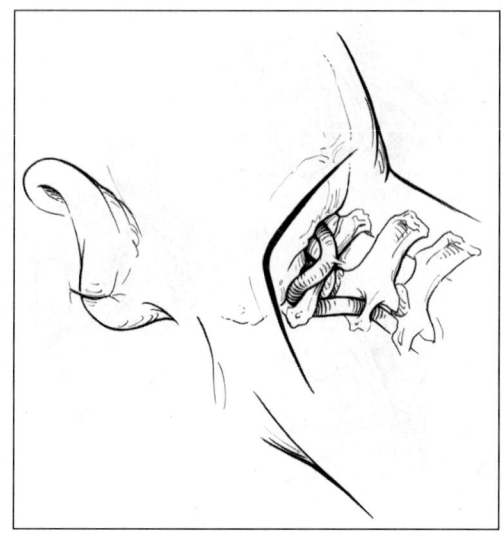

Figure 26-14. The hockey stick incision used to approach the vertebral artery in its suboccipital portion.

the distal ICA graft. The exposure of the distal vertebral artery is the same for all three procedures.

If the VA needs to be bypassed above C1, the anterolateral approach I just described is difficult and sometimes inadequate. To access the artery between the occipital bone C0 and C1, I use a posterior *suboccipital approach*[10] attributed to Druner that I saw in Kirchner's textbook of surgical technique.[11] The incision has a hockey stick shape (Figure 26–14). The semispinalis and splenius capitis muscles are cut (Figure 26–15). The transverse process of the atlas is located by palpation and serves as a reference point for the rest of the operation. The rectus capitis posterior and obliquus capitis superior muscles are cut. The artery is seen resting on the lamina of the atlas and covered by a dense paravertebral plexus that gives it a blue appearance. The vertebral plexus is controlled with bipolar cautery. Once the artery is isolated away from the lamina of C1, enough dissection is made lengthwise to provide room for clamping and anastomosis. There is a good size posterior branch that needs to be divided that hangs over the lamina of the atlas and goes into the musculature of the neck. If it is necessary to bypass the VA at this level, the source for the bypass will be the ICA that can be isolated in its infrapetrosal portion in this approach. For this, we need to mobilize the hypoglossal nerve and the vagus that cover, when approaching posteriorly, the distal segment of the infrapetrosal ICA at this level.

If the segment of VA that partially overhangs the lamina of C1 has been shown to be compressed between the occipital bone and the sharp upper edge of the lamina of C1 during neck extension/rotation, a laminectomy is performed to eliminate the lower of the two elements of compression (Figure 26–16).

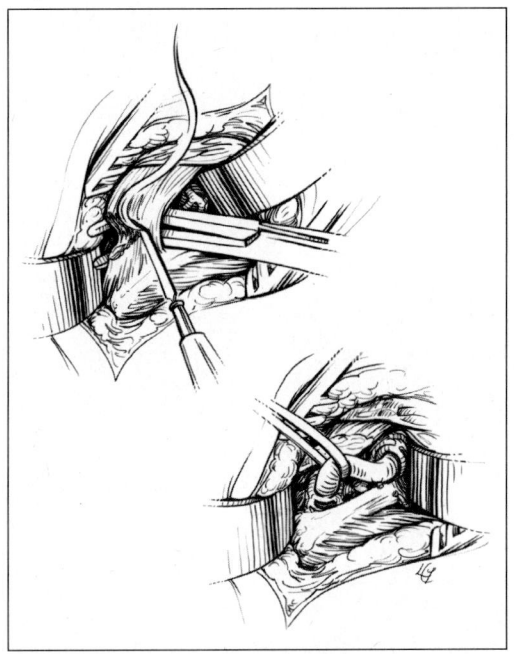

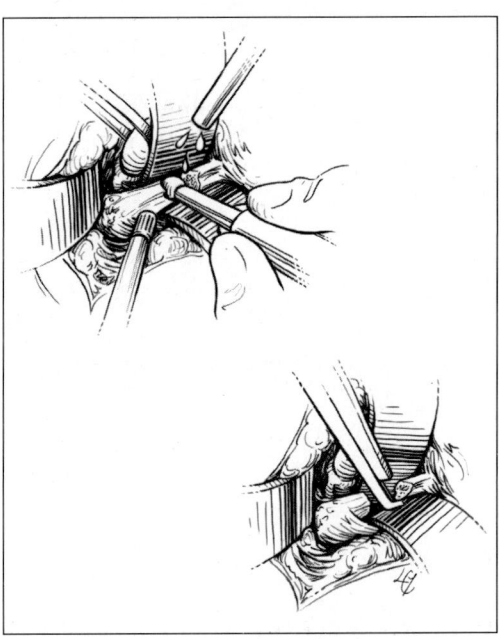

Figure 26-15. Division of the obliquus muscle. Below: lifting the vertebral artery of the lamina of C1 once the periarterial venous plexus has been coagulated.

Figure 26-16. Removal of the segment of the lamina of C2. The artery overlying it is protected with a soft malleable retractor. Completion of the laminectomy.

REFERENCES

1. Berguer R. Surgical reconstruction of the supraaortic trunks and vertebral arteries. In *Vascular & Endovascular Surgery - A Comprehensive Review. 7th Edition.* W.S. Moore, Editor. Sanders-Elsevier. Philadelphia. 2006
2. Berguer R., Kieffer E., *Surgery of the Arteries to the Head.* Springer-Verlag. New York. 1992
3. Berguer R. The short retropharyngeal route for arterial bypass across the neck. *Ann. Vasc. Surg.* 1996;1:127–9
4. Berguer R., Gonzalez J.A. Revascularization by the retropharyngeal route for extensive disease of the extracranial arteries. *J Vasc Surg.* 1994; Vol. 9:217–226
5. Berguer R., Higgins R.F., Reddy, D. Intimal hyperplasia: An experimental study. Arch Surgery 1980;115:332–335
6. Berguer R. Retrojugular approach for exclusion bypass of the carotid bifurcation: a useful method for recurrent or high carotid disease. In *Current Critical Problems in Vascular Surgery,* Vol. 4, F.J. Veith, Editor. Quality Medical Publishing, Inc., St. Louis. 1992
7. Berguer R. Distal vertebral artery bypass: technique, the occipital connection and potential uses. *J Vasc Surg.* 1985; Vol. 2:621–626
8. Berguer R. *High internal carotid exposure. Vascular Surgical Approaches.* Branchereau A., and Berguer R., Editors. Futura Publishing, New York, 1999.
9. Henry, A.K. *External exposure.* Baltimore: Williams & Wilkins 1970
10. Berguer R. Suboccipital approach to the distal vertebral artery. *J Vasc Surg.* 1999; 30: 344–9.
11. Kirchner. *Operative Surgery,* J.B.Lippincott, Philadelphia 1937

27

Hybrid Procedure for Supra-Aortic Trunk Lesions

Michael Monge, M.D.
Mark K. Eskandari, M.D.

The evolution of the endovascular management of supra-aortic trunk lesions has given vascular surgeons a less invasive and lower risk, but durable method, of treating aortic arch vessel disease. In this section, a historical review of the various surgical approaches for the correction of supra-aortic trunk lesions is presented, with their published success and complication rates. Then, the treatment paradigm of both symptomatic and asymptomatic aortic arch vessel athero-occlusive disease is reviewed. The technical aspects of the endovascular correction of these lesions are briefly discussed. In addition, the published literature of the endovascular treatment of supra-aortic trunk lesions is reviewed.

EVOLUTION OF TREATING SUPRA-AORTIC TRUNK DISEASE

Surgical Reconstruction

The treatment of atherosclerotic disease of the common carotid, subclavian, and innominate arteries, collectively known as the aortic arch vessels, has evolved with the advances made in the correction of other vascular lesions. In 1856, the first report of symptomatic subclavian artery occlusion appeared in the literature.[1] Nearly one century later, the surgical repair of a supra-aortic trunk lesion was reported.[2] Shortly thereafter, others reported on the performance of a transthoracic endarterectomy of the innominate artery. However this operation—at the time—was associated with a mortality rate of 22%[3-4] and a major complication rate of 15–26%.[7] A more contemporary series by Berguer et. al. of 100 consecutive transthoracic repairs of supra-aortic trunk lesions showed a combined stroke/death rate reduced to 16%.[5]

In 1957, Lyons and Galbraith described the first carotid-subclavian bypass, and a year later, Debakey et. al. introduced the use of prosthetic grafts to bypass thrombo-obliterative lesions of the aortic arch vessels.[6-7] A decade elapsed before this approach was more broadly utilized and reported.[8] Nevertheless, this approach resulted in an improvement in the mortality rate (5.6%) as compared to the transthoracic repair.[4] The excellent results of extra-anatomic repair of aortic arch vessels have been further substantiated in subsequent series, making it the standard to which other interventions are compared. Berguer et. al. reported a five- and 10-year primary patency rate of 91% and 82%, respectively, with a mortality rate of 0.5% and stroke rate of 3.8%, respectively, in 100 consecutive cervical reconstructions of the supraaortic trunk.[9] Similarly, Perler et. al. reported primary patency rates of 92% and 83% at five and eight years with an extra-anatomic approach.[10]

Extra-anatomic bypass grafting, however, has several associated specific major complications: 1) thoracic duct fistulae, 2) Horner's syndrome, 3) brachial plexus nerve injury, and 4) myocardial infarction. Additionally, skin erosion and infection of the graft, encumbrance of future coronary bypass grafting, and failure to exclude atherosclerotic lesions with future embolic potential, are disadvantages of this approach.

Endovascular Options

Mathias published the first report of percutaneous transluminal angioplasty of aortic arch vessels in 1980.[11] In that same year, Bachman and Kim introduced subclavian artery angioplasty.[12] Subsequent reports demonstrated the safety, efficacy, and efficiency of angioplasty of supra-aortic lesions. In a review of 10 reported series and a total of 423 subclavian and innominate artery angioplasties, there was a 92% initial technical success rate, with a 19% recurrence rate between one and five years of follow-up.[13] Similarly, Kachel et. al., in a review of 774 supra-aortic artery lesions, documented a technical success rate of 95.3% with a 4.0% complication rate.[14]

Stenting of the aortic arch vessels was introduced in the early 1990s after the favorable results of stenting was used as an adjunct to balloon angioplasty of other vascular lesions. Several series[15-17] demonstrated good initial success with stenting of supra-aortic trunk lesions, with acceptable patency rates and low complication rates. Theoretically, stents have the potential to enmesh atheroemboli, promote laminar flow to reduce restenosis, and restrict arterial recoil. Subsequent reports have documented the cost benefit of an endovascular approach to the treatment of arch vessel disease.[18] Endovascular stenting of aortic arch vessels continues to evolve as new techniques and devices are developed.

ETIOLOGY

Multiple inflammatory and infectious disease processes produce stenotic lesions of the supra-aortic trunk, including atherosclerotic disease, Takayasu's arteritis, and radiation-induced atherosclerosis obliterans.

Atherosclerotic occlusive disease, the most common etiology of supra-aortic trunk lesions of the aortic arch vessels, is relatively rare when compared to other vascular lesions. In a report on surgery for aortic arch branch occlusion, 1.7% of 1961 operations were performed on the innominate artery while 4.3% of cases were performed for occlusive lesions of the subclavian arteries.[19]

In the Joint Study on Extracranial Arterial Occlusion, one-third of patients were found to have severe lesions of the supra-aortic trunk by arteriography;[20] 17% of these lesions are located in the innominate and proximal subclavian arteries,[19] of which the left subclavian artery is involved three to four times more often than the right.[21] In a report by Brountzos et. al., 34 of 39 subclavian artery lesions were left-sided.[22] A 1.8% incidence of isolated proximal common carotid artery stenosis has been reported, while a "tandem" lesion of both the carotid bifurcation and common carotid artery has been found in 0.6% of patients undergoing evaluation of cerebrovascular insufficiency.[23]

Atherosclerotic disease of the supra-aortic trunk affects relatively young patients when compared with other vascular lesions.[24] However, significant comorbidities are present in this patient population. In a report of 18 patients undergoing endovascular treatment of atherosclerotic lesions of the aortic arch vessels, coronary artery disease (CAD) was present in 78%, carotid disease in 33%, 44% were diabetic, 67% had a smoking history, and hypertension was present in 61%.[25] Similarly, Brountzos et. al. reported CAD in 52% of patients undergoing percutaneous revascularization of the arch vessels, while 30% had associated disease of the carotid and/or vertebral arteries.[22]

Takayasu's arteritis, a cell-mediated inflammatory process that produces segmental fibrotic stenosis of the aorta and its branches, is the second most common cause of supra-aortic occlusive disease. It has a prevalence of one per 1,000 people in the United States, and six per 1,000 people worldwide.

Although short-term outcomes of PTA and stent procedures to treat Takayasu-related stenoses have been favorable, long-term follow-up has been less encouraging. In their study of patients with Takayasu's arteritis, Liang et. al. reported the occurrence of restenosis or occlusion in three of seven PTA procedures, and five out of seven stent procedures during the follow-up period. The authors attributed the low stent patency rate in Takayasu's arteritis to the long, noncompliant fibrotic lesions, which may not fully dilate, even under injurious inflation pressures.[26] In a separate study of four patients with Takayasu's disease who had undergone stenting of the subclavian or common carotid artery, 10 of 11 stents were occluded at a mean follow-up of 12 months.[27]

Radiation-induced atherosclerosis obliterans is a rare cause of supra-aortic trunk lesions, which is most frequently reported after radiotherapy for breast cancer.[28-29] In a retrospective review, which included 11 centers, 64 patients with radiation-induced supra-aortic trunk disease that had undergone surgical and endovascular reconstruction were identified. Thirteen patients had angioplasty with stent placement of the common carotid or innominate artery preformed. Although no strokes or operative mortality were reported, one restenosis was observed (mean follow-up: 18 months).[30]

INDICATIONS FOR TREATMENT

In general, surgical intervention is indicated when supra-aortic trunk lesions become symptomatic. Symptoms are produced by hypoperfusion of or embolization to the cerebral and upper extremity vascular beds. Lesions of the brachiocephalic trunk may present with upper limb ischemia, digital embolization, and vertebrobasilar insufficiency, manifested by visual disturbances, vertigo, syncope, dysarthria, dysphagia, and ataxia. In a series of 48 patients undergoing stenting of subclavian and innominate arteries, 16.6% of patients exhibited vertebrobasilar insufficiency, 31.3% had upper limb ischemia, while 12.5% had both cerebral and upper limb symptoms.[22] Sullivan et. al. reported that 50% of patients with symptomatic occlusive disease of the innominate artery presented with anterior circulation symptoms, 40% exhibited vertebrobasilar symptoms, and 10% had a combination of symptom complexes.[15]

Not surprisingly, between 0.5% and 1.1% of patients undergoing coronary revascularization have evidence of subclavian artery stenosis.[31-33] Patients with a prior history of internal mammary artery-coronary bypass grafting may present with angina, and in fact, 27 of 83 patients treated for subclavian lesions at The Cleveland Clinic presented with symptoms of internal mammary steal, of which 11 had unstable coronary syndromes.[15]

In addition, patients with an axillary-femoral bypass may exhibit signs of lower limb ischemia from an occlusive lesion of the subclavian artery. Treatment of subclavian artery lesions may also be indicated in patients scheduled to undergo other revascularization procedures. In a series of 48 patients undergoing stenting of subclavian and innominate artery occlusive disease, 12.5% presented with angina before or after LIMA-coronary bypass, while 10.4% complained of leg claudication before or after axillary-femoral bypass grafting.[22]

Treatment of common carotid artery occlusive disease is indicated to improve inflow prior to ipsilateral carotid endarterectomy and bypass procedures involving the carotid arteries. Other indications for surgical intervention of common carotid lesions are nondebilitating stroke with good recovery or TIAs, amaurosis fugax, or critical stenosis of ≥ 75% in an asymptomatic individual with a patent internal carotid artery.[16] Although level I evidence is lacking, many would extrapolate and agree that a symptomatic lesion of ≥ 50% or an asymptomatic arch vessel lesion of ≥ 80% should be corrected either by traditional open surgery or endoluminal therapy. The only caveat is with regard to asymptomatic lesions of the left subclavian artery, and whether it should be treated or not remains a hotly debated topic.

IMAGING STUDIES

Digital subtraction angiography (DSA) remains the "gold standard" for imaging of the aortic arch vessels. However, radiation exposure, the use of nephrotoxic dye, and complications related to the arterial puncture and catheterization are associated with this technique. In addition, there is a potential for stroke with this procedure. As reported by NASCET and ACAS, the risk of stroke with cerebral angiography is 0.7% and 1.2%, respectively.[34-35]

Recently, the use of MRA in the detection, interventional planning, and follow-up of supra-aortic trunk lesions has emerged. When compared to DSA, MRA has a sensitivity and specificity for determining lesion severity of 73–100% and 89–98%, respectively.[36-38] Loewe et. al. demonstrated that the sensitivity and specificity of MRA for exact length measurements of aortic arch lesions was 100% and 96%, respectively.[36] This noninvasive technique, alone or in combination with duplex ultrasonography, has been shown to be cost-effective when compared with preoperative contrast arteriography.[39] Similarly, with improvements in computed tomography (CT) angiography, three-dimensional rendered images provide valuable information about the anatomy and plaque characteristics of the target lesion.

Ultrasonography is important in the diagnosis and follow-up of steno-occlusive disease of the supra-aortic trunk. While this imaging modality is less costly and noninvasive, it lacks the ability to directly characterize lesions, which is required for treatment planning. Ultrasonographic findings in steno-occlusive disease of the innominate artery are reversed or biphasic flow in the right vertebral artery, mid-systolic deceleration in the right carotid arterial system, and an elevated LCCA/RCCA ratio.[40]

Duplex ultrasonography of subclavian arteries with obstructive lesions demonstrates elevated systolic velocity, loss of biphasic waveforms, and poststenotic turbulence.[41] For the detection of a obstructive lesions of $\geq$ 50%, duplex ultrasound has a sensitivity and specificity of 0.73 and 0.91, respectively, and a negative predictive value of 0.97.[42]

TECHNIQUES OF ENDOVASCULAR THERAPY

Several different approaches have been utilized to gain vascular access for the endovascular treatment of supra-aortic trunk lesions. Access via the brachial artery, femoral artery, or cervical carotid has been reported. Advantages and complications are associated with each method, which must be considered during the preoperative planning stage.

Transfemoral (Antegrade) Approach

The transfemoral approach is a similar technique to carotid artery stenting. Using a long 6 or 7 French sheath placed just proximal to the target lesion, the stenosis can then be crossed and treated. This approach allows for the use of a mechanical embolic protection system if desired. Most frequently, a balloon expandable stent is necessary to adequately treat orifical lesions. This allows for accurate placement of the stent, good wall appostion, and strong radial force. Technical success is confirmed by brisk flow through the stented lesions without evidence of thrombosis or dissection. In addition, less than 10% residual stenosis should be observed.[15] With treatment of subclavian and innominate artery lesions, normalization of blood pressure between the two arms should be observed. No access site complications were reported in 40 patients undergoing stenting of the subclavian or innominate artery via a transfemoral approach.[22] Sullivan et. al. reported one pseudoaneurysm occurring in 49 femoral access sites.[15]

Transbrachial or Transaxillary Approach

The retrograde transbrachial approach is useful for occlusive lesions of the left subclavian artery, but may also be used to treat innominate or proximal right subclavian lesions. By approaching the vascular lesion in a retrograde manner, the difficulty of navigating the acute angle of takeoff of this artery is avoided, which may also lessen the risk of aortic dissection. Additionally, the close proximity of the access site to the left subclavian artery orifice may facilitate manipulation of the guidewire and catheter through the lesion. Both open and percutaneous techniques have been described for gaining access via the brachial artery. Typically, the brachial artery is accessed in the antecubital fossa using a micropuncture technique under ultrasound guidance. A 35 cm 5 or 6 French catheter, introduced into the artery over a 0.035-inch guidewire, is advanced to the distal end of the lesion, as described by Criado et. al.[43] Brachial artery access site complications are higher than other methods of vascular access due to the smaller size of the vessel. In two series, operative repair of the brachial artery was necessary following the procedure, either due to thrombosis or pseudoaneurysm.[15,17] Current mechanical embolic protection devices cannot be employed in this circumstance given the retrograde access. As in the transfemoal approach, balloon expandable stents are most frequently used.

Transcarotid Approach

The transcarotid approach is particularly advantageous in cases of small or tortuous brachial, axillary, or iliac arteries. Certainly, a completely percutaneous approach is feasible; however, an added benefit of an open cutdown to the common carotid artery (CCA) is the ability to achieve cerebral protection during the intervention. Several authors have found the retrograde cervical approach useful for the treatment of tandem lesions of the internal carotid bifurcation and common carotid artery at the time of carotid endarterectomy.[44-47] It is also advantageous when treating patients with tortuous aortic arch anatomy, extensive aorto-iliac atherosclerotic disease, and in the 1–2% patients in whom a prior femoral approach has been unsuccessful.[48]

The patient is positioned on the operating table with the neck extended and rotated toward the contralateral side. After general anesthesia is induced, a longitudinal 2-centimeter incision is made at the anterior border of the sternocleidomastoid muscle. After the platysma is incised, the carotid sheath is opened and the CCA encircled with a vessel loop. The vagus nerve, which commonly lies posterior to the artery, must be identified and protected. Next, the patient is systemically heparinized and the CCA cannulated in a retrograde manner using a micropuncture technique. A 5 French sheath is placed. Digital subtraction arteriography is then performed to evaluate the proximal stenosis. A right posterior oblique view is useful to evaluate proximal stenosis of the CCA. Stenosis of the origin of the innominate artery is best evaluated with a left anterior oblique view.[24] A diagnostic pigtail catheter, inserted transfemorally, may facilitate angiographic imaging (Figure 27–1). The guidewire is passed in a retrograde fashion beyond the proximal lesions using fluoroscopic guidance. If the lesion lies at the origin of the common carotid or innominate artery, the stent should be placed 2 or 3 mm into the aortic arch to prevent ostial stenosis using a balloon expandable stent (Figures 27–2A to 27–2C). Prior to inserting the stent, the distal CCA is clamped to prevent intracranial embolization. Once the balloon is removed from the sheath, 20–40 cc of blood is aspirated from the sheath and the CCA clamp is removed to reinstitute antegrade cerebral flow. If necessary, a standard carotid endarterectomy can then be performed.[47] Percutaneous access of the common carotid artery for retrograde stenting

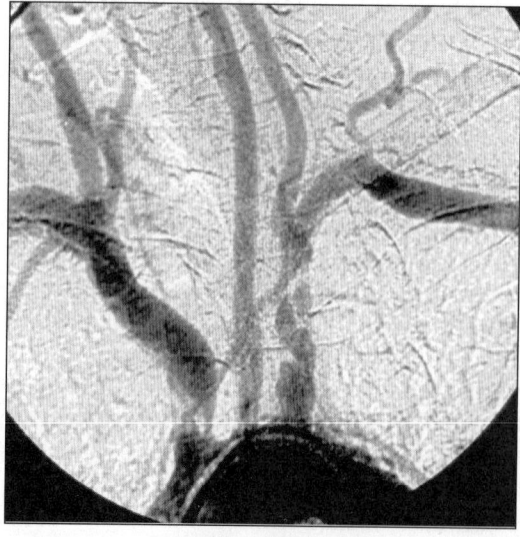

Figure 27-1. Conventional diagnostic arch aortogram via a transfemoral pigtail catheter. This repesents a steep left anterior oblique projection, facilitating a clear view of the right innominate and left subclavian ulcerated stenotic lesions.

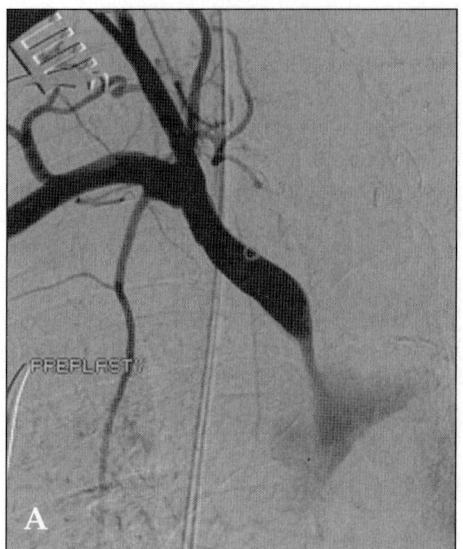

Figure 27-2. Angiogram of a right innominate stenosis approach from right common carotid artery cutdown. **(A)** Imaging shows a severe innominate stenosis, **(B)** after balloon expandable stent placement, and **(C)** completion imaging showing minimal residual stenosis.

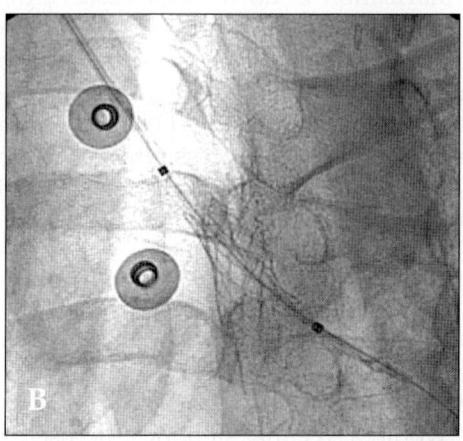

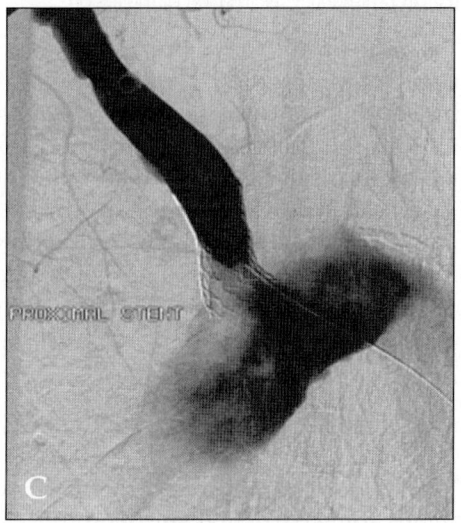

has also been described.[43] However, we prefer the open technique due to the increased incidence of cervical hematoma and potential risk of thrombus formation during post-pull compression with a percutaneous approach.

Grego et. al. reported technical success in 14 of 16 patients undergoing synchronous CEA and retrograde endovascular treatment of aortic arch vessels. In two patients, the innominate lesion could not be traversed with the guidewire.[47] Ruebben et. al. reported a technical success rate of 100% in eight patients treated for isolated stenosis of the innominate artery via a transcervical approach.[49] Levien et. al. published a series in which 43 of 44 patients were successfully treated with balloon angioplasty of brachiocephalic or common carotid artery stenoses at the time of CEA.[50] At our institution, 14 patients have been successfully treated using a retrograde cutdown on the common carotid artery.[51]

Intermediate patency rates of stented aortic arch vessels has been comparable with more traditional surgical interventions. In a review of seven papers with a total of 108

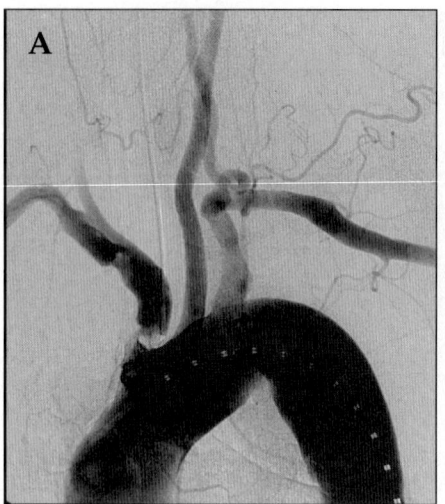
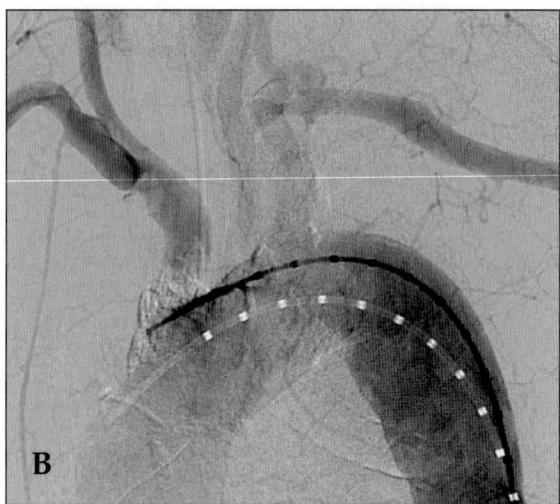

Figure 27-3. Angiogram showing extensive calcified plaque and an associated stenosis of the right innominate artery. **(A)** Arch aortogram showing the lesion and delayed contrast enhancement beyond the stenosis, and **(B)** circumferential calcification of the lesion.

patients undergoing percutaneous revascularization of aortic arch vessels, the combined technical success rate was 97+/-4%. Restenosis occurred in 3+/-5% of patients at a mean duration of follow-up of 20+/-9 months. Although these results are comparable to surgical therapy, the complication rate in the endovascular group was 6+/-5%, significantly lower than the combined complication rate of 16+/-11% in the published surgical series.[25] In a review of the literature, the technical success rate stent placement across supra-aortic trunk lesions ranged from 89–100%. The initial success was higher with stenotic lesions when compared to complete occlusions.

COMPLICATIONS OF ENDOVASCULAR THERAPY

While endoluminal supra-aortic trunk stenting is gaining broader approval, there remains some particular shortcomings. Most would agree that stenotic atherosclerotic lesions can be effectively managed with stent placement; however, total occlusions or heavily calcified lesions should be approached with caution or avoided altogether. This primarily is due to the increased risk of distal embolization, restenosis, stent fracture, or aortic dissection (Figures 27–3A and 27–3B). Other unique complications of endoluminal interventions in this territory are access site complications. and embolization to the anterior or posterior intracranial circulation as well as the visceral vessels and legs.

CONCLUSION

Endoluminal therapy of supra-aortic trunk lesions is a feasible alternative to operative repair with the exception of completely occluded vessels. Agreed upon guidelines for treatment include symptomatic $\geq$ 50% or $\geq$ 80% asymptomatic atherosclerotic lesions, avoidance of heavily calcified plaques, and Takayasu's arteritis. Accepted approaches to the supra-aortic trunk vessels include transfemoral, transbrachial/transaxillary, and transcarotid, with the latter providing the shortest, most direct route to the target vessel, as well as the opportunity to employ embolic protection or do a concomitant carotid endarterectomy.

REFERENCES

1. Savory W. A case of a young woman in whom the main arteries of the both upper extremities, and of the left side of the neck, were throughout completely obliterated. *Med Chir Trans*. 1856;39:205.
2. Shimizu K, Sano K. Pulseless disease. *J Neuropathol Clin Neurol*. 1951;1:37–46.
3. Davis JB, Grove WJ, et. al. Thrombic occlusion of branches of aortic arch. Martonell's syndrome: report-of case treated surgically. *Ann Surg*. 1956;144:124–126.
4. Crawford ES, et. al. Surgical treatment of occlusion of the innominate, common carotid, and subclavian arteries: a 10 year experience. *Surgery*. 1969;65(1):17–31.
5. Berguer R, Morasch MD, Kline RA. Transthoracic repair of innominate and common carotid artery disease: immediate and long-term outcome for 100 consecutive surgical reconstructions. *J Vasc Surg*. 1998;27(1):34–41; discussion 42.
6. Lyons C, Galbraith G. Surgical treatment of atherosclerotic occlusion of the internal carotid artery. *Ann Surg*. 1957;146(3):487–96; discussion 496–8.
7. DeBakey MG, Morris, Jordan G. Segmental thrombo-obliterative disease of the great vessels arising from the aortic arch. *JAMA*. 1958;166:998–1003.
8. Diethrich EB. Occlusive disease of the common carotid and subclavian arteries treated by carotid-subclavian bypass. Analysis of 125 cases. *Am J Surg*. 1967;114(5):800–8.
9. Berguer R, et. al. Cervical reconstruction of the supra-aortic trunks: a 16-year experience. *J Vasc Surg*. 1999;29(2):239–46; discussion 246–8.
10. Perler BA, Williams GM. Carotid-subclavian bypass—a decade of experience. *J Vasc Surg*. 1990;12(6):716–22; discussion 722–3.
11. Mathias K, et. al. Percutaneous transluminal treatment of supraaortic artery obstruction. *Ann Radiol* (Paris). 1980;23(4):281–2.
12. Bachman DM, Kim RM. Transluminal dilatation for subclavian steal syndrome. *AJR Am J Roentgenol*. 1980;135(5):995–6.
13. Becker GJ, Katzen BT, Dake MD. Noncoronary angioplasty. *Radiology*. 1989;170(3 Pt 2): 921–40.
14. Kachel R, et. al. Percutaneous transluminal angioplasty (PTA) of supra-aortic arteries especially the internal carotid artery. *Neuroradiology*. 1991;33(3):191–4.
15. Sullivan TM, et. al. Angioplasty and primary stenting of the subclavian, innominate, and common carotid arteries in 83 patients. *J Vasc Surg*. 1998;28(6):1059–65.
16. Queral LA, Criado FJ. Endovascular treatment of aortic arch occlusive disease. Semin Vasc Surg. 1996;9(2):156–63.
17. Rodriguez-Lopez JA, et. al. Stenting for atherosclerotic occlusive disease of the subclavian artery. *Ann Vasc Surg*. 1996;13(3):254–60.
18. Takach TJ, et. al. Brachiocephalic reconstruction II: operative and endovascular management of single-vessel disease. *J Vasc Surg*. 2005;42(1):55–61.
19. Wylie EJ, Effeney DJ. Surgery of the aortic arch branches and vertebral arteries. *Surg Clin North Am*. 1979;59(4):669–80.
20. Hass WK, et. al., Joint study of extracranial arterial occlusion. II. Arteriography, techniques, sites, and complications. *JAMA*. 1968;203(11):961–8.
21. Williams SJ, 2nd. Chronic upper extremity ischemia: current concepts in management. *Surg Clin North Am*. 1986;66(2):355–75.

22. Brountzos EN, et. al. Primary stenting of subclavian and innominate artery occlusive disease: a single center's experience. *Cardiovasc Intervent Radiol.* 2004;27(6):616–23.
23. Diethrich EB, et. al. Percutaneous techniques for endoluminal carotid interventions. *J Endovasc Surg.* 1996;3(2):182–202.
24. Brountzos EN, Malagari K, Kelekis DA. Endovascular treatment of occlusive lesions of the subclavian and innominate arteries. *Cardiovasc Intervent Radiol.* 2006;29(4):503–10.
25. Hadjipetrou P, et. al. Percutaneous revascularization of atherosclerotic obstruction of aortic arch vessels. *J Am Coll Cardiol.* 1999;33(5):1238–45.
26. Liang P, Hoffman GS. Advances in the medical and surgical treatment of Takayasu arteritis. *Curr Opin Rheumatol.* 2005;17(1):16–24.
27. Sakaida H, et. al. (Stenting for the occlusive carotid and subclavian arteries in Takayasu arteritis). *No Shinkei Geka.* 2001;29(11):1033–41.
28. Budin JA, Casarella WJ, Harisiadis L. Subclavian artery occlusion following radiotherapy for carcinoma of the breast. *Radiology.* 1976;118(1):169–73.
29. Hashmonai M, et. al. Subclavian artery occlusion after radiotherapy for carcinoma of the breast. *Cancer.* 1988;61(10):2015–8.
30. Hassen-Khodja R, Kieffer E. Radiotherapy-induced supra-aortic trunk disease: early and long-term results of surgical and endovascular reconstruction. *J Vasc Surg.* 2004;40(2): 254–61.
31. Kay HR, et. al. Atherosclerosis of the internal mammary artery. *Ann Thorac Surg.* 1976;21(6): 504–7.
32. Singh RN. Atherosclerosis and the internal mammary arteries. *Cardiovasc Intervent Radiol.* 1983;6(2):72–7.
33. Olsen CO, et. al. Review of coronary-subclavian steal following internal mammary artery-coronary artery bypass surgery. *Ann Thorac Surg.* 1988;46(6):675–8.
34. North American Symptomatic Carotid Endarterectomy Trial Collaborators. Beneficial effect of carotid endarterectomy in symptomatic patients with high-grade carotid stenosis. *N Engl J Med.* 1991;325(7):445–53.
35. Executive Committee for the Asymptomatic Carotid Atherosclerosis Study. Endarterectomy for asymptomatic carotid artery stenosis. *JAMA.* 1995;273(18):1421–8.
36. Loewe C, et. al. MRA versus DSA in the assessment of occlusive disease in the aortic arch vessels: accuracy in detecting the severity, number, and length of stenoses. *J Endovasc Ther.* 2004;11(2):152–60.
37. Randoux B, et. al. Proximal great vessels of aortic arch: comparison of three-dimensional gadolinium–enhanced MR angiography and digital subtraction angiography. *Radiology.* 2003;229(3):697–702.
38. Carpenter JP, et. al. Magnetic resonance angiography of the aortic arch. *J Vasc Surg.* 1997;25(1):145–51.
39. Kent KC, et. al. Perioperative imaging strategies for carotid endarterectomy. An analysis of morbidity and cost-effectiveness in symptomatic patients. *JAMA.* 1995;274(11):888–93.
40. Grant EG, et al, Innominate artery occlusive disease: sonographic findings. *AJR Am J Roentgenol.* 2006;186(2):394–400.
41. Kalaria VG, et. al. Duplex ultrasonography of vertebral and subclavian arteries. *J Am Soc Echocardiogr.* 2005;18(10):1107–11.
42. Ackerstaff RG, et. al., Ultrasonic duplex scanning in atherosclerotic disease of the innominate, subclavian and vertebral arteries. A comparative study with angiography. *Ultrasound Med Biol.* 1984;10(4):409–18.
43. Criado FJ, Abul-Khoudoud O. Interventional techniques to facilitate supraaortic angioplasty and stenting. *Vasc Endovasc Surg.* 2006;40(2):141–7.
44. Queral LA, Criado FJ. The treatment of focal aortic arch branch lesions with Palmaz stents. *J Vasc Surg.* 1996. 23(2):368–75.
45. Payne DA, et. al. Cerebral protection during open retrograde angioplasty/stenting of common carotid and innominate artery stenoses. *Br J Surg.* 2006;93(2):187–90.

46. Macierewicz J, et. al. Carotid endarterectomy combined with proximal stenting for multi-level disease. *Eur J Vasc Endovasc Surg.* 2000;20(6):572–5.

47. Grego F, et. al. Synchronous carotid endarterectomy and retrograde endovascular treatment of brachiocephalic or common carotid artery stenosis. *Eur J Vasc Endovasc Surg.* 2003;26(4): 392–5.

48. Yoo BS, et. al. A case of transradial carotid stenting in a patient with total occlusion of distal abdominal aorta. *Cathet Cardiovasc Interv.* 2002;56(2):243–5.

49. Ruebben A, et. al. Feasibility of intraoperative balloon angioplasty and additional stent placement of isolated stenosis of the brachiocephalic trunk. *J Thorac Cardiovasc Surg.* 1998; 115(6):1316–20.

50. Levien LJ, et. al. Retrograde balloon angioplasty of brachiocephalic or common carotid artery stenoses at the time of carotid endarterectomy. *Eur J Vasc Endovasc Surg.* 1998;15(6): 521–7.

51. Peterson BG, et. al. Aortic arch vessel stenting: a single-center experience using cerebral protection. *Arch Surg.* 2006;141(6):560–3; discussion 563–4.

28

Cervical Carotid Bypass

V. Kalakuntla, M.D.
and R. Berguer, M.D., Ph.D.

We reported our series of carotid bypass reconstructions at this symposium in 1998.[1] This presentation covers additional experience with these operations from 1998 to 2002. We discuss here two types of carotid bypass operations: (a) those that are done to replace the common carotid (CCA) segment and (b) those that replace the cervical internal carotid artery (ICA). Common carotid bypasses originating in the aortic arch have restricted indications, pose different technical challenges, and are excluded from this review.

There were 63 carotid bypass operations done on 58 patients over the four-year period covered by this survey. The demographics of this group of patients are shown in Table 28–1. There were 11 CCA and 52 ICA bypass operations (Table 28–2). The material used for the bypass was PTFE in 88% (56/63) of cases. Dacron was used in five patients, autogenous vein in two patients.

Indication for a carotid bypass were severe disease of the CCA, ICA, or both in 56 cases. In 10 of these 56, cases the medical history and the anatomic distribution of the lesions permitted the characterization of the problem as radiation arteritis. A remote carotid operation had been performed on the same side in 34/63 (54%) of patients (Table 28–3). There were 7/63 patients that underwent an ICA bypass at the conclusion of a technically unsatisfactory endarterectomy after noticing a defective wall or following the demonstration of a technical problem in the intraoperative arteriogram. All patients were followed by Duplex at 1, 6, and 12 months, and yearly thereafter. Follow-up data was available in all patients.

TABLE 28-1.

Age	64.3 ± 8.8 SD
Male/Female	34/24
Hypertension	91%
Tobacco (aver. 52 pack/year)	85%
Coronary Disease	47%
Diabetes	29%

TABLE 28-2. SITE AND SIDE OF CAROTID BYPASSES

ICA bypass	52
CCA bypass	11
Bilateral bypasses	3
Contralateral origin	2

TABLE 28-3. PREVIOUS CAROTID OPERATION

Remote, on the same side*	34/63	(54%)
Same setting (poor technical result)	7/63	(11%)

*Five patients had two, and one patient had three, previous carotid endarterectomies at the same site.

COMMON CAROTID ARTERY BYPASS

The indications for this type of reconstruction are severe disease or occlusion of the CCA. The bypasses originated in the ipsilateral (8/11) or contralateral (3/11) common carotid or subclavian (SA) arteries, and their distal anastomosis was made at the carotid bifurcation. The latter required an eversion endarterectomy in preparation for the distal anastomosis in 6/11 patients. Two bypasses originating on the opposite side of the neck crossed the midline using the retropharyngeal pathway.[2]

On the right side, the proximal anastomosis may be done to the SA or to the rim of origin of the CCA from the innominate artery. The latter case is only possible when the distal segment of the latter can be exposed through a cervical incision, generally requiring the excision of the medial clavicular head.

For the last 10 years, we have preferred to access the SA on either side using a more lateral approach than the traditional retroscalene route.[3-6] The artery is identified between the scalenus anticus and the medial trunk of the brachial plexus. Bipolar cautery is used to control the thin veins that course outside the brachial plexus trunks. Only the lateral half of the scalenus anticus needs to be divided to obtain an adequate length of SA. The phrenic nerve is left intact—and identified—as it courses medially. The thyrocervical trunk, proximal to the exposed segment of SA, does not need to be dissected. Control of the SA is obtained with a "J" clamp that obviates the more extensive circumferential dissection needed when separate proximal and distal clamps are used.

The arteriostomy in the SA is made with an aortic punch in its superior wall. Any plaque in the SA at this level is left undisturbed. If the atheromatous intima/media tends to separate from the external elastic membrane, no endarterectomy is attempted and the plaque is affixed to the wall, including it in the anastomotic suture line.

The bypass is constructed with PTFE (6–7 mm). The proximal anastomosis of the graft is suspended ("parachuted") for the first half of its circumference to allow precise placement of the sutures without slack in the thin SA. Once the anastomosis is completed, flow is restablished to the distal SA. The graft is then tunneled to the carotid bifurcation following a path that passes behind the internal jugular vein so that the distal end of the graft meets the carotid bifurcation ascending parallel to the native CCA.[3]

Once flow to the distal SA has been restablished, in the rare case where a shunt is deemed necessary (one case in this series), the proximal end of the shunt is inserted in the proximal part of the graft at this time for brain protection during the distal anastomosis.

The CCA is divided 2 cm. below the flow divider and split along its posterior wall. In cases where there is moderate to severe disease of the carotid bifurcation, we proceed with a type 2 eversion endarterectomy and trim any excess "wings" from the wall. The distal 4–5 cm of CCA are resected to provide room for the prosthetic graft. The distal suture line is an end-to-end anastomosis.[2, 3]

INTERNAL CAROTID BYPASS

The indication for ICA replacement was an unsatisfactory result at the completion of a carotid endarterectomy in 7/52 patients (13%), recurrent disease following a previous endarterectomy or bypass reconstruction in 34/52 (65%), radiation arteritis in 10/52 (19%) and ICA aneurysm in one patient.

We have a series of carotid bypass operations following CCA-ICA resection in conjunction with removal of squamous cell tumor of the neck. These patients underwent replacement of the common and internal carotid arteries with autogenous superficial femoral artery. This specific indication and technique for carotid resection and bypass replacement in head and neck cancer has been the subject of a separate report and these patients have not been included in this review.[7]

The basic principle in ICA bypass is to place the distal anastomosis into previously undissected/nondiseased ICA. This avoids dissection and potential injury to the cranial nerves, a main drawback to reoperations on the ICA.

The bypass is constructed with 6 mm thin-wall PTFE. Rarely a 5 mm thin-wall PTFE will provide a better match. In a previous review of our 15-year experience with bypass replacement of the ICA for restenosing disease following carotid endarterectomy, PTFE fared better than autogenous vein when the bypass was done for intimal hyperplasia.

For these reoperations, the approach is generally different from the one used for conventional carotid endarterectomy. For lesions below the level of C1, we used the retrojugular exposure (30/52 or 58% of ICA bypasses) of the mid-cervical ICA.[8] This approach avoids dissecting the hypoglossal nerve that is left anterior to the plane of dissection. The mid-cervical ICA is isolated behind the digastric muscle, distal to the segment dissected in the course of the previous operation. The upper limit of this approach is roughly the takeoff of the superior laryngeal nerve. The latter, after arising from the vagus nerve, hugs over the ICA before descending behind the internal carotid bulb. The superior laryngeal nerve does not preclude exposing further ICA distal to it. If there is a need for this, the ICA can be divided and transposed anterior to the superior laryngeal nerve, obtaining an additional centimeter of proximal exposure.

For lesions higher than C1, an infratemporal approach is preferred (10/52 patients or 20%).[9] This approach is greatly facilitated by nasotracheal intubation and ipsilateral subluxation of the mandible.[3, 9]

Distal control of the ICA in the infratemporal fossa can pose problems because there is inadequate room for the use of standard carotid clamps and, on the other hand, detachable occluding clips (such as the Heifetz or Yasargil clips used for intracranial aneurysms) are unstable in a crowded and moving field and can be difficult to reposition if they become dislodged. At the level of the infratemporal fossa, we prefer to use short occluding balloon catheters for distal ICA control. Care must be exercised not to advance them beyond the petrous ICA or to overdistend them. The latter may result in rupture of the carotid wall, which is thin at this level, and development of a false aneurysm. On the other hand, if the occluding balloon is placed close to the anastomotic suture line, it may be punctured during the anastomosis. Once the carotid backflow is controlled with the balloon catheter, we place two sutures on opposite sides of the wall in order to retain access and control of the distal cervical ICA should the balloon occlusion be lost by puncture or back migration. Once in the correct place, the balloon catheter is sutured to the field drapes to avoid accidental pulling. The deflated balloon is withdrawn when backbleeding the anastomosis, before pulling the suture snug and tying it.

RESULTS

There were two strokes (3%) following 63 carotid bypass operations (Table 28–4). One patient recovered fully after two days following emergency thrombectomy of a failed bypass graft. There were no deaths. No peripheral nerve injuries were observed.

A restenosis was found by Duplex or postoperative arteriography in 4/63 bypasses within one year (6%). In three of these four patients, the restenosis developed within the bypass graft. One patient developed a recurrent lesion in the intrapetrosal ICA. These restenoses were treated with angioplasty and stenting. A second restenosis in a patient with cardiolipin antibody was managed by replacing the ICA bypass (it has remained free of disease after 28 months). One patient developed a false aneurysm at the distal end of the infrapetrosal ICA that was successfully treated with a stent.

Periodic duplex exam showed patency of the remaining grafts for a mean follow up of 2.8±0.6 SD years. Clinical exams showed patients to be free of neurologic symptoms after a mean length of follow-up of 4.4 ±1.7 SD years.

TABLE 28-4. INMEDIATE OUTCOME

Peripheral Nerve injury		0/63
Stroke*	2/63	(3%)
Death		0/63

*One stroke recovered fully and without evidence of CT infarction after two days, following thombectomy of a failed bypass.

COMMENTARY

In a previous review of our experience with ICA bypass, we recorded a higher restenosis rate in venous bypasses than in bypasses constructed with a PTFE prosthesis. The better outcome for bypasses constructed with PTFE as opposed to those with saphenous vein has also been documented by Lauder, Roddy and Archie.[10-12] Other authors agree with us that a PTFE bypass is preferable to a saphenous vein bypass when performed for reoperations to correct restenosis in patients who have had previous carotid endarterectomy.[11, 13, 14]

As in our earlier review of this matter, the morbidity for ICA bypass is found to be higher than that observed following bifurcation primary carotid endarterectomy.[1] It is worth noting that the patients considered here were failures following carotid endarterectomy or had disease that could not be corrected with the latter. In the light of recent published series, some of these patients—particularly those with high ICA lesions—would be considered today for angioplasty and stent procedures. Our preference for PFTE in the reconstruction of arteries with high flow rates is supported by the high patency rates noted.

We have observed that the most common site for restenosis (in 4/52 ICA bypasses done for recurrent disease) of these grafts is the bend in the proximal inch of the graft as it takes off from the lateral wall of the CCA to follow a vertical course in the neck. All recurrent lesions in the ICA bypasses appeared within 12 months of the operation. It is likely that in these cases, some degree of kinking may have taken place at this site because increased local velocities were already sampled at this site in the postoperative Duplex study. The additional placing of a stent at this site following angioplasty did resolve the progression of recurrent stenosis at this level in three of the four cases.

In one patient (with cardiolipin antibody), the restenosed PTFE bypass graft was replaced with a ring-reinforced PTFE to avoid kinking and the replacement bypass was inserted with enough slack to create a curve of larger radius in its proximal part. This replacement graft has remained fully patent after 28 months.

CONCLUSION

Carotid bypass is preferably performed with PTFE unless there is concern about wound healing or contamination. The morbidity of carotid bypasses—usually reoperations—is higher than that observed in primary carotid endarterectomy but still within acceptable range.

REFERENCES

1. Morasch M, Berguer R. Cervical Carotid Bypass. In: Yao JST, Pearce WH, editors. *Techniques in Vascular and Endovascular Surgery*. Appleton and Lange: Norwalk, CT;1998.
2. Berguer R, Gonzalez JA. Revascularization by the retropharyngeal route for extensive disease of the extracranial arteries. *J Vasc Surg*. 1994;19:217–222.
3. Berguer R, Kieffer E. *Surgery of the Arteries to the Head*. Springer Verlag: New York; 1992.
4. Sullivan TM. Subclavian-carotid bypass to an "isolated" bifurcation: a retrospective analysis. *Ann Vasc Surg*. 1996;10:283–289.
5. Fry WR, Martin JD, Clagett GP, Fry WJ. Extrathoracic carotid reconstruction: the subclavian carotid artery bypass.
6. Chaikoff EL, Smith RB. Surgical management of occlusive disease of the common carotid artery. *Semin Vasc Surg*. 1996;9:111–117.
7. Sessa C, Morasch M, Berguer R, et al. Carotid resection and replacement with autogenous arterial graft during operations for neck malignancy. *Ann Vasc Surg*. 1998;12:229–235.
8. Berguer R. Retrojugular approach for exclusion bypass of the carotid bifurcation: a useful method for recurrent or high disease. In: Veith FJ ed., *Current Critical Problems in Vascular Surgery*., St. Louis: Quality Medical Publishing; 1992.
9. Berguer R. High internal carotid artery exposure. In: *Vascular Surgical Approaches*. Brancherau A, Berguer R, eds. New York: Futura Publishing; 1999.
10. Lauder C, Kelly A, Thompson M et al. Early and late outcome after carotid bypass grafting with saphenous vein. *J Vasc Surg*. 2003;39:1025–1030.
11. Roddy SP, Darling RC, Ozsvath KJ et al. Choice of material for internal carotid artery bypass grafting: vein or prosthetic? Analysis of 44 procedures. *Cardiovasc Surg*. 2002;10: 540–544.
12. Archie JP. Reoperations for carotid artery stenosis: Role of primary and secondary reconstruction. *J Vasc Surg*. 2001;33:495–503.

13. Cormier JM, Cormier F, Laurian C, et al. Polytetrafluoroethylene bypass for revascularization of the atherosclerotic internal carotid artery: late results. *Ann Vasc Surg*. 1987;1:564–571.
14. Camiade C, Maher A, Ricco JB et al. Carotid bypass with polytetrafluoroethylene grafts: a study of 110 consecutive patients. *J Vasc Surg*. 2003:38:1031–1037.

29

Subclavian Artery Reconstruction

Mark D. Morasch, M.D.

Atherosclerotic occlusive disease involving the branches of the aortic arch is common in patients over the age of 65. The Joint Study of Arterial Occlusions reported that one-third of patients undergoing arteriography are found to have significant lesions involving one or more of the vessels supplying blood to the head and arms.[1] Occlusive diseases effecting the supraaortic trunks make up a relatively small fraction of these, however. There are, nonetheless, a number of well-recognized and well-documented ischemic manifestations of occlusive disease effecting the proximal trunk vessels in the cerebral hemispheric, ocular, vertebrobasilar, upper extremity, and cardiac territories.

Despite the fact that the subclavian vessels are relatively difficult to image using noninvasive technology, substantive data has accumulated regarding the natural history of disease over time, and significant experience with surgical reconstruction has accrued over the past four decades. In addition, after two decades of experience with endoluminal therapy for treatment of subclavian artery disease, some useful data have now become available.

HISTORY

Savory was the first to describe a patient with signs and symptoms suggesting occlusive disease involving the supraaortic trunk vessels.[2] Twenty years later, in 1875, Broadbent chronicled a patient who, while living, had no radial pulses and at post-mortem examination, was found to have both brachiocephalic and left subclavian artery occlusions.[3] In 1956, Lyons first reported a series of four subclavian to carotid artery bypasses from a cervical approach[4] and, in 1964, Parrott reported two subclavian to carotid transpositions through a similar exposure.[5] The first reports of subclavian artery angioplasty were published in 1980 by Bachman[6] and by Mathias.[7]

Pathophysiology

Atherosclerosis is, by far, the most common disease affecting the subclavian vessels. Occlusive lesions less commonly result from inflammatory diseases such as Takayasu's arteritis or they can be the result of exposure to therapeutic radiation. The subclavian artery also can dissect or become aneurysmal. Occlusive lesions involving the subclavian vessels develop in a younger age group than atherosclerotic occlusive lesions elsewhere in the extracranial cerebrovascular circulation. Mean and median ages are commonly reported to range from 50 to 61 years. Cigarette smoking is certainly a significant risk factor for the development of atherosclerotic occlusive disease and it is identified as a risk factor in 82% of all patients who require subclavian intervention.[8]

In Berguer's series of 282 transthoracic and cervical revascularizations of the supraaortic trunk vessels, significant disease was present in more than a single vessel in 40% of cases. All three of the trunks were critically diseased in 13%. Revascularization of unifocal disease was necessary in 60% of cases. When disease was limited to one trunk, the left subclavian artery was the vessel most commonly found to be involved with disease.[8,9]

Cerebrovascular symptoms can be the result of emboli or low flow. In addition, patients can present with symptoms of isolated upper extremity ischemia from similar phenomena. When multiple trunk vessels are involved with an occlusive process, patients usually develop symptoms of vertebrobasilar ischemia, which result from diminished posterior circulation perfusion pressures. Single vessel subclavian artery disease is usually asymptomatic unless the lesion is an embolizing one. Alternatively, isolated proximal disease of the subclavian artery can lead to symptomatic subclavian-vertebral steal syndrome although this is quite rare in the absence of disease elsewhere in the cerebrovasculature. Proximal innominate occlusion can result in steal phenomena as well, although the reversed flow generally occurs in the ipsilateral carotid artery.

Patients with subclavian disease may develop varying degrees of arm ischemia ranging from the claudication observed in patients with subclavian steal to limb-threatening ischemia resulting from extensive arterial occlusion or emboli. Patients with subclavian steal syndrome, which results when blockage in the first portion of the subclavian artery causes pressure distally to drop below that at the vertebrobasilar junction, present with posterior cerebrovascular symptoms as blood is siphoned away from the basilar artery (Figure 29–1). Myocardial ischemia from the phenomenon of

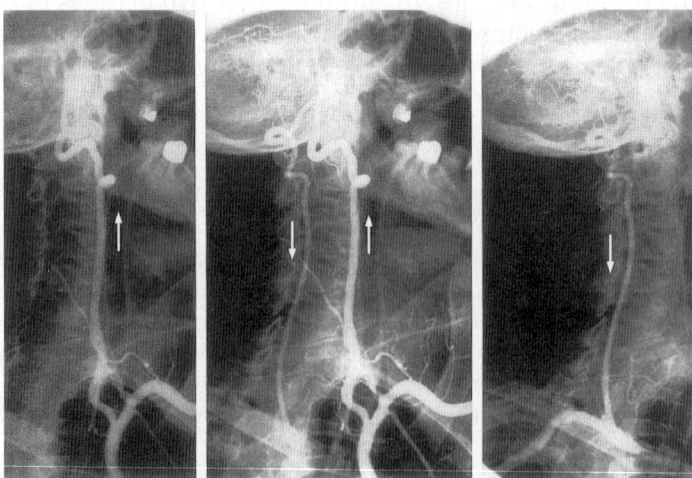

Figure 29-1. Proximal right subclavian artery occlusion accounts for radiographic evidence of subclavian vertebral steal. (From Berguer R, Kieffer E. *Surgery of the Arteries to the Head*. New York: Springer-Verlag New York, Inc., 1992. Reproduced by permission.)

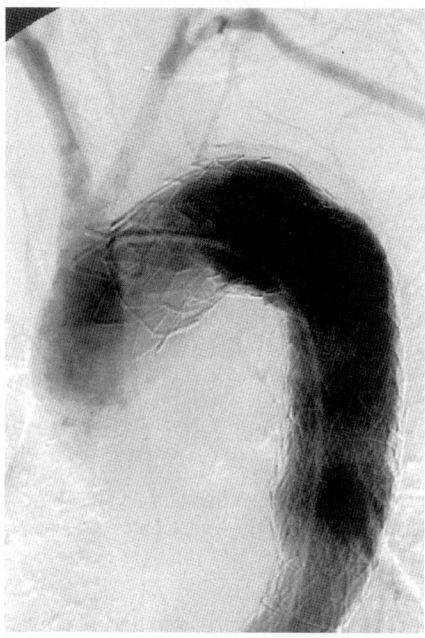

Figure 29-2. Subclavian artery transposed into site of left common carotid in a patient with bovine anatomy followed by thoracic aneurysm repair with an endograft.

coronary steal is another indication for subclavian repair. Coronary steal can develop in patients with innominate or subclavian disease proximal to an internal mammary revascularization of the coronary arteries.

Of particular note, in our institution over the last five years, the most common indication for surgical manipulation of the subclavian artery has been to prepare patients with thoracic and thoracoabdominal aortic aneurysms, dissections, or traumatic tears for an endovascular stent-graft repair. Subclavian artery (and sometimes left common carotid artery) transpositions are not infrequently performed in order to preserve vertebral and left upper extremity flow while extending the proximal neck "landing zone" prior to endograft deployment (Figure 29–2).

An aberrant right subclavian artery arising as the fourth of four supraaortic trunks and passing from left to right across midline and behind the esophagus occurs in approximately 0.5% of the population. Approximately 5% of aberrant retroesophageal subclavian arteries produce symptoms.[10] The most common symptoms are related to swallowing difficulties (dysphagia lusoria). The most frequent type of disease found in an aberrant RSA is atherosclerosis although traumatic, dysplastic, and infectious lesions have also been reported. Treatment generally consists of resection of the aberrant vessel and reconstruction of more normal anatomy by transposing the more distal vessel to a site of origin on the right common carotid artery.

SURGICAL TREATMENT

Cervical reconstruction, as opposed to a transthoracic approach, is the surgical technique of choice for single lesions involving the subclavian artery. Three broad-based approaches have been developed for the treatment of subclavian artery disease, each

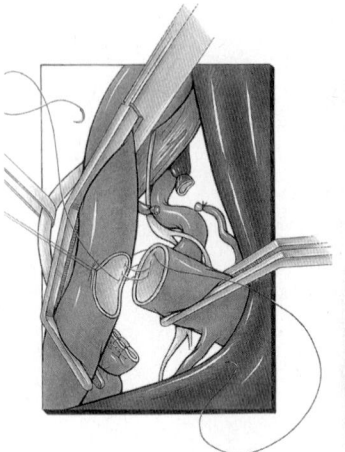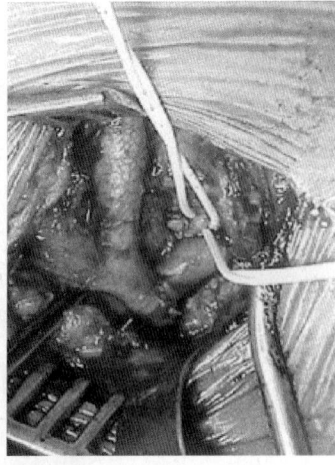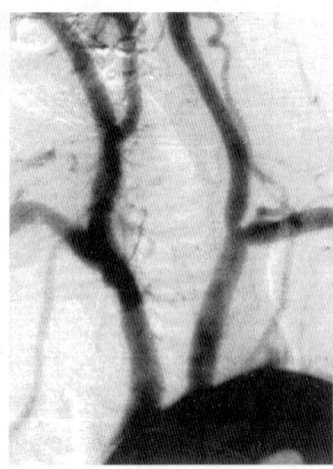

Figure 29-3. A, B, C. Subclavian to common carotid transposition. (Figure 29-3A—From Berguer R, Kieffer E. *Surgery of the Arteries to the Head*. New York: Springer-Verlag New York, Inc., 1992. Reproduced by permission.)

with distinct advantages and disadvantages: arterial transposition, cervical bypass, and endovascular recanalization. Transthoracic repair or multiple remote cervical bypasses can be considered for patients with multiple trunk involvement if there are contraindications to an endovascular approach. When there is a usable ipsilateral "source vessel," an arterial transposition should be the first choice (Figure 29–3).

Transposition

The subclavian artery may be transposed to the adjacent carotid. Not only is preservation of the vertebral artery critical, but it is equally important to mobilize and preserve the valuable internal mammary artery when performing a subclavian transposition. In the reverse, a common carotid to subclavian artery transposition, an adequate length of proximally narrowed common carotid artery can easily be mobilized for reimplantation into the adjacent subclavian artery.

Subclavian transposition is completed through a short, transverse cervical incision made a fingerbreadth above the clavicle. In order to carry out a transposition, the surgical dissection takes place between the two heads of the sternocleidomastoid muscle. After dividing the omohyoid muscle, the jugular vein and the vagus nerve are reflected laterally and the common carotid is mobilized circumferentially and reflected medially. The common carotid should be freed well proximally behind the clavicle and sternum. On the left side, the thoracic duct is identified, ligated, and divided. On the right, multiple cervical lymphatic channels must also be tied. Locating the vertebral vein helps keep the dissection on track. After dividing the vertebral vein, the subclavian artery should be identifiable. Its proximal branches are all carefully dissected and each controlled with a fine vessel loop. Care must be taken when isolating and controlling the vertebral artery as it takes origin from an awkward position on the posterior aspect of the subclavian. In addition, it is important to attempt to leave the sympathetic nerve chain undisturbed so as not to produce an ipsilateral Horner's syndrome. Once heparin has been administered, the distal subclavian artery and its proximal branches are clamped atraumatically and the proximal vessel is controlled with a long right-angled forceps. The vessel is transected as proximal as possible while leaving a short stump to oversew. When the proximal subclavian is patent, it is important to secure the stump immediately after the diseased artery has been divided; if control of a patent transected stump is lost in the chest or mediastinum, the consequences clearly can be devastating. A 5-0 monofilament suture, run back and forth, works best. A tie can also be placed on the proximal subclavian beneath the clamp for extra security. A punch arteriotomy is created on the posterior aspect of the clamped common carotid and the end-to-side anastomosis completed, subclavian to carotid, without tension, using parachute suture techniques. We leave a drain, placed deep to the platysmal closure, overnight.

Bypass

Occasionally, it is not feasible to do a straightforward arterial transposition, so the use of a bypass conduit becomes necessary (Figure 29–4). Arterial transposition is not possible when the vertebral artery takes off early from the subclavian artery. Another indication for carotid-subclavian bypass is proximal subclavian disease in a patient with symptomatic coronary steal from a patent internal mammary artery graft. With the use of a cervical bypass, the arterial clamps can be placed beyond the internal mammary artery to avoid myocardial ischemia. Bypasses are performed, most expediently, through dissection just lateral to the clavicular head of the sternocleidomastoid muscle. The jugular vein is reflected medially in this case, and the common carotid is mobilized laterally with respect to the vein. While protecting the phrenic nerve, the subclavian artery is identified more distally than during transposition by completely dividing the anterior scalene muscle. The bypass is completed to the retroscalene portion of the subclavian artery, usually using prosthetic conduit rather than vein. Prosthetic conduits clearly out-perform autogenous vein with regard to long-term patency.[11-12]

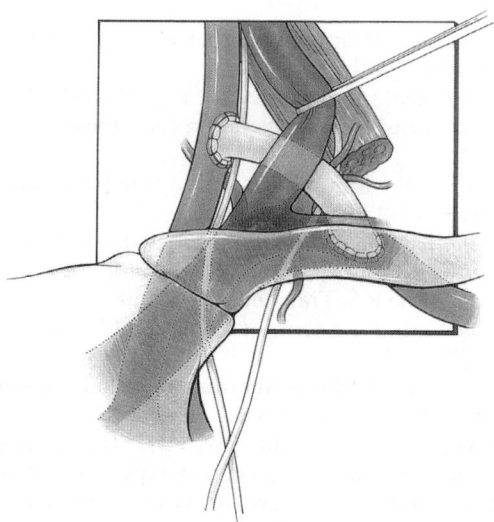

Figure 29-4. Prosthetic carotid-subclavian bypass. (From Berguer R, Kieffer E. *Surgery of the Arteries to the Head*. New York: Springer-Verlag New York, Inc., 1992. Reproduced by permission.)

Endovascular Repair

Balloon angioplasty and stenting of isolated subclavian artery disease is becoming more commonplace. Patients with atherosclerotic occlusive disease as well as patients with inflammatory arteriopathies have been treated with endovascular therapy. Endoluminal therapies can be undertaken in antegrade fashion from the femoral artery or percutaneously and in a retrograde fashion from the brachial artery. In most cases, metallic stents are necessary since most lesions involve the vessel origin and include "spill-over" atherosclerosis from the arch of the aorta much like renal artery atherosclerotic occlusive disease.

CONCLUSION

The indications for subclavian reconstruction are broad but the need for revascularization of this particular vessel is relatively rare. As endovascular recanalization becomes safer, the need for bypass or transposition reconstruction of the subclavian will probably become even less common. On the other hand, as endograft repair of proximal thoracic aneurysms becomes widespread, in order to maintain flow through the subclavian and its important proximal branches, transposition procedures are likely to resurge.

REFERENCES

1. Blaisdell WF, Clauss RH, Galbraith JG, et al. Joint study of extracranial arterial occlusion: IV. A review of surgical considerations. *JAMA*. 1969;209:1889–1895.
2. Savory WS. Case of a young woman in whom the main arteries of both upper extremities, and of the left side of the neck, were through-out completely obliterated. *Med Chir Trans*. 1856;39:205.
3. Broadbent WH. Absence of pulsation in both radial arteries, the vessels being full of blood. *Read*. 1875;165.
4. Lyons C, Galbraith G. Surgical treatment of atherosclerotic occlusion of the internal carotid artery. *Ann Surg*. 1956;146:487–494.
5. Parrott JC. The subclavian steal syndrome. *Arch Surg*. 1964;88:661–665.
6. Bachman DM, Kim RM. Transluminal dilatation for subclavian syndrome. *AJR*. 1980;135: 995–996.
7. Mathias K, Schlosser V, Reimke M. Catheterization of subclavian occlusions. *ROFO Fortschr Geb Rontgenstr Nuklearmed*. 1980;132:346–347 (Ger).
8. Berguer R, Morasch MD, Kline RA, Kazmers A, Friedland MS. Cervical reconstruction of the supra-aortic trunks: A 16-year experience. *J Vasc Surg*. 1999;29:239–248.
9. Berguer R, Morasch MD, Kline RA. Transthoracic repair of innominate and common carotid artery disease: Immediate and long-term outcome for 100 consecutive surgical reconstructions. *J Vasc Surg*. 1998;27:34–42.
10. Beabout JW, Steward JR, Kincaid OW. Aberrant right subclavian artery: Dispute of commonly accepted concepts. *AJR Am J Roentgenol*. 1964;92:855–864.
11. Ziomek S, Quinones-Baldrich WJ, Busuttil RW, et al. The superiority of synthetic arterial grafts over autologous veins in carotid-subclavian bypass. *J Vasc Surg*. 1986;3:140–145.
12. Morasch MD, Berguer R. Supra-aortic trunk revascularization. In Yao JST, Pearce WH, eds. *Modern Vascular Surgery*. New York: McGraw-Hill, 2000, pp. 137–146.

Other Carotid Pathology

30

Endovascular Treatment of Carotid Dissection

Saad Ali, M.D., Daniel Surdell, M.D., and Ali Shaibani, M.D.

A tear in the wall of the carotid artery leading to the entry of blood within the layers of the arterial wall is a phenomenon well described in literature, yet not completely understood. Carotid dissection has an estimated incidence of two and a half to three per 100,000[1] and accounts for 10% to 25% of ischemic strokes in the young and middle-aged.[2] Recent studies have attempted to better elucidate the genetic and environmental factors involved in this condition. With technical advancements, new approaches for diagnosis and treatment of this condition have also emerged. In this chapter, we will focus on the recent trend toward endovascular management of extracranial carotid dissection, including the indications, the technique, and outcome of this form of therapy.

The mainstay of carotid dissection treatment has been pharmacological in the form of antiplatelet medications and anticoagulants. The natural history of carotid dissections is such that most often healing (i.e., restoration of vascular morphology) occurs spontaneously, up to 90% in spontaneous dissections[3] and 60% in traumatic dissections.[4] The goal of medical treatment, then, is the prevention of thrombus formation on the injured endothelial surface and to avoid artery-to-artery embolism that may result in cerebral ischemia.[5] Studies have suggested that more than 90% of infarcts following dissection are thromboembolic,[6] and hence the use of antiplatelet and anticoagulant drugs is promoted; however, there is no randomized controlled trial to support this form of treatment, and the optimum dosage, duration, efficacy, and safety remain to be established.[7]

A significant proportion of cases remain in which carotid dissection persists, progresses,[8] or recurs.[9] Studies with long-term follow-ups demonstrate that 40% of dissections and up to 100% of pseudoaneurysms do not heal with anticoagulation therapy (i.e., do not return to a morphologically normal shape).[4] More relevant, however, than a negative morphological outcome[10,11] is assessing the risk of stroke that remains despite medical management. In addition, anticoagulants have their own complication rates (hemorrhage in 2% per year),[12] and may be contraindicated (i.e., in patients with multiple trauma, intracranial hematomas, and penetrating injures), and thus should be prescribed after careful contemplation. Risk stratification for stroke, therefore, is the key, and treatment options, whether medical or nonmedical, should be considered in accordance. Surgical treatment of carotid dissection has included direct surgical repair, proximal carotid ligation, extracranial-intracranial carotid artery bypass, and carotid endarterectomy; however, with dissection often extending to the skull base and sometimes lack of good collateral circulation and damaged tissue planes, these procedures can be technically demanding and are associated with high morbidity.[13]

Over the years, endovascular management has developed as the preferred approach[14] over surgery, allowing patency to be reestablished from within the carotid lumen. The stent provides centrifugal force to allow the dissected segment to be apposed against the vessel wall, obliterate the false lumen, and treat the stenosis. This reduces the likelihood of cerebral ischemia from embolism or thrombosis.

INDICATIONS

Indications and criteria for stent-assisted angioplasty for dissection include:[15-19]

1. Clinical failure of medical therapy (recurrent TIAs, fluctuating neurological signs, or neurological deterioration)
2. Impending stroke attributable to significant stenosis or occlusion with poor collateral circulation and reduced parenchymal perfusion on the angiographic capillary phase or CT and MR imaging
3. Contraindication to anticoagulation because of intracranial or systemic hemorrhage
4. Evidence of symptomatic thromboembolic occlusion of cerebral vessels
5. Contralateral carotid stenosis or occlusion
6. Need for elective occlusion of the contralateral ICA for other pathology
7. Need to avoid flow increase through the anterior communication artery because of an associated aneurysm

Endovascular therapy has been employed in these various settings of carotid dissection and has shown excellent results; however, support for this approach is almost entirely based on published individual experiences and case series, and controlled trials are necessary before accepting it as a standard of therapy. For simplicity, carotid dissection from the endovascular perspective can be divided into nonflow-limiting dissections without embolism, nonflow-limiting dissections with embolic sequelae, flow-limiting dissection with ischemia, flow-limiting dissections with ischemia as well as embolic sequelae, and last, dissecting aneurysms, which may present with a combination of the previous.

NONFLOW-LIMITING DISSECTIONS WITHOUT EMBOLISM

A nonflow-limiting tear without embolism is the most common consequence of carotid dissection. Once diagnosis is established using cross-sectional imaging such as CT or MR angiography or conventional angiography, only medical management is required in the form of systemic heparinization or warfarin, and spontaneous resolution of the lesion occurs in the majority of cases.[3,4] Anticoagulation, however, may be contraindicated at times, particularly in the setting of traumatic dissection. These patients often have multiple trauma and penetrating injuries with associated hematomas, and are at high risk of bleeding. Occurrence of life-threatening gastrointestinal and intracerebral hemorrhages have been documented in literature following anticoagulation therapy in patients with carotid dissection.[20] On the other hand, the traumatized brain is already vulnerable to ischemia—due to coexisting raised intracranial pressure, hemodynamic compromise, shearing forces, and the like—and further emboli from the dissection may lead to severe neurologic dysfunction and death.[21] Therefore, in cases of contraindication to anticoagulants, the safety and efficacy of antiplatelet agents alone need to be assessed, as well as possible endovascular or surgical treatment, even prior to the development of embolic symptoms. Several authors have reported using endovascular treatment as the initial therapy of choice if contraindication to medical therapy exists.[15,17,22] Cohen et al. described successful stent-assisted arterial reconstruction following traumatic dissection in three patients who had a contraindication to heparin or warfarin, and had negligible to mild carotid stenosis.[23] Although patients in these series have demonstrated excellent neurological outcome, only a randomized controlled study can establish whether patients treated with early stenting will have a better outcome than those treated with anticoagulation despite a contraindication. In our practice, such patients are usually placed on aspirin and monitored closely. In the event of any thromboembolic phenomenon, endovascular treatment is performed.

NONFLOW-LIMITING DISSECTIONS WITH EMBOLISM

Nonflow-limiting dissections with embolism are another category of carotid dissection cases. For management purposes, the embolus in these cases can be classified as small or large. In the event of large vessel embolization (such as ICA terminus, MCA trunk, and M2 branches), endovascular management involves intra-arterial thrombolysis or mechanical removal of the embolus (see Figures 30-1A–F). The precise indications for thrombolysis in embolic stroke from dissection are similar to other causes of artery-to-artery embolization and are beyond the scope of this chapter. These patients are subsequently treated with systemic anticoagulation.

Small vessel emboli resulting in very small strokes do not warrant intra-arterial stroke therapy and are best managed with anticoagulation alone. Failure of medical therapy represents another scenario warranting endovascular therapy. Medical treatment failure is defined as the presence of recurrent transient ischemic attacks, fluctuating neurological signs, or neurological deterioration despite anticoagulant or antiplatelet therapy. Stenting presumably removes the source of recurrent emboli[24] while maintaining the patency of the injured vessel. There are numerous studies describing successful endovascular management of dissection in these refractory cases[17-19,22,24,25] with only rare reports of subsequent TIAs and strokes following endovascular therapy.[24,25] However, long-term follow-up data in these series has been limited. Enlarging or progressive dissection despite medical therapy is another indication where stenting has been shown to be valuable in nonflow-limiting dissection cases.[20] Surgical therapy is an option in these "failure of medical treatment" cases, whether in the form of direct surgical repair, proximal carotid ligation, extracranial-intracranial carotid artery bypass, or carotid endarterectomy. It is, however, associated with a 9%

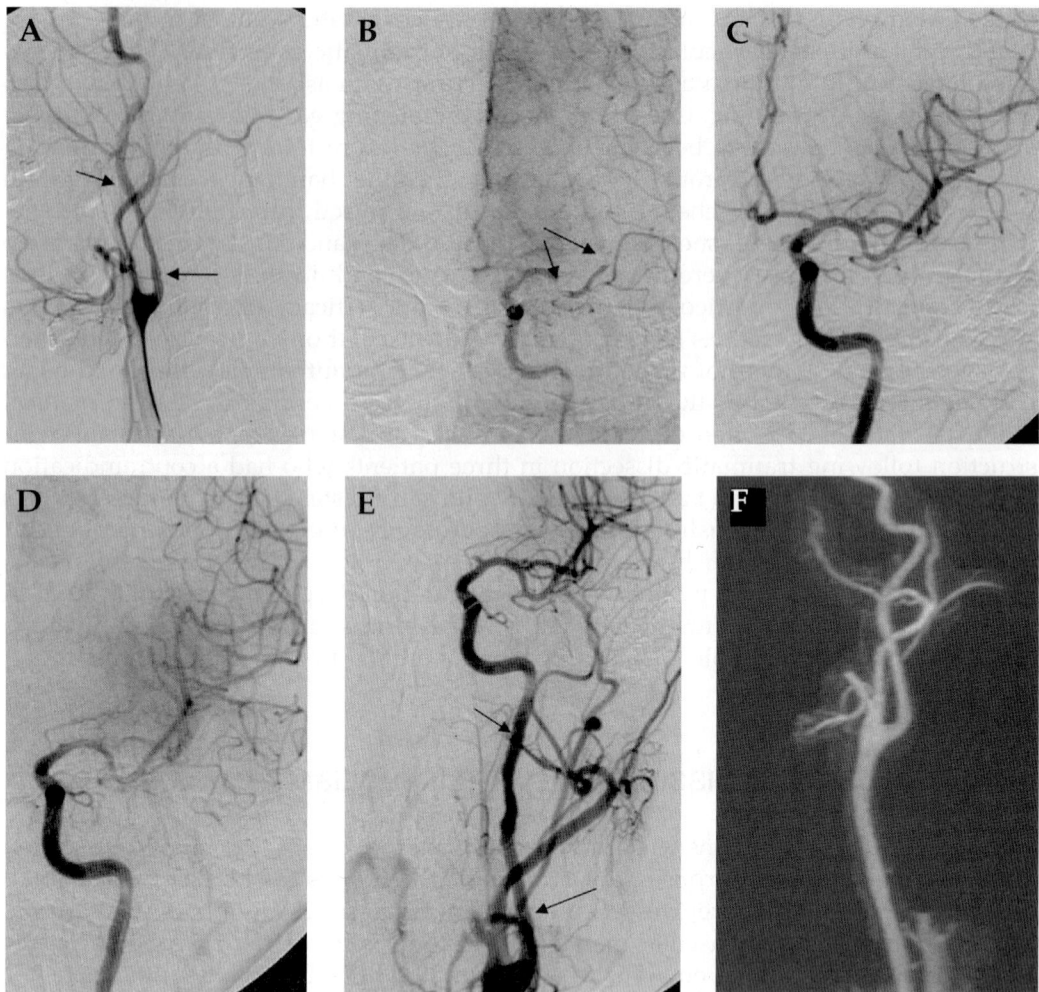

Figure 30-1. Fifty-year-old male found down in his office with clinical signs of left MCA territory stroke. **(A)** Left CCA angiogram demonstrating a nonflow-limiting dissection of the left ICA (arrows). **(B)** Anteroposterior view of left CCA angiogram demonstrating embolic occlusion of the MCA trunk and posterior division (arrows). **(C, D)** Anteroposterior view of left ICA angiogram showing successful thrombolysis of the MCA occlusion. **(E)** Final left CCA angiogram demonstrating the patent left MCA and nonflow-limiting dissection (arrows) of the left ICA. **(F)** Three-month follow-up contrast-enhanced MRA demonstrating resumption of smooth lumen of left ICA, consistent with healing.

to 12% incidence of death and stroke[24,26] and should be considered when the patient is not eligible for endovascular therapy.[14]

FLOW-LIMITING DISSECTIONS WITHOUT EMBOLIC PHENOMENON

In a subset of carotid dissection cases, pressurized blood enters through the dissected medial defect into the false lumen, and causes compression and occlusion of the true lumen. In these patients, spontaneous healing does not occur,[4] and although anticoagulation may prevent thromboembolic events, the flow limitation is enough to produce ischemia. Patients present with clinical or radiological signs of inadequate collateral supply or neurologic deterioration despite anticoagulation (as discussed above in failure of medical therapy) with recurrent TIAs from reduced flow. Stenting in these situations allows apposition of the dissected segment and vessel wall to occlude the false lumen and remove the stenosis in the true lumen, and consequently restore cerebral blood flow (see Figures 30-2A–F).

In a case series of traumatic dissections in 10 patients, Cohen et al. showed a mean improvement in stenosis with angioplasty and stenting from 69% to 8% without neurological or clinical complications.[19] These patients did not develop in-stent de novo stenoses or stent thrombosis on subsequent follow-up. In another study, Malek et al. used similar stenting technique in 10 spontaneous, iatrogenic, and traumatic dissection cases, and showed improvement in dissection-related stenosis from approximately

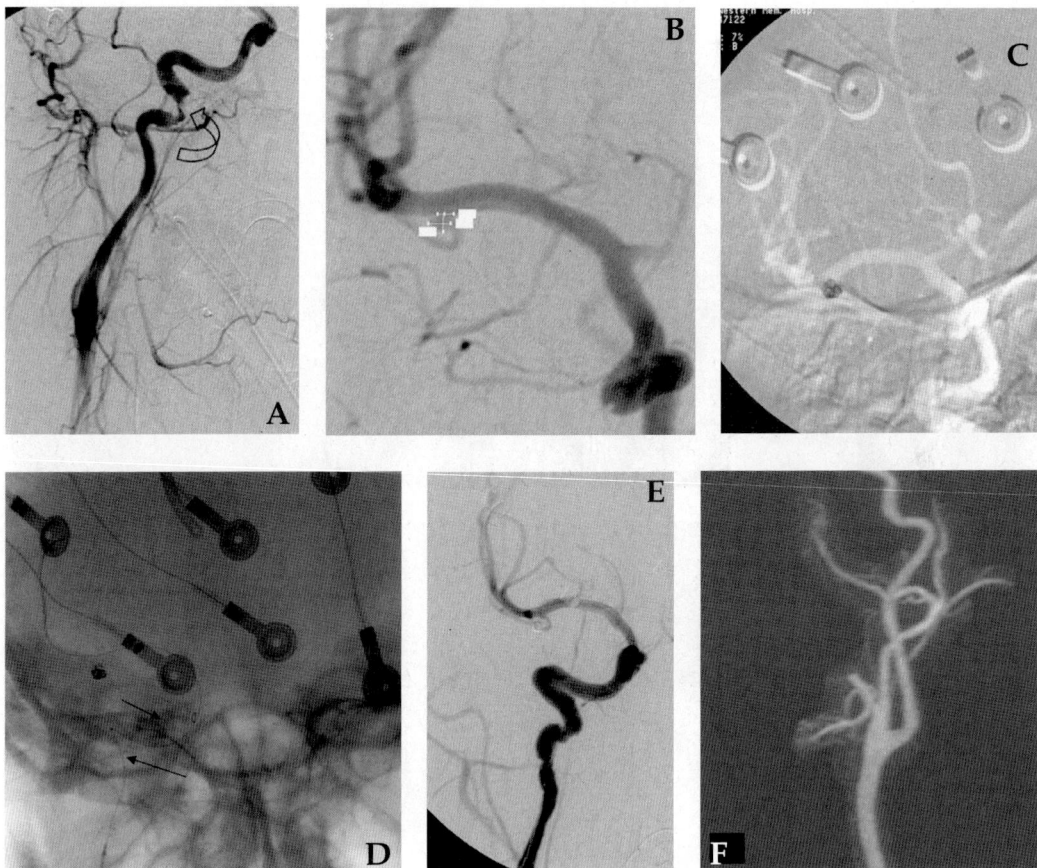

Figure 30-2. Forty-two-year-old female with subarachnoid hemorrhage, Hunt and Hess grade V, and subsequent fall. The presumed rupture site was the largest aneurysm arising from the MCA trunk. **(A)** Right CCA angiogram demonstrating a flow-limiting dissection (curved arrow) of the right ICA just below the skull base. **(B, C)** Right ICA angiogram and road map demonstrating the MCA aneurysm pre- and post-coiling. The aneurysm was treated before treating the dissection to avoid a sudden increase in flow that would possibly have caused a rupture. **(D)** Proximal and distal stent markers (arrows) after placement of a Neuroform stent covering the dissection. **(E)** Right ICA angiogram after stent placement demonstrating a much better luminal diameter with some arterial spasm. **(F)** One-month follow-up contrast-enhanced MRA demonstrating a normal right ICA.

74% to 5.5%.[18] This series described significant improvement in neurological status of their patients as quantified with the Rankin score and Barthel index. They reported no further TIAs or strokes in patients or any case of stent occlusion or stenosis on follow-up angiography or sonography.

Emergent stenting has been advocated in the setting of impending or evolving stroke after carotid dissection. In these scenarios, prognosis is usually poor and heparin has not been shown to alter the course.[27] One study described three cases in which radiological and clinical evidence was used to emergently stent nontraumatic carotid dissections.[28] Patients were selected for therapy based on the initial identification of large ischemic penumbral tissue with a diffusion-perfusion mismatch on MRI or by finding delayed capillary filling on parenchymography during angiography (see Figures 30-3A–F and 30-4A–D). In addition, stenosis, causing reduced flow, was identified at the dissection site with carotid duplex and MRA. After stent insertion, there

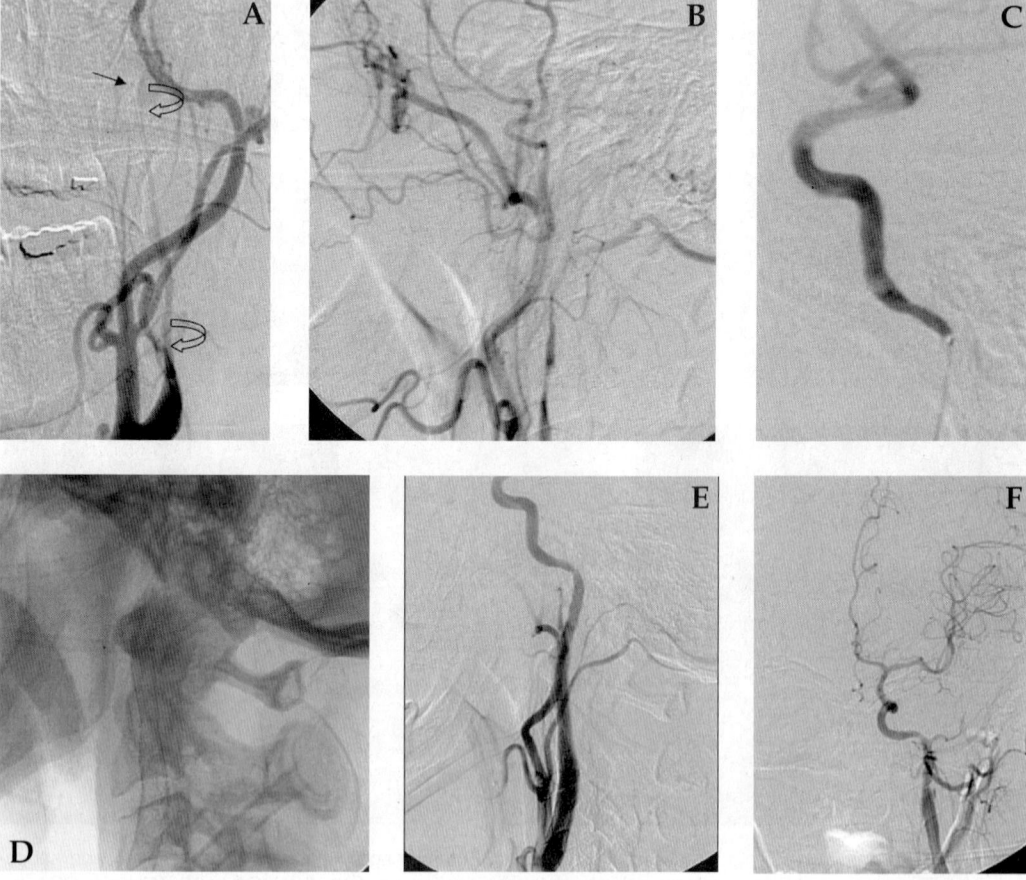

Figure 30-3. Forty-five-year-old female presenting with three TIAs despite anticoagulation therapy (please refer to Figure 30-4 for MR perfusion images). **(A, B)** Anteroposterior and lateral views of left CCA injection demonstrating the dissection of the cervical left ICA (between two curved arrows), which ends at the skull base. A normal proximal petrous ICA is seen (straight arrow). **(C)** Microcatheter injection in the normal petrous ICA after careful navigation through the true lumen. **(D)** Two overlapping stents covering the entire dissected segment. **(E, F)** Lateral and anteroposterior views of left CCA injections after stent placement depicting normal anterogade flow.

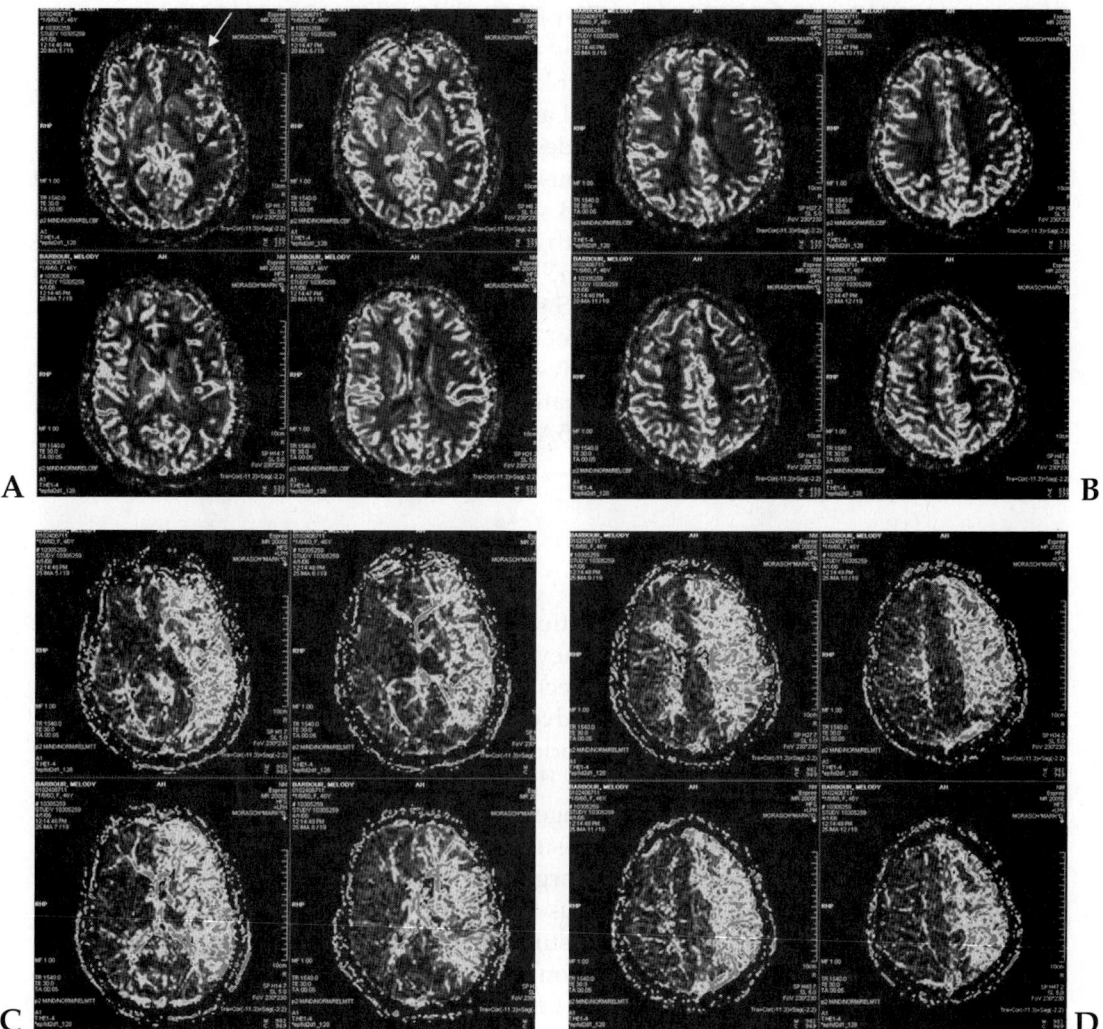

Figure 30-4. MR perfusion imaging of the brain pretreatment (same patient as Figure 30-3). **(A, B)** Relative cerebral blood flow (rCBF) maps demonstrating decreased CBF in the left middle cerebral artery (MCA) and anterior cerebral artery (ACA) territories (arrow). **(C, D)** Relative mean transit time (rMTT) maps demonstrating significantly increased transit times (i.e., slow flow) in the left MCA and ACA territories (increased more in the MCA than ACA).

was a prompt resolution of ischemic symptoms with no subsequent complications. Similar success with emergent stenting has also been reported by other authors.[16,29,30] Although these reports suggest the efficacy and safety of immediate stenting to restore lumen integrity, one also has to stress that eligible patients are only those who on neuroimaging show a viable, hypoperfused ischemic penumbra. If CT or MR imaging demonstrates infarction accounting for the neurological deficit without any additional tissue at risk, reestablishing the flow may not be of any benefit and only increase the risk of hemorrhagic conversion of the stroke.

FLOW-LIMITING DISSECTIONS WITH EMBOLIC PHENOMENON

There is also the rare scenario where stroke results from carotid dissection causing both flow limitations from stenosis as well as embolism. Endovascular management in these situations would theoretically include immediate stenting to restore the patency of the carotid artery as well as simultaneous intra-arterial thrombolysis to dissolve the embolus. Recently, Abboud et al. reported such a case where a patient, who had been on prior anticoagulation for dissection with a mural hematoma occluding the ICA, developed hemiplegia from MCA embolism.[31] The patient was eligible for intravenous or intra-arterial tPA (based in the NIHSS score, time-frame, and so on), but would have likely not improved as the ICA occlusion would have been left in place. Consequently, stenting was done to resolve the ICA occlusion and intra-arterial tPA was infused to recanalise the MCA. The patient's symptoms completely resolved with this combined approach[31] (see Figures 30-5A–I).

DISSECTING ANEURYSMS

Dissecting aneurysms are another indication for endovascular therapy. We consider their management separately, though they may present with a combination of the above categories. Unlike subintimal dissections that result in stenosis of the arterial lumen, dissections between media and adventitia cause aneurysmal dilatation of the artery. They are often referred to as "pseudoaneurysms" when, in fact, their walls are composed of tunica media and adventitia.[14] Again, medical, endovascular, and surgical therapy are all options for their management. Endovascular and surgical therapy are often considered if patients have persistent symptoms of ischemia despite medical therapy, if the aneurysm continues to enlarge and cause significant mass effect, or if it contains persistent intraluminal thrombus that may represent a source and risk for thromboembolic complications. Unlike surgery, endovascular management allows separation of the aneurysm from circulation and preservation of the parent artery (see Figures 30-6A–F). There are three options for endovascular repair of dissecting carotid aneurysms: carotid occlusion, combined stent placement and coiling of the aneurysm, and stent-grafts. Endovascular occlusion of the carotid artery is safe, provided a test occlusion ensures collateral flow; in general 75% of patients are able to tolerate internal carotid occlusion.[32] Considering, however, that many of these patients are young, it is preferable to use a flow-preserving procedure. Klein et al. described the use of a combination of uncovered stents and coils in the treatment of posttraumatic aneurysms.[33] Another technically simpler and less risky alternative is to use covered stents. They, however, require bulky delivery systems and may be difficult to navigate. Also, as compared to bare stents, covered stents may be more thrombogenic and have a poorer long-term patency rate, although long-term data remain limited.[34] Occasionally, two or more porous stents can be placed using a "stent-in-stent" technique to reconstruct the carotid artery.[16-18] This technique allows for decreased porosity of the stent and possible spontaneous thrombosis of the excluded aneurysm lumen, especially if the "neck" is small.

Biffl et al. demonstrated that in cases of grade III BCI (blunt carotid injury causing aneurysm formation), only 8% of aneurysms healed with heparin therapy while 89% healed with endovascular stents.[35] In a smaller series, Duke et al. assessed long-term

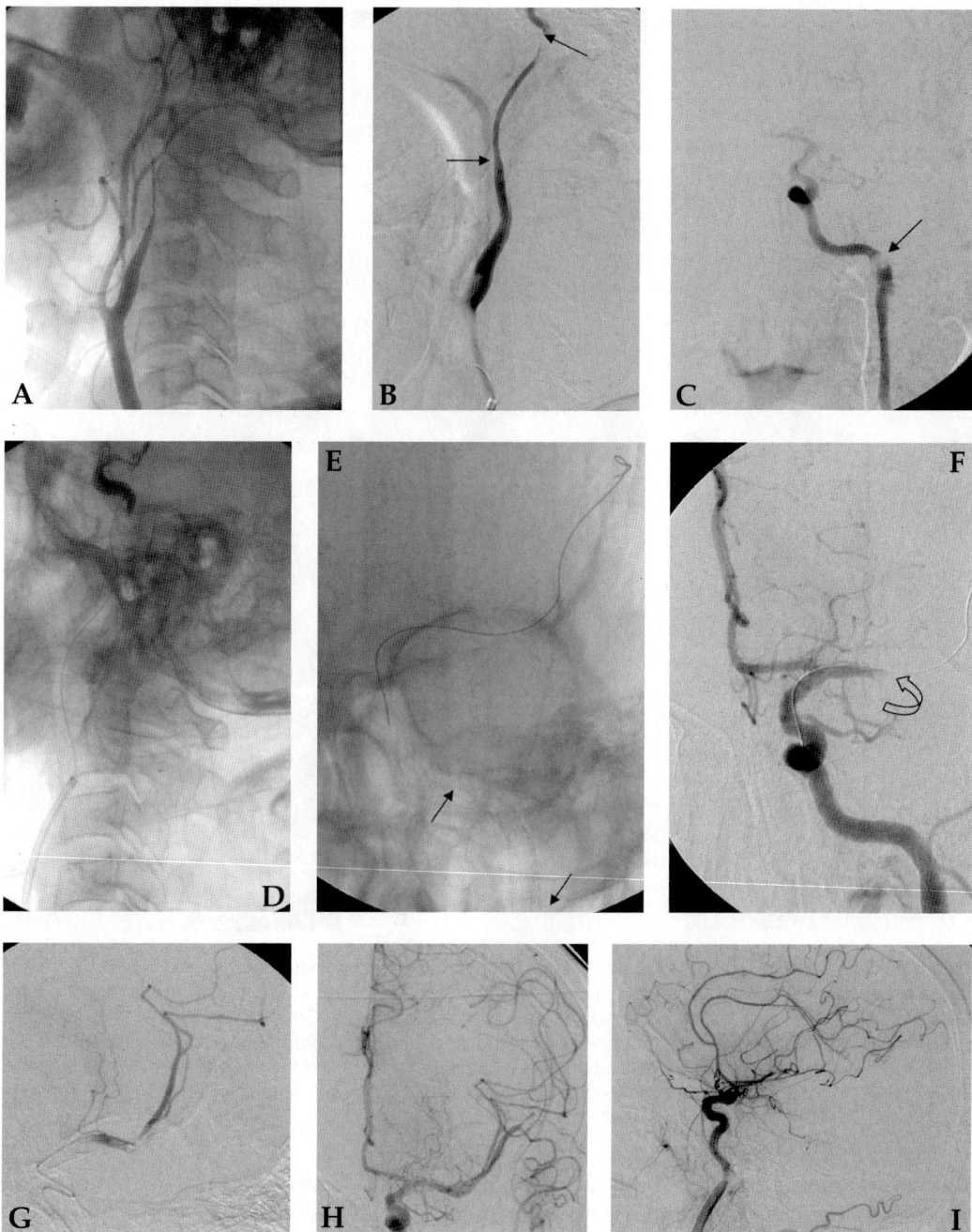

Figure 30-5. Fifty-eight-year-old male with clinical signs of left MCA territory infarct. **(A, B)** Lateral view of left CCA angiogram demonstrating a dissection (arrow) of the left CCA extending to the skull base. **(C)** Anteroposterior view of left ICA angiogram demonstrating an intraluminal clot (arrow) just above the left ICA dissection. **(D)** Microcatheter angiogram in cavernous left ICA after careful navigation through the true lumen. **(E, F)** Anteroposterior view of pre- and postcontrast injection left ICA angiogram showing the deployed stent (arrows) and reconstruction of the normal lumen of the left ICA. Embolic occlusion of the left MCA trunk is seen (curved arrow). **(G)** Microcatheter injection in left MCA trunk. **(H, I)** Anteroposterior and lateral views of left ICA angiogram demonstrating successful opening of the MCA trunk and posterior division following chemical and mechanical thrombolysis.

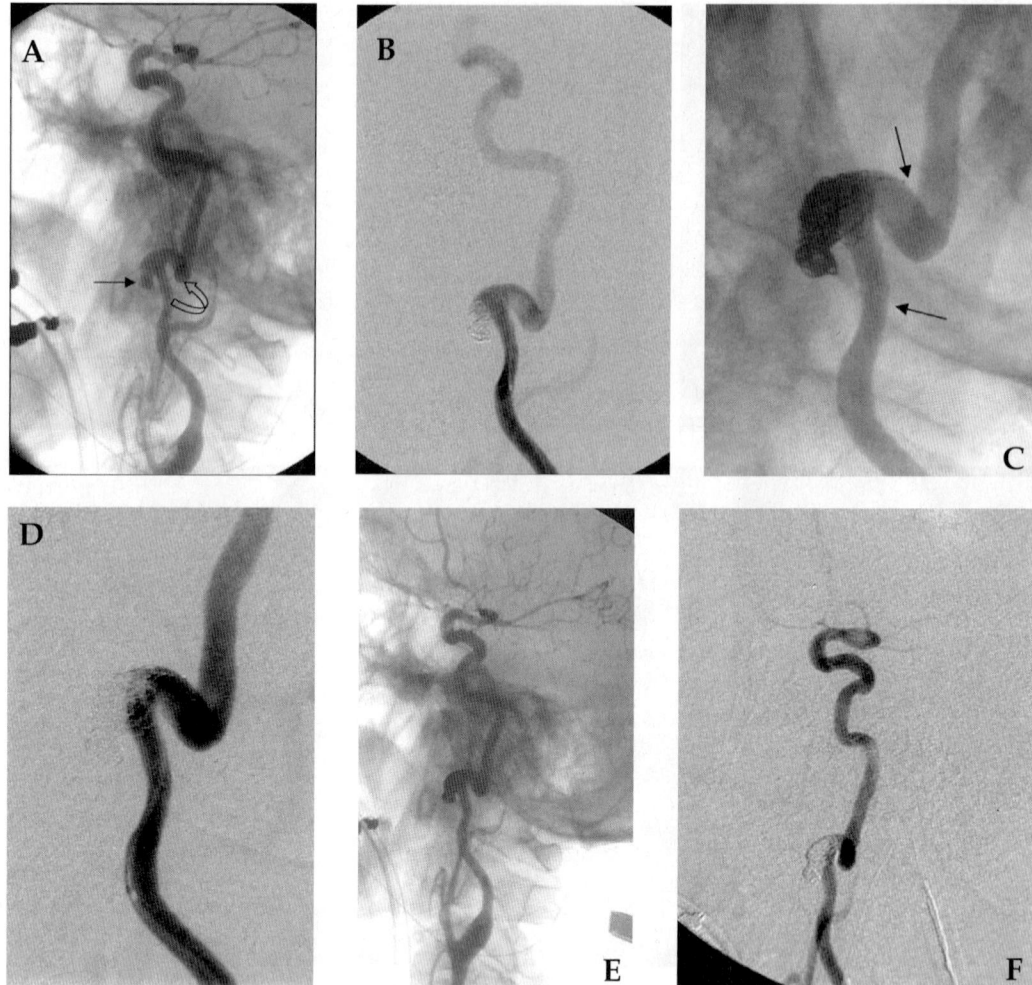

Figure 30-6. Sixty-eight-year-old male with history of recent left-sided amaurosis fugax and clot in the central retinal artery. Workup demonstrated an old dissecting aneurysm of the left ICA with intraluminal thrombus. **(A)** Lateral left CCA arteriogram showing significant tortuosity of the cervical ICA (curved arrow) with a dissecting aneurysm (straight arrow). **(B)** Left ICA arteriogram during stent-assisted coiling of the aneurysm. **(C, D)** Left ICA arteriogram demonstrating the proximal and distal stent markers (arrows) and the coil mass within the dissecting aneurysm. **(E, F)** Final left ICA control arteriogram demonstrating a good angiographic result.

follow-up and reported no ischemic complications over several months following stent placement for traumatic aneurysms.[20] In dealing with these blunt carotid injuries, it has been pointed out by some that to avoid the risk of stroke from manipulation of catheters, the acutely injured carotid artery should not be manipulated within 48–72 hours of the event, and to wait seven days before attempting stenting.[36] However, if any of the indications listed previously for emergency treatment exist, then endovascular treatment shoud be initiated. Also, adjunctive anticoagulation[35] or antiplatelet therapy[20] is necessary to prevent thrombotic complications from stents themselves.

A pertinent question in the treatment of chronic dissecting aneurysms is the definition of "healing." As alluded to above,[4] only a minority of arteries with a dissecting aneurysm will return to a "normal" morphology. The presence of an aneurysmal section of the artery in and of itself is not necessarily a risk factor for stroke, especially if the intimal lining has healed and there is no intraluminal thrombus or significant flow stagnation. Touze et al. followed 32 patients with dissecting carotid aneurysms on antiplatelet (aspirin) therapy, and showed that despite 19 of these failing to resolve or decrease in size over the next three years, none of these patients suffered a transient ischemic attack, stroke, or clinical symptoms suggestive of aneurysmal rupture or compression.[11] As the risk of ischemic complications is small and a favorable outcome can be expected on antiplatelet therapy alone, a very careful assessment is necessary before exposing patients with dissecting aneurysms to the risks of endovascular or surgical therapy.

TECHNIQUE

All patients undergoing stent placement will require antiplatelet agents preprocedurally. If possible, a three-day to five-day regimen of ASA (81 or 325 mg) and Plavix (75 mg) is given. If emergency therapy is indicated, a loading dose of Plavix (600 mg) and ASA (81 mg) can be given orally prior to the procedure, or crushed and given by NG tube. Alternatively, an ASA suppository can be given, and supplemented by IV Toradol, which seems to work well in most cases (author's own anecdotal experience). The patients are heparinized, with the goal of achieving an ACT of 250–300.

After placing a standard guide sheath (5–7 French depending on stent size) and/or guide catheter (6 Fr), a standard neuro microcatheter (.014–0.018 lumen) is very carefully navigated over a soft neuro micro-wire (0.014), through the true lumen and into the normal lumen beyond the dissection. The position of the microcatheter in the true lumen is documented by a microcatheter angiogram.

The length of the dissected segment is measured. Self-expanding stents are used in all cases unless unavailable in the required diameter. The stent diameter is usually oversized by 1–2 mm compared to the normal arterial diameter. If the normal diameter of the dissected carotid artery is difficult to assess, the contralateral carotid diameter is used. In cases where the dissected length is longer than the available stent and overlapping stents are needed, stenting is performed distally to proximally. Generally, pre-and postdilation are not necessary unless the dissection was superimposed on a preexisting stenosis.

Carefully magnified control arteriograms are performed with special attention to the stent lumen to detect in-stent thrombus development. This can be treated with a small dose of a glycoprotein IIb-IIIa inhibitor or a small dose of tPA. A standard cerebral arteriographic run is then performed to assess for any distal thromboembolism.

Postprocedurally, the patients are monitored in the neuro-ICU for 24–48 hours. Postprocedural medications include daily ASA (81mg) and Plavix (75 mg). If the patient has significant other injuries where the combination of ASA and Plavix is thought to be dangerous, then ASA (325 mg) alone will often suffice.

COMPLICATIONS

Although relatively safe to perform, angioplasty and stenting in carotid dissections is associated with several potential complications. First, the stent needs to be appropriately sized and placed correctly to ensure vessel patency. At times, multiple stents may be needed that may further increase the risks of the procedure. Second, during angioplasty, thrombotic debris can embolize. Risks of this occurrence can be reduced by antiplatelet medications before and systemic heparinization during the procedure. If embolization does occur, intra-arterial thrombolysis may be needed. Third, vessel rupture can occur. Though rare, it can be disastrous, and one needs to gradually inflate the angioplasty balloon and smoothly unsheathe the stent deployment device to prevent such an occurrence. Fourth, restenosis can occur after angioplasty and stenting, either acutely due to thrombosis, or in the subacute or chronic phase, from myointimal hyperplasia[37] and progressive atherosclerosis.

In the 10-case series reported in the literature of patients with carotid dissections treated with endovascular stent angioplasty,[17-19,22,24,25,28,38-40] (which include a total of 90 patients, 37 of whom had spontaneous dissections), no deaths occurred intraprocedurally or as a consequence of the treated vessel. Two strokes have been reported, one from a hemorrhagic conversion of a prior ischemic stroke 13 days after the procedure[24] and another with a stroke from reocclusion of the vessel 22 days after the procedure.[25] Also, three TIAs have been reported intraprocedurally and two TIAs reported occurring several months after the stenting and angioplasty.[25] Thus, with these few neurologic sequelae reported, endovascular therapy seems to be a safe option when medical therapy is insufficient or inappropriate. Needless to say, however, long-term followups have been limited in many of these reports, and randomized controlled trials are needed to establish the efficacy and safety of these procedures.

To conclude, while medical therapy is the optimal treatment for carotid dissection, endovascular techniques seem to be safe and effective means of managing refractory cases. There are applications in both flow-limiting and nonflow-limiting dissections, as well as dissections that may or may not exhibit embolic sequlae. Percutaneous stenting restores cerebral blood flow and prevents flow-related and embolic complications. Though the technique is relatively simple and the reported complications are few, large trials would help to better establish the true efficacy and safety. As improvements in stent technology and delivery tools occur over time, one can expect a larger role of endovascular therapy in carotid dissection, as well as other vascular conditions.

REFERENCES

1. Schievink WI, Mokri B, Whisnant JP. Internal carotid artery dissection in a community. Rochester, Minnesota, 1987–1992. *Stroke*. 1993;24:1678–1680.
2. Ducrocq X, Lacour JC, Debouverie M, et al. [Cerebral ischemic accidents in young subjects. A prospective study of 296 patients aged 16 to 45 years]. *Rev Neurol (Paris)*. 1999;155: 575–582.
3. Hart RG, Easton JD. Dissections of cervical and cerebral arteries. *Neurol Clin*. 1983; 1:155–182.
4. Fabian TC, Patton JH, Jr., Croce MA, et al. Blunt carotid injury. Importance of early diagnosis and anticoagulant therapy. *Ann Surg*. 1996;223:513–522; discussion 522–515.
5. Stapf C, Elkind MS, Mohr JP. Carotid artery dissection. *Annu Rev Med*. 2000;51:329–347.
6. Lucas C, Moulin T, Deplanque D, et al. Stroke patterns of internal carotid artery dissection in 40 patients. *Stroke*.1998;29:2646–2648.
7. Lyrer P, Engelter S. Antithrombotic drugs for carotid artery dissection. *Stroke*. 2004;35: 613–614.

8. Houser OW, Mokri B, Sundt TM, Jr., et al. Spontaneous cervical cephalic arterial dissection and its residuum: angiographic spectrum. *AJNR Am J Neuroradiol*. 1984;5:27–34.

9. Schievink WI, Mokri B, O'Fallon WM. Recurrent spontaneous cervical-artery dissection. *N Engl J Med*. 1994;330:393–397.

10. Ohtoh T, Ono Y, Iwasaki Y, et al. Non-traumatic recurrent dissection and its spontaneous repair in the circle of Willis: report of two autopsy cases. *Neuropathology*. 2003;23:195–198.

11. Touze E, Randoux B, Meary E, et al. Aneurysmal forms of cervical artery dissection : associated factors and outcome. *Stroke*. 2001;32:418–423.

12. Levine MN, Raskob G, Hirsh J. Hemorrhagic complications of long-term anticoagulant therapy. *Chest*. 1989;95:26S–36S.

13. Schievink WI, Piepgras DG, McCaffrey TV, Mokri B. Surgical treatment of extracranial internal carotid artery dissecting aneurysms. *Neurosurgery*. 1994;35:809–815; discussion 815–806.

14. Schievink WI. Spontaneous dissection of the carotid and vertebral arteries. *N Engl J Med*. 2001;344:898–906.

15. DeOcampo J, Brillman J, Levy DI. Stenting: a new approach to carotid dissection. *J Neuroimaging*. 1997;7:187–190.

16. Biondi A, Katz JM, Vallabh J, et al. Progressive symptomatic carotid dissection treated with multiple stents. *Stroke*. 2005;36:e80–82.

17. Bejjani GK, Monsein LH, Laird JR,et al. Treatment of symptomatic cervical carotid dissections with endovascular stents. *Neurosurgery*. 1999;44:755–760; discussion 760–751.

18. Malek AM, Higashida RT, Phatouros CC, et al. Endovascular management of extracranial carotid artery dissection achieved using stent angioplasty. *AJNR Am J Neuroradiol*. 2000;21:1280–1292.

19. Cohen JE, Ben-Hur T, Rajz G, et al. Endovascular stent-assisted angioplasty in the management of traumatic internal carotid artery dissections. *Stroke*. 2005;36:e45–47.

20. Duke BJ, Ryu RK, Coldwell DM, Brega KE. Treatment of blunt injury to the carotid artery by using endovascular stents: an early experience. *J Neurosurg*. 1997;87:825–829.

21. Server A, Dullerud R, Haakonsen M, et al. Post-traumatic cerebral infarction. Neuroimaging findings, etiology and outcome. *Acta Radiol*. 2001;42:254–260.

22. Liu AY, Paulsen RD, Marcellus ML, et al. Long-term outcomes after carotid stent placement treatment of carotid artery dissection. *Neurosurgery*. 1999;45:1368–1373; discussion 1373–1364.

23. Cohen JE, Ben-Hur T, Gomori JM, et al. Stent-assisted arterial reconstruction of traumatic extracranial carotid dissections. *Neurol Res*. 2005;27 Suppl 1:S73–78.

24. Edgell RC, Abou-Chebl A, Yadav JS. Endovascular management of spontaneous carotid artery dissection. *J Vasc Surg*. 2005;42:854–860; discussion 860.

25. Kadkhodayan Y, Jeck DT, Moran CJ, et al. Angioplasty and stenting in carotid dissection with or without associated pseudoaneurysm. *AJNR Am J Neuroradiol*. 2005;26: 2328–2335.

26. Muller BT, Luther B, Hort W, et al. Surgical treatment of 50 carotid dissections: indications and results. *J Vasc Surg*. 2000;31:980–988.

27. Bogousslavsky J, Despland PA, Regli F. Spontaneous carotid dissection with acute stroke. *Arch Neurol*. 1987;44:137–140.

28. Cohen JE, Leker RR, Gotkine M, et al. Emergent stenting to treat patients with carotid artery dissection: clinically and radiologically directed therapeutic decision making. *Stroke*. 2003;34:e254–257.

29. Janjua N, Qureshi AI, Kirmani J, Pullicino P. Stent-supported angioplasty for acute stroke caused by carotid dissection. *Neurocrit Care*. 2006;4:47–53.

30. Sbarigia E, Battocchio C, Panico MA, et al. Endovascular management of acute carotid artery dissection with a waxing and waning neurological deficit. *J Endovasc Ther*. 2003; 10:45–48.

31. Abboud H, Houdart E, Meseguer E, Amarenco P. Stent assisted endovascular thrombolysis of internal carotid artery dissection. *J Neurol Neurosurg Psychiatry*. 2005;76:292–293.

32. Linskey ME, Sekhar LN, Horton JA, et al. Aneurysms of the intracavernous carotid artery: a multidisciplinary approach to treatment. *J Neurosurg*. 1991;75:525–534.

33. Klein GE, Szolar DH, Raith J, et al. Posttraumatic extracranial aneurysm of the internal carotid artery: combined endovascular treatment with coils and stents. *AJNR Am J Neuroradiol*. 1997;18:1261–1264.

34. Beregi JP, Prat A, Willoteaux S, et al. Covered stents in the treatment of peripheral arterial aneurysms: procedural results and midterm follow-up. *Cardiovasc Intervent Radiol*. 1999; 22:13–19.

35. Biffl WL, Moore EE, Offner PJ, et al. Blunt carotid arterial injuries: implications of a new grading scale. *J Trauma*. 1999;47:845–853.

36. Singh RR, Barry MC, Ireland AJ, Bouchier-Hayes DM. Current diagnosis and management of blunt internal carotid artery injury. *Eur J Vasc Endovasc Surg*. 2004;27:577–584.

37. Crawley F, Brown MM, Clifton AG. Angioplasty and stenting in the carotid and vertebral arteries. *Postgrad Med J*. 1998;74:7–10.

38. Albuquerque FC, Han PP, Spetzler RF, et al. Carotid dissection: technical factors affecting endovascular therapy. *Can J Neurol Sci*. 2002;29:54–60.

39. Hurst RW, Haskal ZJ, Zager E, et al. Endovascular stent treatment of cervical internal carotid artery aneurysms with parent vessel preservation. *Surg Neurol*. 1998;50:313–317; discussion 317.

40. Kubaska SM, 3rd, Greenberg RK, Clair D, et al. Internal carotid artery pseudoaneurysms: treatment with the Wallgraft endoprosthesis. *J Endovasc Ther*. 2003;10:182–189.

31

Carotid Body Tumors and Cervical Schwannoma Tumors

Thomas A. Whitehill, M.D., Jayer Chung, M.D.

CAROTID BODY TUMORS

The liberal use of arteriography, CT arteriography, MRI/MRA, and modern surgical techniques has reduced the risk of postoperative stroke in carotid body tumor resection from approximately 30% to less than 2% over the past 25 years. However, the incidence of cranial nerve injury continues to remain high in modern series, ranging from 15% to 35%.[1,2] As there are no suitable alternatives to surgical resection, carotid body tumors need to be approached using the most precise techniques possible by well-experienced and well-prepared surgical specialists.

Diagnosis

Duplex ultrasound is the best initial investigation for diagnosis. It can demonstrate splaying of the carotid bifurcation by the tumor ("lyre" sign) and the characteristic mixed-signal color flow image ("firestorm") within the usually well-vascularized tumor. The measured end diastolic velocities within the external carotid artery may be very high because it feeds the tumor. Fine-cut (3 to 5 mm), rapid-sequenced computed tomographic angiography (CTA) with computer reconstructions is quite valuable to confirm the diagnosis, define the distal extent of the tumor, and delineate carotid artery anatomy with its vascular supply to the tumor. This study can also exclude or detect metastatic deposits up to the base of the skull and identify bilateral disease. CTA is replacing the more invasive catheter-based angiography or DSA for preoperative surgical planning. MRI/MRA can be equivalent to CTA at selected centers with interest in this modality for vascular diagnostics. MR imaging may be superior to CT scanning for demonstrating the relationship of the carotid body tumor to adjacent structures.

Percutaneous needle biopsy (or FNA) has been historically associated with far too many hemorrhagic complications and should only be mentioned to condemn its use to diagnose any neck mass associated with the carotid arteries.

Cranial nerve function should be evaluated carefully prior to operation. This evaluation must include indirect or fiberoptic laryngoscopic evaluation of vocal cord movement. An occasional patient will have a preexisting asymptomatic cord palsy or paresis, with no history to suggest a cause. Additionally, an operative cord palsy or paresis may be present and go undetected by the patient and the surgeon in the postoperative period, only to become evident after nerve damage following a second operation for a bilateral tumor (or CEA). The obvious consequences of bilateral cord palsy include airway obstruction, and the need for immediate endotracheal reintubation and possible tracheostomy. Catecholamine screening should be reserved for those individuals who present with a history suggesting endocrine activity, and for those patients with bilateral tumors or a family history of carotid body tumors, both of which are thought to be more likely to predispose to neurosecretory activity.

Treatment Options

Untreated carotid body tumors usually grow very slowly and will ultimately wrap around the internal and external carotid arteries, extend upward to the base of the skull, and entrap neighboring cranial nerves. The larger the tumor, the more likely the cranial nerves will be involved with a correspondingly higher incidence of nerve damage during surgery. Most vulnerable are the superior laryngeal, the hypoglossal, the glossopharyngeal, the vagus, and the recurrent laryngeal nerves. Untreated tumors, even though benign on histological examination can, by their bulk, compress the trachea, erode into the base of the skull, and extend intracranially, requiring a combined suboccipital-cervical dissection. Increasing size can also interfere with normal functions such as speech, swallowing, and respiration. All tumors, once discovered, should be surgically removed unless the host is too old or has too many comorbidities to tolerate a cervical procedure.

Radiation therapy, chemotherapy, and percutaneous embolization have been tried with neither consistent nor durable success. Carotid body tumors are generally radioresistant. Radiation exposes the carotid arteries to radiation arteritis, accelerated atherosclerosis, and even necrosis. Delayed surgical excision after radiation is even more difficult. Catheter-based tumor embolization can temporarily reduce the vascularity of the tumor, and some surgeons have used it preoperatively with mixed results. It carries the risk of embolization or thrombosis of the ICA as well as extension of clots into the more distal cerebral circulation. Carotid body tumors aggressively redevelop and recruit collateral vessels after ligation or embolization of their vessels of supply much like AVMs do. As such, tumor embolization by itself is not a viable alternative to operative resection. Partial surgical resection is also unsuccessful because of tumor regrowth and the possibility of tumor spillage with resultant metastatic spread. Partial resection has been used in attempts to remove huge tumors where potential nerve damage was thought to be unacceptable and blood loss associated with total resection thought to be life threatening.[3]

Preoperative Embolization

Preoperative catheter-based embolization of carotid body tumors does not significantly improve outcome in patients undergoing resection of tumors measuring up to 5 cm.[4] It is an important adjunct to consider when treating selected patients with larger carotid body tumors (>6 cm) to reduce blood loss and to decrease the technical problems with their resection. Postembolization surgical exploration proceeds more smoothly, the blood loss is usually less, and patients may have decreased morbidity from cranial nerve injury.[5] This adjunctive procedure should take place the day before anticipated surgical resection and only be carried out by skilled interventionalists due to the high propensity for attendant ICA embolization and stroke.

Operative Planning and Surgical Technique

The anatomic and basic technical details of operations for carotid body tumors are similar to those for carotid endarterectomy. Because blood loss can be substantial, an autotransfusion device should be available, reducing the requirements for bank blood. Planning for harvest of a suitable saphenous vein should be done since complicated arterial reconstruction may be required. Carotid shunts should be available if clamping of the ICA is necessary because of unexpected carotid injury, low carotid back-pressure, intraoperative EEG changes, or other indication of inadequate cerebral perfusion. In addition to normal electrocautery, bipolar coagulation is invaluable. A nerve stimulator may sometimes be useful to help with cranial nerve identification. Heparinzation is not used unless a period of prolonged carotid occlusion is necessary or unavoidable. Blood pressure should be maintained at normal levels throughout the case; an arterial monitoring catheter is indispensable. Loop magnification is essential. The total conduct of the operation is characterized by patience, persistence, and precision.

Positioning and Preparation

As for carotid endarterectomy, the patient is placed supine with the head of the table slightly elevated. This tends to decrease venous pressure, which is an aid in dissection and diminishes bleeding. The head, supported in a head ring or foam "doughnut," is mildly extended and turned toward the side opposite the tumor.

Temporomandibular Subluxation

Extremely large tumors extending toward the base of the skull may require temporary subluxation of the temporomandibular joint to facilitate distal carotid exposure. If the tumor extends distal to a line between the angle of the mandible and the tip of the mastoid, it is considered inaccessible (at or above the level of C-2 vertebral body) using standard carotid exposure techniques. Preoperative identification of patients who require exposure of this distal internal carotid artery is important because temporomandibular subluxation (TMS) requires satisfactory nasotracheal intubation anesthesia before the cervical incision is made.[6] Such subluxation maneuvers are usually performed in cooperation with an oral surgeon or ENT surgeon. It is important to only sublux, and not dislocate, the ipsilateral mandible as dislocation may damage the temporomandibular joint cartilage.[7] This technique transforms a triangular operating field into a rectangular one (Figure 31–1).

Once satisfactory general nasotracheal anesthesia is obtained, and before prepping and draping, unilateral mandibular subluxation is performed. In dentate patients, the subluxed position is held in place by IVY loop interdental diagonal wiring of an ipsilateral mandibular cuspid or bicuspid tooth to a contralateral maxillary cuspid or bicuspid tooth using 25-gauge stainless steel wire. Gentle manual anterior mandibular subluxation is performed while the diagonal wires are tightened. In edentulous

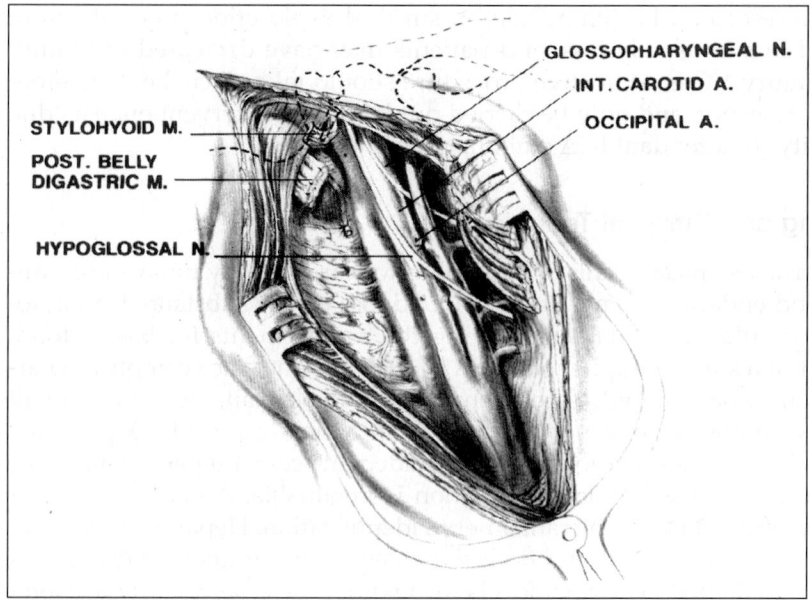

Figure 31-1. Exposure of the distal right internal carotid artery after temporomandibular subluxation, division of the posterior belly of the digastric muscle and styloid muscles, and ligation and division of the occipital artery, (From Dossa C, et al. *J Vasc Surg* 1990;12:319–325, with permission of C.V. Mosby/Elsevier Publishing.)

patients, TMS stabilization is maintained by intermaxillary-mandibular wiring around two 3/32 inch Steinmann pins drilled intraorally at the gingival margins into the ipsilateral mandible and contralateral maxilla. The first Steinmann pin is placed by retracting the ipsilateral lower lip and drilling the pin through the oral mucosa into the mandible 2 cm from the midline, anterior to the mental foramen, and 1 to 2 cm from the alveolar crest, aiming at the contralateral mandibular angle. In a similar fashion, a second pin is drilled into the contralateral maxilla. This pin is placed 2 cm from the midline and 1 to 2 cm above the alveolar crest. When the pins are adequately placed, the tips can be palpated beneath the mucosa. Both pins are trimmed so that approximately 1 cm protrudes. Loops of 25-gauge stainless steel wire are attached to the pins and then tightened as the ipsilateral mandible is gently subluxed. Note that a slight shift of the standard anatomic landmarks occurs due to this movement of the mandible. Such subluxation maneuvers can be performed in 10 to 15 minutes.[7-8] Older techniques, which include maxillomandibular arch bar fixation, circummandibular/transnasal wiring, and mandibular osteotomy or partial mandibulectomy, are more time-consuming, have associated complications, and have been largely abandoned in distal carotid surgery. Nasal intubation for resection of a distal tumor may, by itself, increase distal access by allowing for increased mandibular mobility, even without TMS. If nasotracheal intubation and TMS is not being utilized, general endotracheal anesthesia is almost always required. The exception is for a very small tumor that lies low in the neck that might be addressable under local anesthesia/cervical field block in a very calm and cooperative patient.

Incision Selection and Initial Exposure

A longitudinal incision placed anterior and parallel to the medial border of the stern-ocleidomastoid muscle usually gives adequate exposure for resection of small- and medium-sized tumors. Larger tumors (> 4cm) are more easily excised using a modified-T neck incision or an S-shaped sweeping pre-auricular incision (Figure 31–2). This latter incision, in front of the ear with anterior parotid gland mobilization and facial nerve preservation, can facilitate very distal ICA exposure.[9] The alternate postauricular extension of the distal end of the incision avoids injury to the ramus mandibularis of the facial nerve. but extreme distal ICA exposure may be hindered. Cutaneous nerves that cross the incision are divided, but the greater auricular nerve should be preserved.

Exposure is developed and deepened from the mastoid process to the lower limit of the incision through dissection and lateral retraction of the sternocleidomastoid muscle. The internal jugular vein is now dissected away from the underlying tumor and carotid arteries. An increased number of small venous tributaries draining the tumor may be encountered at this level. The common facial vein and any other anterior tributaries are ligated and divided. The facial vein is often quite attenuated as it is being stretched by the underlying tumor mass. Self-retaining retractors of choice can safely be used to maintain a static field. Lymph nodes present at this level of dissection are usually not sent for histologic evaluation unless they appear abnormal, enlarged, or contiguous with the carotid body tumor.

Avoidance of cranial nerve injury may be achieved by meticulous dissection over and around the tumor and by the use of bipolar electrocautery to minimize conductive heat injury to adjacent nerves. Fine mosquito clamp dissection and 4-0 silk ligation also work very well when in proximity to nerves. The vagus and hypoglossal nerves must be identified and protected during this phase of the dissection. The vagus nerve

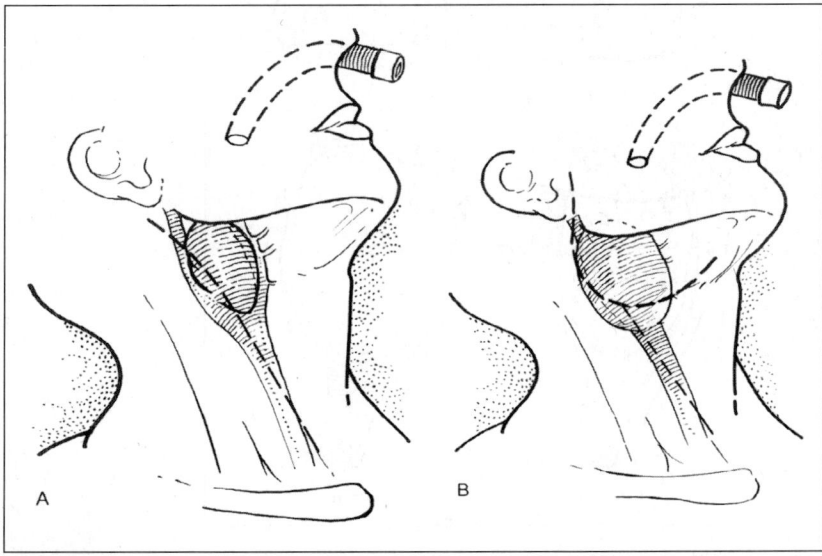

Figure 31-2. Possible neck incisions for carotid body tumor resection. **(A)** - Incision for smaller tumors (<3-4 cm). **(B)** Incision for medium and larger tumors (>4-5 cm), and those requiring more distal exposure. (From Hallett JW, et al. *J Vasc Surg* 1988;7:284–291, with permission of C.V. Mosby/Elsevier Publishing.)

is carefully identified throughout its course. The hypoglossal nerve can usually be identified lying on top of the tumor, and easily dissected off the tumor and fully preserved. However, sometimes its course is within the tumor and it can only be dissected out at a later stage of the operation. The descending limb of the ansa cervicalis nerve running with the hypoglossal nerve is usually visible overlying the tumor and can be sacrificed.

Vascular Dissection—Carotid Arteries

For most carotid body tumors, the tumor begins at or just below the level of the carotid bifurcation with the internal and external carotid branches splayed apart by the tumor. In the simplest form, the carotid vessels are clearly identifiable throughout (Shamblin I), but in more complex tumors, the arteries may be embedded in and surrounded by the tumor (Shamblin II & III)[9-10] (Figure 31–3). The internal and external carotids will come close together again above the tumor. It is important to identify the internal carotid at that level before commencing the dissection in order to avoid vascular injury in this difficult-to access area. The first tenet of vascular surgery, which is to obtain distal and proximal arterial control, should be followed. However, control of the external carotid artery may be especially difficult because it gives rise to the blood supply of the tumor. The superior thyroid artery can be ligated, if necessary, for exposure and mobilization of the bifurcation.

After vascular control has been obtained, the tumor should be mobilized circumferentially to assess the extent of disease. These tumors do not have a capsule and do not shave off the arterial wall easily. Resection should not be carried out in a subad-

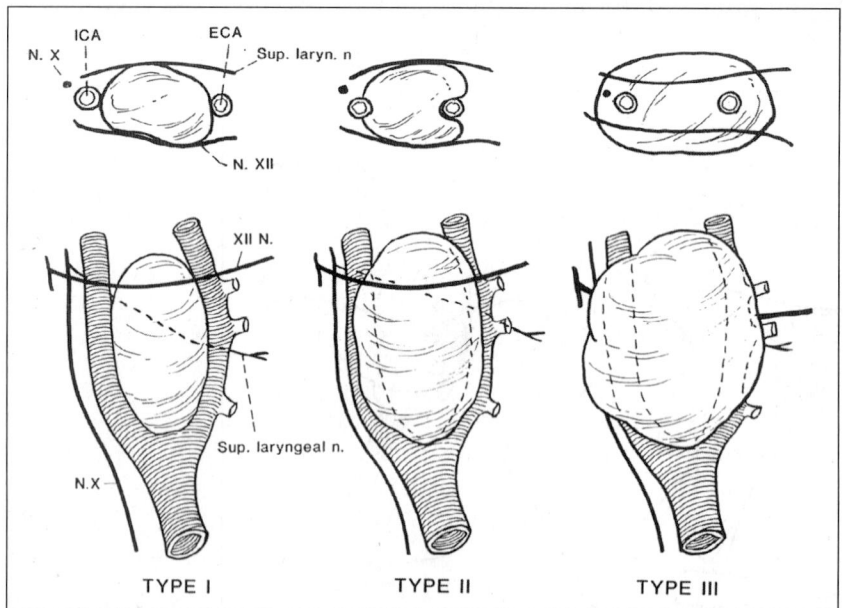

Figure 31-3. The Shamblin classification of difficulty of surgical resection. Group I tumors are localized and easily resected. Group II includes tumors adherent to or partially surrounding the carotid arteries. Group III completely surround or encase at least one of the arteries. (From Hallett JW, et al. *J Vasc Surg* 1988; 7:284–291, with permission of C.V. Mosby/Elsevier Publishing.)

ventitial plane as earlier writers have recommended. This can lead to a weakened arterial wall, predisposing the patient to intraoperative hemorrhage or postoperative carotid blowout. Instead, the plane of dissection should be periadventitial. Here again, a fine mosquito and careful technique pays the most dividends. The tumor should be removed beginning at its inferior extent and progressing cephalad. As most of the blood supply to the tumor is derived from the external carotid artery or its branches, the dissection proceeds along that vessel first. Numerous small vessels will course between the external carotid and the tumor; here, the bipolar cautery is invaluable. Larger feeder vessels are ligated with fine silk ties and divided. Each such division renders the tumor somewhat less vascular. These small and fragile vessels cannot be sought for and ligated until the tumor is peeled off the carotid and they are exposed during the course of dissection. Meddlesome bleeding and oozing can be controlled with bipolar cautery or the intermittent application of a topical hemostatic agent such as gelfoam with thrombin.

If the tumor completely surrounds the vessels, it is usually necessary to divide the tumor in order to reach and continue to the correct plane of dissection. Again, any such dissection is best carried out on the external carotid side of the tumor. The dissection will then proceed over the external carotid to its anterior surface, then to its posterior surface. It is very important not to twist the tumor too far around during its resection as this may torque and occlude the internal carotid artery, and result in cessation of flow to the brain. The carotid lumen is most easily entered during the final stages of tumor resection from the vessels in the "saddle" between the internal and external carotid arteries. The tumor is most densely adherent here, especially posteriorly, owing to the site of tumor origin and a higher density of tumor blood supply. In more difficult cases, early ligation and division of the external carotid artery may reduce blood flow to the tumor and facilitate further resection of the tumor (Figure 31–4). The clamped external carotid artery can then be used as a handle to assist in mobilization of the shrinking tumor.[11] Reconstruction of the external carotid artery following tumor resection is not necessary, and the external carotid stump is oversewn with polypropylene suture.

The Distal Aspects of the Exposure

When the carotid body tumor is confined within the bifurcation (at or below the angle of the mandible) there is fortunately no further need to focus on these more difficult aspects of distal exposure. However, for very distal or extensive tumors, this is the most important and demanding part of the operation. To achieve this exposure, the facial nerve is first identified by dissecting along the sternocleidomastoid muscle until the posterior belly of the digastric is displayed. Dissection is then carried out in the angle above this and between the posterior belly of the digastric and the mastoid process. The nerve stimulator can be valuable in identifying this nerve. Identification of the facial nerve is important to ensure its safety during the remainder of the dissection. The posterior belly of the digastric muscle can then be divided, preferably at its insertion into the mastoid groove. This will improve distal exposure of the ICA by 1 cm and allow exposure of the more distal ICA to within 2 cm of the base of the skull. Further dissection is facilitated by division of the crossing occipital branch of the external carotid artery, its accompanying vein, and the many small muscular branches of the external carotid artery that supply the upper sternocleidomastoid muscle. Careful ligation and division of these vessels and the many delicate

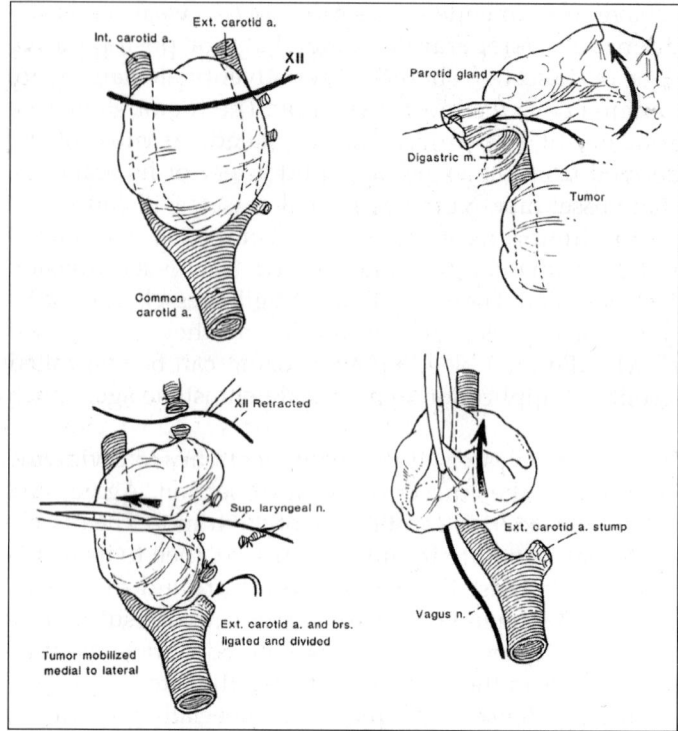

Figure 31-4. Techniques for removal of a large carotid body tumor. The external carotid artery has been divided and oversewn to improve removal of the tumor. (From Hallett JW, et al. *J Vasc Surg* 1988;7:284–291, with permission of C.V. Mosby/Elsevier Publishing.)

veins in the area (this may include a large retro-mandibular vein) will ensure a dry operative field in which the critical cranial nerves can be easily identified and protected. The stylohyoid muscle, above, and parallel to the digastric, should also be divided. This permits exposure and resection of the underlying stylomandibular ligament and styloid process with resultant access to the most distal internal carotid artery. Division of the styloid group of muscles (styloglossus, stylopharyngeus, and stylohyoid) and resection of the styloid process can extend exposure by another 5 mm.[7] The glossopharyngeal nerve is at risk for injury during these maneuvers. The nerve courses between the internal carotid artery and internal jugular vein, lying deep to the styloid process and attached muscles. Should even more superior isolation of the internal carotid artery be required, exposure and gentle retraction of the facial nerve are necessary. Excision of the tail of the parotid gland will assist soft tissue exposure behind the mandible. The preauricular extension of the cervical incision facilitates safe exposure of the facial nerve. For this surgical approach, a combined team of vascular surgeon, neurosurgeon, and/or ENT surgeon may be appropriate.[12]

ICA Resection, Bypass, and Ligation

If the proper plane between the tumor and the carotid artery cannot be developed because of transmural tumor invasion of the arterial wall, carotid resection may be required. When this is necessary, a segment of greater saphenous vein harvested from the thigh can be used as an interposition graft. When required, carotid artery reconstruction at the time of carotid body tumor resection can be performed safely.[13]

Occasionally, with very large tumors, the distal ICA cannot be exposed and arterial reconstruction is impossible. In this case, sacrifice of the ICA may be required. However, ligation of the internal common carotid artery results in a stroke incidence ranging from 23% to 50% and a mortality rate of 14% to 64%. When carotid ligation is anticipated preoperatively, temporary balloon occlusion of the carotid artery in the awake patient during preoperative arteriography may predict the outcome of ligation.[3] This may be critically important in operative planning, and certainly, in patient preparation and operative informed consent.

Final Style Points

Quite often, more of the tumor volume exists posteromedial or behind the carotid bifurcation. Pushing the tumor completely through the bifurcation or pulling it anteriorly through the bifurcation may improve exposure angles and make some elements of dissection easier. When the posterior surface of the tumor is being separated from the deeper parapharyngeal tissues, it is very important to avoid injury to the superior and inferior laryngeal nerves and the glossopharyngeal nerves, which are immediately posterior to most moderate-sized tumors (Figure 31–5). The nerves are often not easy to identify and must be assumed to be in danger. The superior and inferior laryngeal branches of the vagus supply the muscles of the larynx, and varying degrees of dysphonia result when they are injured.[9] Dissection of the posterior and

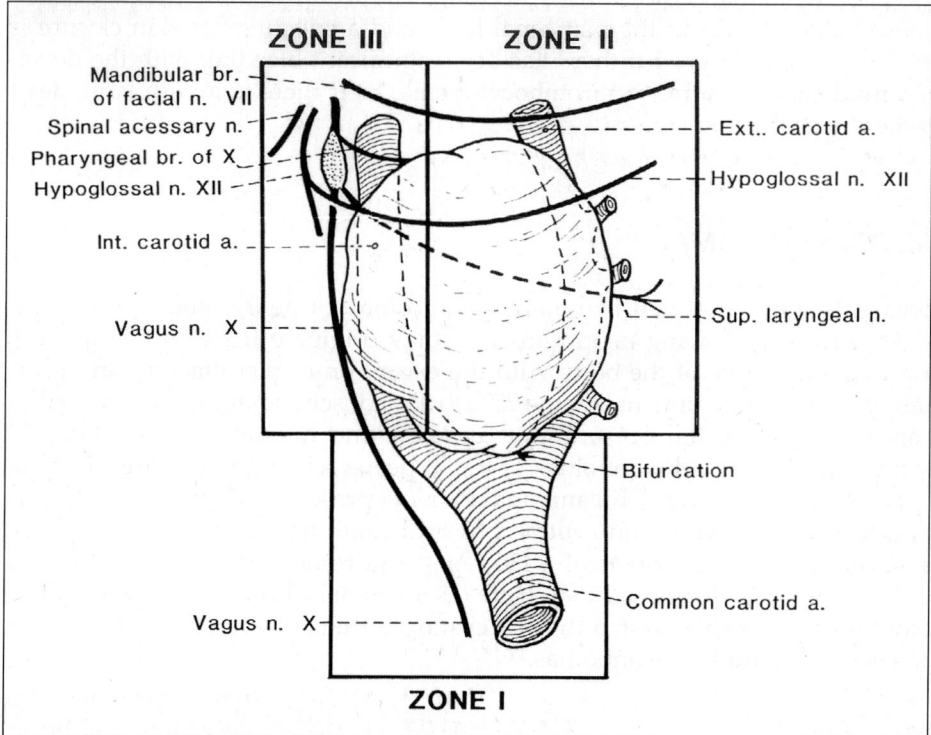

Figure 31-5. Dissection zones about a carotid body tumor with Zone III being the most dangerous. (From Hallett JW, et al. *J Vasc Surg* 1988;7: 284–291, with permission of C.V. Mosby/ Elsevier Publishing.)

medial aspects of the tumor must take place right against the tumor to avoid injury to these nerves. At times, the branches of the laryngeal nerve are embedded or invested within the tumor. and it will be impossible to spare them if complete resection of the tumor is to be completed. Excessive downward traction on the tumor during the final stages of resection can also cause indirect injury to the glossopharyngeal nerve. The carotid sinus nerve (nerve of Hering) courses to the glossopharyngeal nerve, and will transmit downward traction to the glossopharyngeal until it is sectioned at the upper end of the tumor. Many of the draining veins of carotid body tumors are also in this most cephalad substance of the tumor. Careful ligation and division are more effective than cautery at this critical location. Retraction of incompletely cauterized veins toward the base of the skull can present an unnecessary technical challenge in an anatomically critical area. If the most cephalad aspects of the tumor are dissected and ligated early on, the tumor may swell and become quite turgid due to a lack of draining veins with ongoing arterial inflow. This makes tumor resection quite difficult and blood loss will increase.

Once the tumor has finally been separated from the vessels, it will appear smaller and firmer. Most of the bleeding ceases at this stage although an occasional vessel in the tumor bed requires cauterization with bipolar coagulation, Ensure that the cranial nerves are not close by. Once the tumor resection is complete, most of the nagging bleeding stops; topical thrombin and gelfoam, or a similar hemostatic agent, can be added as an aid to gain complete wound hemostasis. Additional time and attention spent on wound hemostasis at this point is worth it to avoid the morbidity of "takeback" surgery for avoidable postoperative bleeding. The wound is then closed with interrupted absorbable sutures in the platysmal layer and a subcuticular skin closure is completed. Drains are only used if there has been significant bleeding with the development of a mild coagulopathy or thrombocytopenia, or if there is a very large dead space after the resection.

CERVICAL SCHWANNOMAS

Schwannomas, also known as neurilemmomas, neuromas, or neurinomas, are uncommon nerve sheath slow-growing neoplasms that may originate from any peripheral, cranial, or autonomic nerve of the body with the exception of the olfactory and optic nerves. Malignant change is unusual. Some 25% to 45% of schwannomas are located in the head and neck, and often present as diagnostic and management challenges. Cervical sympathetic chain schwannomas or vagal nerve schwannomas are the most common type of head and neck schwannoma. Patients present with an asymptomatic unilateral neck mass discovered on routine physical examination, an enlarging neck mass, hoarseness, or the acute onset of a Horner's syndrome. Often, these unilateral neck masses are clinically diagnosed incorrectly as an enlarged cervical lymph node, a carotid body tumor, a brachial cyst, a thyroid cyst or nodule, or even a parotid cyst or tumor in the case of parotid schwannomas.[14]

Diagnosis

With the lack of symptoms and physical examination findings, imaging plays the central role in diagnosing and distinguishing parapharyngeal space neoplasms. Over the past 15 years, CT and MRI scanning have emerged to become the standard imaging modalities used. MRI provides superior soft tissue contrast resolution and is now considered the study of choice. On MRI, schwannomas are well-circumscribed homogeneous masses that exhibit high-signal intensity on T2-weighted images and a relatively homogeneous low-signal intensity on T1-weighted images. In contrast with carotid body tumors, there are no vascular flow voids seen in schwannomas. In addition to facilitating diagnosis, preoperative MR imaging provides information on tumor size, location, extent, and surrounding anatomy, thereby aiding surgical planning.[14-15]

Preoperative imaging characteristics can facilitate the differentiation of the likely nerve of origin of a parapharyngeal space schwannoma. Schwannomas of the cervical sympathetic chain are shown to displace both the carotid and jugular vessels anteriorly and laterally without separating them. Vagal nerve schwannomas are found to displace the carotid arteries medially as they displace the internal jugular vein laterally. A vagal nerve schwannoma may also displace all of the sheath vessels posteriorly without splaying them. Consistent with the first section of this chapter, any splaying of the carotid bifurcation revealed by an imaging study is usually indicative of a carotid body tumor. Overall, the anatomic detail that is now afforded by these scanning modalities facilitates effective preoperative counseling and planning regarding the expected sequelae of surgical resection.[16]

Operative Planning and Surgical Technique

Like carotid body tumors, these neoplasms are relatively radioresistant, so complete surgical resection remains the treatment of choice. The accepted contemporary treatment of schwannomas is microneurosurgical resection. However, surgery is not always recommended because of the indolent nature of the tumor and the risk of postoperative neural deficits. Their slow growth, low recurrence rate, and usual noninvasive nature often allow for an observational approach. If surgical treatment is pursued, the transcervical surgical approach to the parapharyngeal space is the current preferred operation. It the schwannoma is completely removed, recurrence rates are extremely low.

Because schwannomas arise outside the involved fascicle, they tend to compress the nerve fascicles to the periphery as they enlarge, and can usually be dissected free of all adjacent structures except the parent fascicle. Most authors have recommended careful intracapsular excision of the tumor to minimize postoperative deficits. Microneurosurgery to facilitate intraoperative microscopic diagnosis of the schwannoma and achieve more superior nerve preservation has been described. This involves microscopic enucleation of the tumor after opening the epineurium without disrupting nerve continuity. Even as all attempts are made to preserve the nerve of origin, structural preservation may not necessarily lead to preservation of its functional integrity.[14] Occasionally, a section of the affected nerve of origin requires sacrifice with nerve reconstruction (especially facial). In most cases, however, patients should be prepared for the anticipated dysfunction of the involved nerve after schwannoma resection. As an example, patients with suspected vagal nerve schwannomas should be referred to a laryngologist and speech or swallowing specialist in the preoperative period to discuss postoperative rehabilitation options.

REFERENCES

1. Nora JD, Hallett JW, O'Brien PC, et al. Surgical resection of carotid body tumors: Long-term survival, recurrence, and metastasis. *Mayo Clin Proc.* 1988;63:348–352.
2. Sajid MS, Hamilton G, Baker DM, et al. A multicenter review of carotid body tumor management. *Eur J Endovasc Surg.* 2007;34:127–30.
3. Krupski WC. Management of Extracranial Cerebrovascular Disease. In: Rutherford RB, ed. *Vascular Surgery.* Philadelphia: WB Saunders; 2005:2066–2073.
4. Litle VR, Reilly LM, Ramos TK. Preoperative embolization of carotid body tumors: When is it appropriate? *Ann Vasc Surg.* 1996;10:464–468.
5. Smith RF, Shetty PC, Reddy DJ. Surgical treatment of carotid paragangliomas presenting unusual technical difficulties: The value of preoperative embolization. *J Vasc Surg.* 1988;7:631–637.
6. Simonian GT, Pappas PJ, Padberg FT, et al. Mandibular subluxation for distal internal carotid exposure: Technical considerations. *J Vasc Surg.* 1999;30;1116–1120.
7. Dossa C, Shepard AD, Wolford DG, et al. Distal internal carotid exposure: A simplified technique for temporary mandibular subluxation. *J Vasc Surg.* 1990;12:319–325.
8. Fisher DF, Clagett GP, Parker JI, et al. Mandibular subluxation for high carotid exposure. *J Vasc Surg.* 1984;1:727–733.
9. Hallett JW, Nora JD, Hollier LH, et al. Trends in neurovascular complications of surgical management for carotid body and cervical paragangliomas: A fifty-year experience with 153 tumors. *J Vasc Surg.* 1988;7:284–291.
10. Shamblin WR, ReMine WH, Sheps SG, et al. Carotid body tumor (chemodectoma): Clinicopathologic analysis of ninety cases. *Am J Surg.* 1971;122:732–739.
11. Krupski WC, Effeney DJ, Ehrenfeld WK, et al. Cervical chemodectoma: Technical considerations and management options. *Am J Surg.* 1982;44:219–224.
12. Kasper GC, Welling RE, Wladis AR, et al. A multidisciplinary approach to carotid paragangliomas. *Vasc Endovascular Surg* 2006;40:467–474.
13. Smith JJ, Passman MA, Attlio JB, et al. Carotid body tumor resection: Does the need for vascular reconstruction worsen outcome? *Ann Vasc Surg.* 2006;20:435–439.
14. Furukawa M, Furukawa MK, Katoh K, et al. Differentiation between schwannoma of the vagus nerve and schwannoma of the cervical sympathetic chain by imaging diagnosis. *Laryngoscope.* 1996;106:1548–52.
15. Saito DM, Glastonbury CM, El-Sayed IH, et al. Parapharyngeal space schwannomas: Preoperative imaging determination of the nerve of origin. *Arch Otolaryngol Head Neck Surg.* 2007;133:662–667.
16. Kang GCW, Soo KC, Lim DTH. Extracranial non-vestibular head and neck schwannomas: A ten-year experience. *Ann Acad Med Singapore.* 2007;36:233–40.

32

Contemporary Management of Carotid Stenosis: Carotid Endarterectomy is Here to Stay

Thomas A. Abbruzzese, M.D., Richard P. Cambria, M.D.

Carotid artery angioplasty and stenting (CAS) was originally presented as an alternative therapy for patients with extracranial cerebrovascular disease who were deemed too "high risk" for carotid endarterectomy (CEA). Early single center experiences of CAS at least provided a "proof of concept" that CAS can be performed safely in properly selected patients.[1-3] Ironically, perhaps, a decade later as trial data emerge, the feared stroke risk associated with endovascular manipulation of the carotid bifurcation has, in fact, been realized, and the ongoing debate centers around the safety profile of the two procedures. Interventionalists, whose perspective at times appears no more sophisticated than, "if its percutaneous endovascular, it must be better," and who often have little or no direct experience with CEA, concluded that CAS should replace CEA as the treatment of choice in the majority of patients with critical carotid stenosis. Herein we review the evidence for CEA and CAS to provide a rationale for our view that, given the current data, CEA remains the preferred treatment for the majority of patients who require treatment of carotid stenosis.

DEFINING THE PROBLEM

Eighty percent of strokes are ischemic in nature, and of these, thromboembolic complications from carotid bifurcation disease accounts for up to 24%. The clinical goal of any treatment of carotid bifurcation stenosis, be it medical, surgical, or endovascular, is the prevention of stroke. Annually, 700,000 Americans will experience a stroke.[4] Approximately 500,000 of these are first events and 200,000 are recurrent. Stroke is the third leading cause of death in the Unites States, accounting for one out of every 16 deaths in 2004.[5] The clinical sequelae of an initial stroke are significant, and mortality varies with age, gender, ethnicity, and etiology. For men and women over 40 years of age, the five-year survival rate after an initial stroke is 53% for men and 49% for

317

women. For those over 70 years of age, the outlook is grim, with only 42% of patients surviving five years. In terms of morbidity, in 1999, more that 1.1 million American adults reported significant impairment of function and difficulty in completing activities of daily living due to the effects of stroke.[6] The estimated direct and indirect cost of stroke for 2007 is $62.7 billion. The mean lifetime cost of an individual stroke, including inpatient care, rehabilitation, and follow-up care for residual neurological deficits, is estimated at $140,048.[7]

Given the magnitude of the socioeconomic and clinical impact of stroke, and since the only effective treatment is prophylactic, the enormity of treatment directed at carotid stenosis is logical. While important, other tenets of stroke prevention such as risk factor modification, optimal medical therapies, and anticoagulant therapy for cardiac arrhythmia, are not further considered herein.

CAROTID ENDARTERECTOMY — STATE OF THE ART

The efficacy and durability of CEA in the prevention of stroke in both symptomatic and asymptomatic patients, as compared to medical therapy alone, has been validated in large, multicenter, randomized trials.[8-11] For symptomatic patients, the North American Symptomatic Carotid Endarterectomy Trial (NASCET) and the European Carotid Surgery Trial (ECST) demonstrated a significant reduction in the rate of stroke in patients with internal carotid artery stenosis =70% (although the studies differed in their calculation of carotid stenosis severity). These studies demonstrated that the absolute risk reduction in major ipsilateral stroke was 11% at two years (NASCET) and 14% at three years (ECST—80–99% stenosis cohort). The 30-day mortality after CEA was 0.6% (NASCET) and 1.2% (ECST), and the combined 30-day rate of stroke or death was 5.8% (NASCET) and 6.3% (ECST), respectively. All results were highly significant when compared to medical therapy alone, which largely consisted of aspirin and selective risk factor modification. CEA achieved a significant benefit over medical therapy by six months. A later report from NASCET showed that this observed reduction in stroke and death from CEA in symptomatic patients was durable and extended to patients with more moderate (50–99%) internal carotid artery stenosis.[12]

While there is consensus regarding the role of CEA in symptomatic carotid stenosis, debate continues about its application in asymptomatic carotid stenosis, irrespective of a body of level-1 evidence supporting CEA in such patients. This debate centers around the risk/benefit ratio in individual patients, the lack of studies addressing comprehensive medical therapies, and the natural history of asymptomatic carotid stenosis. Several observational studies have shown that stroke risk increases in proportion to the degree of carotid stenosis.[13-17] One such recent report is the ongoing Asymptomatic Carotid Stenosis and Risk of Stroke (ACSRS) study, which has reported the results of the first 1,115 patients recruited, with follow-up ranging from 6–84 months.[17] Patients were eligible for this natural history study if they were found to have >50% stenosis on carotid duplex examination, a normal neurological examination, and had never experienced any ipsilateral hemispheric or retinal symptoms. Patients were still eligible if they had previously experienced contralateral symptoms, but had not experienced these symptoms in the six months prior to study enrollment. In the case of bilateral carotid artery stenosis, the more severely stenotic side was considered the ipsilateral side for the purposes of the study. After a mean follow-up of 37.1 months, the rate of ipsilateral hemispheric stroke was 3.2% for stenosis <60% (approximately 1% per year) and 4.7% for stenoses from 60–99% (approximately 1.5% per year). These rates are similar to the 2% per year rate in asymptomatic carotid stenosis culled from NASCET trial data.[18] The ACSRS investigators also noted that the risk of stroke was three times greater for patients with a history of contralateral transient ischemic attacks and 2.1 times greater for patients with renal insufficiency. Studies like the ACSRS contributed to the debate regarding the optimal treatment of asymptomatic patients with carotid stenosis.

Randomized controlled trials comparing CEA to medical therapy in asymptomatic patients include the Asymptomatic Carotid Atherosclerosis Study (ACAS) and the Asymptomatic Carotid Surgery Trial (ACST).[10-11] Both studies involved patients with ≥60% carotid artery stenosis and showed that CEA provided an absolute risk reduction of 6% (ACAS) and 3.7% (ACST) in major ipsilateral stroke after five and 3.4 years, respectively. The rate of stroke and death was reduced by 6% (ACAS) and 5% (ACST). The 30-day mortality was 0.4% (ACAS) and 1.2% (ACST), and the rate of any stroke or death at 30 days after CEA was 2.3% and 2.8%, respectively. Life-table analysis demonstrated that CEA provided significant benefit over medical therapy by two years, with a halving of stroke risk at five years. Notably, in ACST, a large number of patients (1,241 of 3,120 randomized patients) actually completed five years of follow-up.

The results of the NASCET, ECST, ACAS, and ACST trials helped establish CEA as the "gold standard" treatment for asymptomatic patients with carotid stenosis ≥80% and symptomatic patients with stenosis =70%, provided that the perioperative major morbidity and mortality rates remain less than 3% in asymptomatic and 6% in symptomatic patients.[19] Despite the "positive" results of the large CEA trials, surgical complication rates, especially in the symptomatic trials, would be considered unacceptable in contemporary practice. Refinements in surgical techniques,[20] and in particular processes of care such as routine preoperative use of antiplatelet therapy,[21] liberal use of regional anesthesia in patients at risk of systemic complications,[22-23] and recently, exploitation of the pleiotropic effects of statin use[24] have contributed to the current state of the art of CEA. Furthermore, data accumulated across a spectrum of hospitals and surgeons indicate that such safety and efficacy is not restricted to large single-center reports. Matsen and colleagues, in a review of statewide experience in Maryland and California, reported perioperative stroke rates of 0.29–0.65% for asymptomatic and 0.90–2.29% for symptomatic patients annually over the period of 1996–2003 in 23,237 patients.[25] In a report from the National Surgical Quality Improvement Program (NSQIP) database, Stoner et. al. reported a combined (asymptomatic and symptomatic patients) 30-day rate of stroke and death of 3.4% in 13,622 patients.[22] Halm also reported a 2.3% rate of 30-day stroke and death in asymptomatic patients, 2.9% in patients presenting with transient ischemic attacks, and 7.1% in patients who had a prior stroke.[23] For octogenarians, Teso et. al. reported 30-day rates of stroke of 1.2% and death of 0.6% for a combined stroke and death rate of 1.8%; such results are clearly superior to those reported after CAS in octogenarians.[26] Finally, local experience and expertise will always influence treatment decisions in any individual environment. Over a 20-year interval involving some 3,000 patients, the stroke/death rate accompanying CEA has been a consistent 1.5% at our institution.[27] These data in summary serve as an appropriate reference standard for procedural morbidity against which CAS should be compared.

CAROTID ARTERY ANGIOPLASTY AND STENTING

The evolution of CAS over more than a decade has been largely steeped in technical developments directed at making procedural safety approach that of CEA. Fundamental considerations such as whether luminal expansion of bifurcation plaque affords equivalent early and late stroke protection as plaque excision have never been addressed. The intuitively logical concern that endovascular manipulation of complex carotid plaque would result in unacceptable risk of embolic stroke has, in fact, been realized in the evolution of CAS (Table 32-1). The first consideration is the certain consensus that CAS without distal protection (at least for native plaque lesions) is a reckless endeavor. Multiple examples (CAVATAS, WALLSTENT, and even the initial EVA-3S patients) can be cited wherein unacceptable—even horrific—risk of stroke related to CAS were reported.[28-30] We would even question how ethical physicians and surgeons could be party to such efforts!

One of the first prospective, randomized trials comparing carotid angioplasty to CEA was the Carotid and Vertebral Artery Transluminal Angioplasty Study (CAVATAS), which did not use distal embolic protection.[28] A total of 251 patients were randomized to the endovascular arm and 253 to CEA. The 30-day rate of stroke or death was an unacceptably high 10% for both groups, at least in part related to treatment delays after randomization. Moreover, 18.5% of patients in the endovascular group developed severe restenosis at one year, compared to 5.1% of patients after CEA (p<0.0001). Unfortunately, the absence of distal embolic protection, combined with the fact that 74% of the endovascular group had angioplasty without stenting, makes this study of historical interest only.

The WALLSTENT study was a multicenter, randomized trial of CAS versus CEA in symptomatic patients.[29] A total of 219 patients were enrolled, 107 were randomized to CAS and 112 to CEA. The 30-day rate of any stroke or death was significantly higher in the CAS group than the CEA group (12.1% vs. 4.5%, respectively, p = 0.049). After a follow-up of one year, the combined rate of ipsilateral stroke/procedure death/vascular-related death was 12.1% in the CAS group and 3.6% for CEA (p = 0.022). The authors concluded that CAS was not equivalent to CEA in symptomatic patients.

The first major, randomized trial comparing CAS with embolic protection versus CEA was the Stenting and Angioplasty with Protection in Patients at High Risk for Endarterectomy Trial (SAPPHIRE).[31] This trial, published in 2004, enrolled a total of 334 patients: 167 were randomized to CAS, using a self-expanding nitinol stent (Smart or Precise; Cordis Endovascular, Warren, NJ) with a distal embolic protection device (Angioguard or Angioguard XP; Cordis Endovascular, Warren, NJ), or CEA. To be eligible for enrollment, symptomatic patients had to have a stenosis >50% and asymptomatic patients had to have a stenosis >80% as identified on duplex examination. In addition, patients had to have at least one systemic or local anatomic criteria making them "high risk" for CEA. For example 30% of randomized patients were "high risk" based on the treatment of recurrent (after CEA) stenosis. Overall, the 30-day rate of stroke, myocardial infarction, or death (stroke/MI/death) was 4.4% for CAS and 9.9% for CEA (p = 0.09). For symptomatic patients, the perioperative rate of stroke/MI/death was 2.1% for CAS and 9.3% for CEA (p = 0.18). In asymptomatic patients, the perioperative rate of stroke/MI/death was 5.4% for CAS and 10.2% for CEA (p = 0.20). There was no difference in the primary outcome at one year in symptomatic patients, but was significantly higher in asymptomatic patients after CEA (9.9% for CAS vs. 21.5% for CEA, p = 0.02). The authors concluded that CAS with distal embolic

TABLE 32-1 OUTCOME RESULTS FOR THE MAJOR STUDIES COMPARING CAROTID ARTERY ANGIOPLASTY/STENTING (CAS) AND CAROTID ENDARTERECTOMY (CEA), AS WELL AS RESULTS FOR THE MAJOR NONRANDOMIZED CAS STUDIES AND CAS POSTAPPROVAL REGISTRIES. *DATA INCLUDE MYOCARDIAL INFARCTION (MI); NR, NOT REPORTED.

Study	30-day stroke or death		30-day disabling stroke or death		1-year stroke or death		30-day stroke, death or MI		Modality favored		
	CAS N (%)	CEA N (%)	CAS N (%)	CEA N (%)	CAS N (%)	CEA N (%)	CAS N (%)	CEA N (%)	CAS	Neutral	CEA
Randomized Controlled Trials											
CAVATAS	25 (10)	25 (10)	16 (6.4)	15 (5.9)	36 (14.3)	34 (13.4)	25 (10)	28 (11.1)		✓	
WALLSTENT	13 (12.1)	5 (4.5)	NR	NR	13 (12.1)	4 (3.6)	13 (12.1)	5 (4.5)			✓
SAPPHIRE	8 (4.8)	9 (5.4)	NR	NR	22 (13.2)	33 (19.8)	8 (4.8)	16 (9.3)		✓	
SPACE	46 (7.7)	38 (6.5)	38 (4.7)	22 (3.8)	NR	NR	NR	NR			✓
EVA-3S	25 (9.6)	10 (3.9)	9 (3.4)	4 (1.5)	31 (11.7)	16 (6.1)	NR	NR			✓
NR											
Non-randomized Studies and Registry Data											
ARCHeR	40 (6.9)		9 (1.5)		56 (9.6)*		48 (8.3)				
CREATE	22 (5.2)		18 (4.2)		NR		26 (6.2)				
CAPTURE	200 (5.7)		101 (2.9)		NR		220 (6.3)				
CASES-PMS	NR		NR		NR		71 (4.8)				

protection is not inferior to CEA in patients with severe carotid artery stenosis and significant comorbidities.

In an accompanying editorial, we detailed the flaws in SAPPHIRE.[32] In particular, although a total of 747 patients were enrolled in the study, only 334 (45%) were ultimately randomized, 167 to CAS and 167 to CEA. Of the 413 patients not randomized, 406 were enrolled into a stent registry after study surgeons determined that endarterectomy "could not be safely performed" in these patients, and they underwent CAS outside of the study. Moreover, the rates of perioperative and one-year events were unacceptably high in the surgical group, particularly for asymptomatic patients, when compared to the major randomized trials of CEA. Furthermore, the only difference was related to a higher rate of periprocedural non-Q wave myocardial infarction in the CEA group; in that regard, the troponin "smoke and mirror" data of SAPPHIRE has been soundly refuted by data from many other trials including ACST, EVA-3S, and even CAPTURE. The relatively small sample size and design concerns of the SAPPHIRE trial preclude major conclusions regarding the efficacy of CAS in comparison to CEA. Finally, a year after SAPPHIRE was published, its principal investigator was dismissed from his academic position when it was revealed he had a major conflict of interest.

The Stent-Supported Percutaneous Angioplasty of the Carotid Artery versus Endarterectomy (SPACE) is a randomized trial comparing CAS and CEA in patients with symptomatic carotid artery stenosis.[33] A total of 1,200 patients were enrolled: 605 were randomized to CAS and 595 to CEA. The 30-day rate of ipsilateral ischemic stroke or death was 6.8% with CAS and 6.3% for CEA, and was not significantly different between groups. Of note, although not statistically significant, there was a clear trend in the secondary end-points of disabling ipsilateral stroke or death, disabling ipsilateral stroke, any stroke, or any stroke or death that favored CEA over CAS. Subgroup analysis demonstrated that there was a higher event rate for patients = 75 years of age for both CAS (11%) and CEA (7.5%). Women also experienced a higher rate of stroke or death with CAS than with CEA (7.7% versus 6.0%, respectively). The authors concluded that SPACE failed to prove the noninferiority of CAS versus CEA in symptomatic patients at 30 days.

The Endarterectomy versus Angioplasty in Patients with Severe Symptomatic Carotid Stenosis (EVA-3S) trial is a multicenter, randomized, noninferiority trial comparing CAS and CEA in symptomatic patients with 60–99% stenosis of the internal carotid artery.[30] A total of 527 patients were randomized to the study: 262 were assigned to the CAS group and 265 to CEA. CAS was performed with distal embolic protection in 227 (92%) of patients. The 30-day rate of stroke or death was 9.6% after CAS and 3.9% after CEA (relative risk 2.5, p = 0.01). At six months of follow-up, the rate of any stroke or death was significantly higher after CAS than after CEA (11.7% versus 6.1%, p = 0.02). Further analysis showed that the differences between groups were not related to either the number of study patients enrolled or CAS operator experience, a variable that many advocates of CAS have decried in this trial. Furthermore, the study demonstrated that CAS and CEA had equivalent (<1%) rates of periprocedural, non-stroke complications including myocardial infarction, although the individual rates varied as expected with the nature of the differences between these two procedures. The study investigators concluded that the rates of stoke and death were higher after CAS than CEA in symptomatic patients at one and six months.

The ARCHeR (ACCULINK for Revascularization of Carotids in High-Risk Patients) trial compared CAS with distal embolic protection with historical rates of cerebrovascular events after CEA in high-risk patients.[34] This trial is actually a sequential series of three prospective, nonrandomized studies that were designed to demonstrate noninferiority of CAS versus CEA in the one-year composite end-point of stroke, death, or myocardial infarction. A total of 581 patients were enrolled in the three studies: ARCHeR-1 (n = 158), ARCHeR-2 (n = 278), and ARCHeR-3 (n = 145). Patients were eligible for enrollment if they were symptomatic with a stenosis (50% or asymptomatic stenosis (80% by angiography, and had one or more "high-risk" criteria. The high-risk criteria were determined by literature review as was the "historical control," consisting of the 30-day rate of stroke/death/MI plus one year rate of ipsilateral stroke, which being derived from several decades-old CEA studies (many including combined CEA/CABG patients) was estimated at 14.4% for "high-risk" CEA. This included a 15% rate in patients with medical/surgical comorbidities and an 11% rate in patients with unfavorable anatomy. Procedural success was high (98.8%) and distal embolic protection was used in 69.4% of procedures. The 30-day rate of stroke, death, or myocardial infarction of CAS was 8.3% overall, 13.1% in symptomatic and 6.8% in asymptomatic patients. Based on these results, the authors concluded that CAS was not inferior to "historical control" CEA in the treatment of "high-risk" patients. The almost laughable flaw in the study relates, of course, to the historical control estimate of surgical end-points used for comparison to CAS. I personally believe the editors of *The Journal of Vascular Surgery* published this article to illustrate the ridiculous distortion of scientific method sometimes employed by advocates of CAS to make unacceptable results appear palatable! The design flaws of the ARCHeR studies indicate that no reasonable comparisons can be drawn regarding the safety and efficacy of CAS as compared to CEA from them.

Recently, data from post-market CAS registries have become available. Safian and colleagues reported the results from the CREATE, Carotid Revascularization with ev3 Arterial Technology Evolution, registry of 419 patients who underwent CAS using the ev3 Protégé stent and SPIDER distal embolic protection system (ev3; Plymouth, MN).[35] The primary end-point was a composite of 30-day rate of ipsilateral stroke, procedure-related contralateral stroke, death, and myocardial infarction in so-called "high-risk" patients. In total, 17% of patients were symptomatic and 83% asymptomatic. The 30-day rate of any stroke, death, or myocardial infarction was 6.2%. There were eight deaths, 14 nonfatal strokes, and four myocardial infarctions. The authors concluded that CAS is a reasonable alternative for some patients with severe carotid stenosis and high-risk features for CEA; in our opinion, the complication rates were unacceptable.

The CAPTURE registry is a post-approval study by Guidant Corporation of CAS in high-risk patients using the Guidant ACCULINK stent with ACCUNET distal embolic protection system (Guidant Corporation; Haverhill, MA).[36] Patients were eligible for the study if they had symptomatic stenosis >50% (less than 10% of all patients) or asymptomatic stenosis >80%, and all enrollees were intended to be "high risk." Over 3,500 patients have been enrolled in the registry. Mean age was 73 years of age and 24% of patients are octogenarians. The majority (86%) of patients was asymptomatic. The primary end-point was 30-day rate of stroke, death, or myocardial infarction, which occurred in 6.3% of patients overall, 13% in symptomatic patients and 5.4% in asymptomatic patients. In octogenarians, the rates of stroke, death, or myocardial infarction were 9.4%, significantly higher than the 5.3% rate observed in younger patients. There was no difference in outcomes when analyzed by operator experience.

Cordis Corporation presented their post-approval registry data to CMS in March of 2006 from their Carotid Artery Stenting with Embolic Protection in Patients at High

Surgical Risk for Carotid Endarterectomy (CASES-PMS).[37] The CASES-PMS was designed to assess the safety and efficacy of CAS with distal embolic protection in high-risk patients using the Cordis PRECISE carotid stent with the ANGIOGUARD distal embolic protection system. Similar to the CAPTURE registry, the composite end-point was 30-day rate of death, stroke, and MI, and eligibility was symptomatic stenosis >50% or asymptomatic stenosis >80%. A total of 1,479 patients was enrolled at the time of the report, 78% of whom were asymptomatic. The 30-day rate of stroke, death, or myocardial infarction was 4.8% for all patients, 5.9% for symptomatic patients, and 4.5% for asymptomatic patients. There was no difference in outcome when analyzed by operator experience.

DISCUSSION

What consensus then can be formulated based on the data reviewed herein, and the emerging data on CAS? First, our opinion (and seemingly difficult to refute this point) is that CAS is a procedure in evolution and definitive data as to its utility (or lack thereof) are, as yet, unavailable. Different strategies for distal embolic protection such as internal carotid artery flow reversal could improve the unacceptable complication rates observed in symptomatic and octogenarian patients. Alternatively, CEA is a mature procedure, supported by Level-1 data, and performed with an enviable degree of safety and efficacy in a multitude of reports across a spectrum of operators and hospitals.[22,25,26] Indeed, even aggressive endovascular surgeons (such as ourselves) are reluctant to embrace CAS since the available data indicate its safety/efficacy profile compares poorly to what has consistently been achieved with CEA. Soon, large administrative database studies will appear indicating that in examination of the ultimate "hard end-point," namely periprocedural death, CAS is statistically inferior to CEA.[38]

Fundamentally, the position advocated herein is entirely consistent with the Society for Vascular Surgery (SVS) position paper submitted to the Centers for Medicaid and Medicare Services (available on the CMS website) in public comment referable to a reconsideration of the restrictive national coverage policy for CAS. Appeal for such reconsideration was made by corporate interests. The important elements of this document advocate the positions that:

1. CAS should not be performed in octogenarians (excepting enrollment in CREST) based on the large body of data indicating unacceptable risk of CAS in such patients. With respect to age (age ≥80 is frequently used as a "high-risk" criteria in CAS trials), data from randomized trials such as Carotid Revascularization Endarterectomy versus Stenting Trial (CREST) and SPACE as well as the CAPTURE registry consistently demonstrate unacceptable rates of stroke and death in octogenarians.[33,36,39] Data from the first 1,479 patients from CREST, presented at the 2007 International Symposium on Endovascular Therapy in Hollywood, Florida, demonstrated a linear association in the 30-day rates of stroke and death with patient age.[39] Patients ≥60 years old had a 30-day rate of stroke/death of 2.2%, while those ≥70 years had a rate of 5.4%, and octogenarians had the highest rate, which was 11.3%. SPACE reported a 30-day rate of stroke/death of 11% and the rate was 7.4% in CAPTURE (86% of whom were asymptomatic). Stanziale et. al. reported results from a prospective CAS registry including 384 patients, 87 of whom were > 80 years of age.[40] When

TABLE 32-2. ANATOMIC AND PHYSIOLOGIC FACTORS ASSOCIATED WITH HIGHER CAROTID ENDARTERECTOMY COMPLICATION RATES.

High Risk Anatomic Factors

Contralateral laryngeal nerve palsy.
Presence of a tracheostomy stoma
Prior radical neck dissection
Radiation damage to the neck from previous radiation therapy
Recurrent carotid artery stenosis s/p CEA
High cervical lesions (above C2)
Low cervical lesions (below the clavicle)
Severe tandem lesions

High Risk Physiologic Factors

Unstable angina
Recent myocardial infarction (>24 hours and < 4 weeks)
NYHA Class III/IV congenstive heart failure
Severe left ventricular dysfunction
Open heart surgery within 6 weeks
Severe pulmonary disese
Unstable angina
Contralateral carotid artery occlusion
Age > 80 years

compared to younger patients, octogenarians had a significantly higher 30-day rate of stroke, death, or myocardial infarction (9.2% versus 3.4%, p = 0.02). These data in summary led to formation of the SVS position that CMS should not cover CAS outside of a randomized controlled trial setting.

2. Coverage of CAS in patients with anatomic "high-risk" considerations for CEA (Table 32–2). In a systematic review of the literature, Narins and Illig studied the benefit of CAS and CEA in the presence of a variety of anatomic and physiologic high-risk characteristics.[41] Of the anatomic risk factors studied, CAS was preferred over CEA in the presence of prior neck irradiation, prior radical neck surgery, or in patients with a tracheostomy stoma. They also concluded that CAS may be better than CEA in the setting of a high carotid bifurcation, restenosis after previous CEA, and severe neck immobility as these factors tend to be associated with increased CEA complication rates, although the author's admitted that the benefit was likely to be marginal. Of the physiologic risk factors evaluated, CAS was preferred in patients with contralateral recurrent laryngeal nerve dysfunction and significant cardiac or pulmonary disease. They found that CEA was the preferred option for patients >80 years of age as well as in patients with difficult vascular access, difficult aortic arch anatomy, difficult carotid anatomy, or in clinical scenarios that preclude the use of distal embolic protection. Indeed, this review has not addressed specific anatomic features that even advocates of CAS indicate are circumstances that pose a higher risk for CAS as compared to CEA.[42] Our own position is that noninvasive imaging such as computed tomographic angiography can and should delineate such patients.

3. There should be no expansion of coverage in "systemic high-risk" asymptomatic patients. Patients with advanced comorbidities so as to limit longevity

and/or preclude safe CEA in general should not have intervention for asymptomatic lesions. Furthermore, much of what has been written and/or argued about such patients ignores processes of care that have been demonstrated to facilitate safe CEA in patients who might be at risk for a general anesthetic. Two large studies (i.e., sufficiently powered to demonstrate the effect) have demonstrated the efficacy of regional anesthesia in such circumstances.[22,23] Other circumstances frequently cited as "high risk" for CEA such as imminent need for coronary artery bypass graft surgery are effectively managed with combined CEA/CABG.[43] Interestingly, a consortium of professional societies (in addition to the SVS) have logged position papers opposing expansion of coverage to "systemic high-risk" asymptomatic patients. These include the American Congress of Neurosurgery, the American Academy of Neurology, and even the Stroke Council of the American Heart Association!

CONCLUSION

In consideration of an evidence-based approach, CEA (versus CAS) is the preferred treatment for carotid stenosis. Nearly every study of CAS demonstrates a higher rate of stroke and death than is considered acceptable for CEA; this is particularly true for octogenarians and all asymptomatic patients, regardless of age (Table 32–1). The patient cohort that seems to benefit most from CAS are younger, good-risk patients, but the attendant higher rate of stroke and death, as compared to CEA, makes CAS a poor choice even in this group. A meta-analysis of five trials found insufficient evidence to support a widespread change in clinical practice away from recommending CEA as the treatment of choice for suitable carotid artery stenosis, and recommended that CAS only be offered in a trial setting to patients who are otherwise suitable for CEA.[44] Recently, CMS released its final decision on CAS that limits coverage to patients who are deemed "high risk" for CEA and have symptomatic stenosis ≥70%, symptomatic stenosis between 50% and 70%, or asymptomatic stenosis ≥80% in the setting of a clinical trial.[45] Until further data become available to change this landscape, we believe that CEA remains the treatment of choice for the vast majority of symptomatic and asymptomatic patients who require treatment for carotid stenosis.

REFERENCES

1. Diethrich EB, Ndiaye M, and Reid DB. Stenting in the carotid artery: Initial experience in 110 patients. *J Endovasc Surg.* 1996;3:42–62.
2. Yadav JS, Roubin GS, Iyer S, et al. Elective stenting of the extra-cranial carotid arteries. *Circulation.* 1997;95:376–381.
3. Shawl F, Kadro W, Domanski MJ, et al. Safety and efficacy of elective artery stenting in high-risk patients. *J Am Coll Cardiol.* 2000;35:1721–1728.
4. American Heart Association Statistics Committee and Stroke Statistics Subcommittee, Heart Disease and Stroke Statistics-2007 Update. *Circulation.* 2007;115:e69–e171.
5. Health, United States, 2006. National Center for Health Statistics. Available at: http://www.cdc.gov/nchs/hus.htm and ftp://ftp.cdc.gov/pub/Health_Statistics/NCHS/Publications/Health_US/hus06tables/Table037.xls. Accessed March 12, 2007.

6. Centers for Disease Control and Prevention (CDC). Prevalence of disabilities and associated health conditions among adults: United States, 1999. *MMWR Morb Mort Wkly Rep.* 2001;50:65–76.

7. Taylor TN, Davis PH, Torner JC, et al. Lifetime costs of stroke in the United States. *Stroke.* 1996;27:1459–1466.

8. North American Symptomatic Carotid Endarterectomy Trial Collaborators: Beneficial effect of carotid endarterectomy in symptomatic patients with high-grade carotid stenosis. *N Eng J Med.* 1991;325:445–453.

9. European Carotid Surgery Trialists' Collaborative Group: Randomised trial of endarterectomy for recently symptomatic carotid stenosis: final results of the MRC European Carotid Surgery Trial (ECST). *Lancet.* 1998;351:1379–1387.

10. The Executive Committee for the Asymptomatic Carotid Atherosclerosis Study: Endarterectomy for asymptomatic carotid artery stenosis. *JAMA.* 1995;273:1421–1428.

11. The MRC Asymptomatic Carotid Surgery Trial (ACST) Collaborative Group: Prevention of disabling and fatal strokes by successful carotid endarterectomy in patients without recent neurological symptoms: randomized controlled trial. *Lancet.* 2004;363:1491–1502.

12. North American Symptomatic Carotid Endarterectomy Trial Collaborators: Benefit of carotid endarterectomy in patients with symptomatic moderate or severe stenosis. *N Eng J Med.* 1998;339:1415–1425.

13. Johnson JM, Kennelly MM, Decesare D, et al. Natural history of asymptomatic carotid plaque. *Arch Surg.* 1985;120:1010–1012.

14. Chambers BR, Norris JW. Outcome in patients with asymptomatic neck bruits. *N Eng J Med.* 1986;315:860–865.

15. Mackey AE, Abrahamowicz M, Langlois Y, et al. Outcome of asymptomatic patients with carotid disease. *Neurology.* 1997;48:896–903.

16. Nadareishvili ZG, Rothwell PM, Beletsky V, et al. Long-term risk of stroke and other vascular events in patients with asymptomatic carotid artery stenosis. *Arch Neurol.* 2002;59:1162–1166.

17. Nicolaides AN, Kakkos SK, Griffin M, for the Asymptomatic Carotid Stenosis and Risk of Stroke (ACSRS) Study Group. Severity of asymptomatic carotid stenosis and risk of ipsilateral hemispheric ischaemic events: Results from the ACSRS study. *Eur J Vasc Endovasc Surg.* 2005;30:275–284.

18. Inzitari D, Eliasziw M, Gates P, et al. The causes and risk of stroke in patients with asymptomatic internal carotid artery stenosis. *N Eng J Med.* 2000;342:1693–1700.

19. Biller J, Feinberg WM, Castaldo JE, et al. Guidelines for carotid endarterectomy, a statement for healthcare professionals from a special writing group of the Stroke Council, American Heart Association. *Circulation.* 1998;97:501–509.

20. Bond R, Rerkasem K, AbuRahma AF, et al. Patch angioplasty versus primary closure for carotid endarterectomy. *Cochrane Database Syst Rev.* 2004;2:CD000160.

21. Kresowik TF, Bratzler DW, Kresowik RA, et al. Multistate improvement in process and outcomes of carotid endarterectomy. *J Vasc Surg.* 2004;39:372–80.

22. Stoner MC, Abbott WM, Wong DR, et al. Defining the high-risk patient for carotid endarterectomy: an analysis of the prospective National Surgical Quality Improvement Program database. *J Vasc Surg.* 2006;43:285–295.

23. Halm EA, Hannan EL, Rojas M et al. Clinical and operative predictors of outcomes of carotid endarterectomy. *J Vasc Surg.* 2005;42:420–428.

24. Brooke BS, McGirt MJ, Woodworth GF, et al. Preoperative statin and diuretic use influence the presentation of patients undergoing carotid endarterectomy: Results of a large single-institution case-control study. *J Vasc Surg.* 2007;45:298–303.

25. Matsen SL, Chang DC, Perler BA, et al. Trends in in-hospital stroke rate following carotid endarterectomy in California and Maryland. *J Vasc Surg.* 2006;44:488–495.

26. Teso D, Edwards RE, Frattini JC, et al. Safety of carotid endarterectomy in 2,443 elderly patients: Lessons from nonagenarians-are we pushing the limit? *J Am Coll Surg.* 2005;200:734–741.

27. LaMuraglia GM, Stoner MC, Brewster DC, et al. Carotid endarterectomy at the millennium: What interventional therapy must match. *Ann Surg*. 2004;240:535–546.

28. The CAVATAS Investigators: Endovascular versus surgical treatment in patients with carotid stenosis in the Carotid and Vertebral Artery Transluminal Angioplasty Study (CAVATAS): a randomized trial. *Lancet*. 2001;357:1729–1737.

29. Alberts MJ. Results of a multicenter prospective randomized trial of carotid artery stenting vs. carotid endarterectomy. *Stroke*. 2001;32:325. (abstract)

30. Mas JL, Chatellier G, Beyssen B, for the EVA-3S Investigators. Endarterectomy versus stenting in patients with symptomatic severe carotid stenosis. *N Eng J Med*. 2006;355:1660–1671.

31. Yadav JS, Wholey MH, Kuntz RE, for the Stenting and Angioplasty with Protection in Patients at High Risk for Endarterectomy Investigators (SAPPHIRE): Protected carotid-artery stenting versus endarterectomy in high-risk patients. *N Eng J Med*. 2004;351: 1493–1501.

32. Cambria RP. Stenting for carotid-artery stenosis. *N Eng J Med*. 2004;351:1565–1567.

33. The SPACE Collaborative Group. 30 day results from the SPACE trial of stent-protected angioplasty versus carotid endarterectomy in symptomatic patients: a randomized non-inferiority trial. *Lancet*. 2006;368:1239–1247.

34. Gray WA, Hopkins LN, Yadav S, for the ARCHeR Trial Collaborators. Protected carotid stenting in high-surgical-risk patients: the ARCHeR results. *J Vasc Surg*. 2006;44:258–269.

35. Safian RD, Bresnahan JF, Jaff MR, et al. Protected carotid stenting in high-risk patients with severe carotid artery stenosis. *J Am Coll Cardiol*. 2006;47:2384–2389.

36. Gray WA, Yadav JS, Verta P, et al for the CAPTURE Trial Collaborators. The CAPTURE registry: Results of carotid stenting with embolic protection in the post approval setting. *Catheteriz Cardiovasc Interv*. 2007;69:341–348.

37. Phurrough S, Salive M, McClain S, et al. Proposed decision memo for percutaneous transluminal angioplasty (PTA) of the carotid artery concurrent with stenting (CAG-00085R3). Centers for Medicare and Medicaid Services. Published online at www.cms.hhs.gov. Dated: February 1, 2007.

38. McPhee JT, Hill J, Eslami MH, et al. Increased national in-hospital mortality following carotid stenting a compared to carotid endarterectomy. To be presented at the 2007 Annual Vascular Meeting, Baltimore, MD. Published online at http://www.vascularweb.org/_CONTRIBUTION_PAGES/Annual_Meeting/Abstracts/2007/mcphee_increased_national_in_hospital.html.

39. Gray WA. What the CREST data tells us. Presented at the 2007 International Symposium on Endovascular Therapy, Hollywood, Florida. January 29, 2007.

40. Stanziale SF, Marone LK, Boules TN, et al. Carotid artery stenting in octogenarians is associated with increased adverse outcomes. *J Vasc Surg*. 2006;43:297–304.

41. Narins CR and Illig KA. Patient selection for carotid stenting versus endarterectomy: A systematic review. *J Vasc Surg*. 2006;44:661–672.

42. Roubin GS, Iyer S, Halkin A, et al. Realizing the potential of carotid artery stenting: Proposed paradigms for patient selection and procedural technique. *Circulation*. 2006;113: 2021–2030.

43. Akins CW, Hilgenberg AD, Vlahakes GJ, et al. Late results of combined carotid and coronary surgery using actual versus actuarial methodology. *Ann Thorac Surg*. 2005;80: 2091–2097.

44. Coward LJ, Featherstone RL, and Brown MM. Safety and efficacy of endovascular treatment of carotid artery stenosis compared with carotid endarterectomy: A Cochrane systematic review of the randomized evidence. *Stroke*. 2005;36:905–911.

45. Phurrough S, Salive M, McClain S, et al. Decision memo for percutaneous transluminal angioplasty (PTA) of the carotid artery concurrent with stenting (CAG-00085R3). Centers for Medicare and Medicaid Services. Published online at www.cms.hhs.gov. Dated: April 30, 2007.

33

Carotid Artery Stenting versus Open Surgery: Stent

Jon S. Matsumura, M.D.

Carotid endarterectomy (CEA) has been thoroughly evaluated in several large randomized clinical trials that established the utility of the intervention for patients with carotid disease. These pivotal studies included the North American Symptomatic Carotid Endarterectomy Trial, the European Carotid Surgery Trial, the Asymptomatic Carotid Atherosclerosis Study (ACAS), and the Asymptomatic Carotid Surgery Trial (ACST).[1-4] The results of these studies have established the indications for CEA in patients with symptomatic stenosis of >/ = 50%, and asymptomatic stenosis of >/ = 60%. Carotid artery stenting (CAS) is in an earlier phase of development, with publication of some smaller randomized trials, most of which were stopped prior to completion. In the context of a debate, this "Pro-Stent" chapter will review proposed credentialing volumes and outcomes assessment for CAS, then analyze the results of early carotid trials from that perspective. The chapter will also review current understanding of risk factors for CAS and emerging optimal techniques for CAS.

COMPETENCY STATEMENTS

Several competency statements for CAS have been published with varied clinical, technical, radiologic, and cognitive skill sets. Creager et. al.[5] and Rosenfield et. al.[6] cover clinical competence for general interventional treatment of peripheral vascular disease, specifically carotid stenting, and these are endorsed by cardiology, medicine, and vascular surgery societies. Quality improvement guidelines by Barr et. al.[7] and competency standards by Connors et. al.[8] are endorsed by neurology and radiology societies. These documents advocate different skill set requirements that, not surprisingly, align with the training programs of the respective societies, but both sets of documents are in agreement on the importance of outcomes assessment and comparison to risk-adjusted standards. This is an important similarity to stress, as all specialties have recognized that CAS is a complex procedure with significant risks to the patient, and have determined that outcomes assessment is important in credentialing.

Further, a European group has published a consensus document for the Italian Consensus Carotid Stenting (ICCS)/Stroke Prevention and Educational Awareness Diffusion (SPREAD) group, which represents over 30 scientific societies and patient organizations. They address volume thresholds of experience after achieving basic skill for catheter-based intervention, which are much larger than the previous standards. These thresholds are at least 150 procedures of supra-aortic vessel engagement within two years, of which at least 100 as the primary operator; and at least 75 carotid stenting procedures, of which at least 50 as the primary operator, within a two-year fellowship. A minimum requirement to maintain technical skill is 50 carotid stenting procedures per year.[9] They recommended "CAS, if performed with adequate procedural quality levels, should be used instead of CEA in the presence of severe vascular or cardiac comorbidities or specific conditions" defined as high risk for CEA.

Both ACAS and ACST included quality thresholds for operators to become eligible investigators, and this requirement in study design has continued in treatment recommendations regarding carotid interventions. Interestingly, quality thresholds were not routinely used in many CAS trials.

Finally, Medicare, in their most recent national coverage decision (CAG-00085R3, April 30, 2007), has required facility certification every two years that requires attestation of specific standards. These include data analysis of CAS with a "clearly delineated program for granting carotid stent privileges and for monitoring the quality of the individual interventionalists and the program as a whole." Medicare "places significant importance" in each facility's data analysis plan. It is obvious that several organizations have determined that operator volume and quality are essential considerations in CAS.

CAS TRIALS

Each clinical trial had unique eligibility criteria and protocols for management of CAS patients. Further, each clinical trial established its own eligibility criteria for physician-investigators to perform CAS. It is illuminating to review the trials with attention to investigator qualifications.

In the Carotid and Vertebral Artery Transluminal Angioplasty Study (CAVATAS),[10] interventionalists were generally radiologists who had training in neuroradiology and angioplasty. Their experience was reviewed and centers with fewer prior cases received training and assistance from more experienced centers. Eighty-eight percent of patients in CAVATAS were symptomatic. In those randomized to angioplasty, 74% had angioplasty without stenting (only 26% had stents) and none had embolic protection. Thirty-day stroke (defined as symptoms more than seven days)/death rate was 10% in both the CEA and angioplasty arms. Although restenosis was more common in the angioplasty arm, there was no difference in stroke rate up to three years after randomization. While this trial was a randomized trial that showed similar results, CAS technology and experience have matured significantly with routine use of stenting. In fact, a second follow-up trial with routine stenting (CAVATAS-2) is underway although embolic protection is not routinely recommended in the second trial.

In Carotid Revascularization using Endarterectomy of Stenting Systems (CaRESS) Phase I, total previous interventionalist CAS experience was at least 20 cases with a stroke/death rate <6% and at least five cases with distal balloon embolic protection.[11,12] It is important to note that this trial had a quality threshold and not only a volume criteria. Later, the training cases with distal balloon were included in the Phase I results. Patients were both high and low risk for CEA, and 32% were symptomatic. Thirty-day stroke/death rate was 2.1% with CAS and 3.6% with CEA. At one year, stroke/death rate was 10.0% with CAS and 13.6% with CEA.

The lead-in phase for the Carotid Revascularization Endarterectomy vs Stenting Trial (CREST) trial required interventionalists to submit results from 10–30 CAS cases.[13,14] A quality threshold was used of 30-day stroke/death rate <6% for symptomatic patients and satisfactory performance in the lead-in phase. The lead-in portion of the trial included patients at high and low risk for CEA, and a mix of asymptomatic and symptomatic patients. Thirty-day stroke/death rate was about 4.6%, with subsequent periodic reports appearing. The results of the randomized phase are not available, but might be expected to be superior to this since the lead-in phase included the learning curve and some investigators who did not eventually get approved.

The Stenting and Angioplasty with Protection in Patients at High Risk for Endarterectomy (Sapphire) trial randomized patients at high risk for CEA to have CAS or CEA.[15] As the name implies, CAS patients received stenting with routine cerebral protection. Interventionalists were required to have <6% periprocedural stroke/death. The total experience of each interventional physician was a median of 64 cases with a range of 20–700 CAS procedures. Sapphire had one of the highest preexisting CAS volumes along with a quality threshold. In comparison, the annual volume of each surgeon was a median of 30 cases with a range of 15–100 CEA procedures. Thirty-day intent-to-treat stroke/death/MI rate was 4.8% with CAS and 9.8% with CEA.

The Stent-supported Percutaneous Angioplasty of the Carotid artery versus Endarterectomy (SPACE) trial randomized 1,200 symptomatic patients to CAS or CEA.[16] The interventionalists had to show proof of 25 consecutive successful PTA or stenting procedures. To improve enrollment, this threshold was lowered part way into the trial. Vascular surgeons had to document 25 consecutive CEA with mortality and morbidity rates for those procedures. Ten sites failed the quality standards. Twenty-seven percent of CAS patients had embolic protection. Thirty-day ipsilateral stroke/death rate was 6.84% with CAS and 6.34% with CEA. CAS stroke/death/MI rates in patients > 75 years were 11% compared to 6% in younger patients. This trial was stopped after the second interim analysis, noting inadequate power due to funding limitations and slow enrollment rates. It is noteworthy that any noninferiority trial that has inadequate enrollment and is stopped will "fail" to show noninferiority.

The Endarterectomy Versus Angioplasty in patients with Symptomatic Severe carotid Stenosis (EVA-3S) trial randomized 527 symptomatic patients.[17] EVA-3S selected interventionalists that 1) had performed 12 CAS, 2) 35 stenting procedures in supra-aortic trunks, including 5 CAS, or 3) had supervision by an experienced tutor, and at least two CAS with any new device. Surgeons had to perform at least 25 procedures in the year before enrollment. This alone may constitute a quality threshold as few surgeons would keep a large referral practice if results were poor. Prior to July 2003 when the DSMB required routine embolic protection, 21.6% of CAS patients did not have protection devices. The 30-day stroke/death rate was lower (P = .03) at 7.9% with embolic protection compared to 25% without embolic protection. Seventeen percent of patients had single antiplatelet preprocedure therapy. Although EVA-3S reported no significant difference in 30-day stroke/death rates in patients treated by investigators who were experienced interventionalists (10.5%), tutored during training (7.1%), and tutored after training (12.3%), enrollment rates were quite low from November 2000 to

September 2005 when the trial was stopped. The size of this trial may limit the power of post hoc subset analysis. The 30-day stroke/death rate was lower (P = .01) at 3.9% with CEA compared to 9.6% with CAS. Poor results with CAS were also seen in the stopped Leicester and Wallstent trials that clearly involved very inexperienced interventionalists.

The Capture trial is the largest database of contemporary CAS procedures with routine embolic protection.[18] Although it is an uncontrolled registry, its size has enough statistical power for multivariate analysis in order to identify variables that predicted adverse outcomes. Unlike population-based studies, Capture has independent neurologic assessment as recommended in society endorsed guidelines. Based on initial univariate analysis if P<.25, a multivariate model was created using stepwise regression. Missing data were not imputed; only patients with complete data for all selected variables were included. The final multivariate model consisted of the parameters that have a P<.05 and were: age ≥ 80 years, symptomatic status, predilation without EPD and multiple stents. This type of exploratory analysis is helpful in identifying patient factors and techniques associated with higher risk for stroke with CAS.

Because each trial has different primary endpoints, heterogeneity of patient risk profiles, differences in operator experience, use of embolic protection, and inclusion/exclusion criteria, it is difficult to reconcile or even compare the outcomes. Yet taken together, it appears clear that operator qualification and routine use of embolic protection are key factors in determining CAS outcomes. As knowledge has been gained of factors that make patients higher risk for carotid artery stenting (such as arterial tortuosity and advanced age), it is apparent that prior CAS experience helps identify and select patients who are high risk for CAS, just as high risk for CEA parameters have previously emerged. It is possible that specific patient subsets will be identified where one treatment or the other is preferred.

Quality improvement programs that have improved outcomes with CEA should have similar effects on CAS. As CAS undergoes the same maturation processes that CEA did, CAS must be evaluated in larger randomized trials in which investigator experience and quality are equally vetted with standardized techniques and devices. CREST and the Asymptomatic Carotid stenosis, stenting versus endarterectomy Trial (ACT 1) are underway to provide these evaluations.

CONCLUSION

CAS is a new procedure and undergoing evolution. Earlier studies with inexperienced interventionalists, primitive equipment, and unselected application in all patients have shown suboptimal outcomes with CAS. Many studies were flawed and stopped early. Careful vetting of physician qualifications, routine use of embolic protection, and exclusion of patients who are high risk for CAS as well as those high risk for CEA are likely to provide a more fair comparison between CAS and CEA. It is likely that the procedures may be complimentary, for CAS trials themselves may have improved recent results with CEA by treating patients at high risk for CEA. Larger randomized clinical trials must be completed comparing operators with similar prior outcomes. In the meantime, vascular surgeons should learn CAS as it is likely to be an alternative and complementary to CEA.

REFERENCES

1. North American Symptomatic Carotid Endarterectomy Trial Collaborators. Beneficial effect of carotid endarterectomy in symptomatic patients with high-grade carotid stenosis. *N Engl J Med*. 1991;325(7):445–53.
2. European Carotid Surgery Trialists' Collaborative Group. Randomised Trial of Endarterectomy for Recently Symptomatic Carotid Stenosis: Final Results of the MRC European Carotid Surgery Trial (ECST). *Lancet*. 1998;351:1379–87.
3. Executive Committee for the Asymptomatic Carotid Atherosclerosis Study. Endarterectomy for Asymptomatic Carotid Artery Stenosis. *JAMA*. 1995;273:1421–28.
4. MRC Asymptomatic Carotid Surgery Trial (ACST) Collaborative Group. *Lancet*. 363: May 2004. 1491–1502.
5. Creager MA, Goldstone J, Hirshfeld HW Jr., et al. ACC/ACP/SCAI/ SVMB/SVS clinical competence statement on vascular medicine and catheter-based peripheral vascular intervention. *J Am Coll Cardiol*. 2004;44:941–57.
6. Rosenfield K, Cowley MJ, Jaff MR, et al. SCAI/SVMB/SVS clinical competence statement on carotid stenting: training and credentialing for carotid stenting. *J Am Coll Cardiol*. 2005;45:165–74.
7. Barr JD, Connors JJ, Sacks D, et al. Quality improvement guidelines for the performance of cervical carotid angioplasty and stent placement. *J Vasc Interv Rad*. 2003;14:1079–93.
8. Connors JJ, III, Sacks D, Furlan AJ, et al. Training, competency, and credentialing standards for diagnostic cervicocerebral angiography, carotid stenting, and cerebrovascular intervention. *Am J Neuroradiol*. 2004:25;1732–41.
9. Cremonesi A, Setacci C, Bignamini A, et al. Carotid artery stenting. First consensus document of the ICCS-SPREAD joint committee. *Stroke*. 2006;37:2400–09.
10. CAVATAS Investigators. Endovascular versus surgical treatment in patients with carotid stenosis in the carotid and vertebral artery transluminal angioplasty study: a randomized trial. *Lancet*. 2001;35:1729–37.
11. CARESS Steering Committee. Carotid revascularization using endarectomy or stenting systems (CARESS): phase I clinical trial. *J End Ther*. 2003;10:1021–30.
12. CARESS Steering Committee. Carotid revascularization using endarectomy or stenting systems (CARESS): phase I clinical trial: 1 year results. *J Vasc Surg*. 2005;42:213–9.
13. Hobson RW II, Howard VJ, Roubin GS et al. Carotid artery stenting is associated with increased complications in octogenarians: 30-day stroke and death rates in the CREST lead-in phase. *J Vasc Surg*. 2004;40:1106–11.
14. Hobson RW II, Howard Virginia, Roubin GS et al. Credentialing of surgeons as interventionalists for carotid artery stenting: Experience from the lead-in phase of CREST. *J Vasc Surg*. 2004;40:952–7.
15. Yadav JS, Wholey MH, Kuntz RE, et al. Protected carotid-artery stenting versus endarterectomy in high-risk patients. *N Engl J Med*. 2004;351:1493–501.
16. The SPACE collaborative Group. 30 day results from the SPACE trial of stent-protected angioplasty versus carotid endarterectomy in symptomatic patients: a randomized non-inferiority trial. *Lancet*. 2006:368.
17. Mas JL, Chatellier G, Beyssen B et al. Endarterectomy versus stenting in patients with symptomatic severe carotid stenosis. *N Engl J Med*. 2006;355:1660–71.
18. Gray W. CAPTURE 3500 Update. TCT 2006 oral presentation.

Index